Neurology

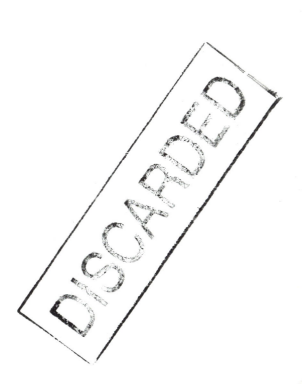

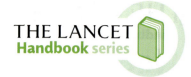

THE LANCET
Handbook series

For Elsevier:

Publisher: Heidi Harrison
Development Editor: Siobhan Campbell
Production Manager: Andy Hannan/Yolanta Motylinska
Design: Andy Chapman
Typesetting and production: Helius

THE LANCET
Handbook of Treatment in
Neurology

EDITED BY
Charles Warlow BA MB BChir MD FRCP FMedSci

Professor of Medical Neurology, University of Edinburgh,
Edinburgh, UK

Honorary Consultant Neurologist, Western General Hospital,
Edinburgh, UK

Honorary Consultant Neurologist, Falkirk and District Royal Infirmary,
Falkirk, UK

FOREWORD BY
Graeme J. Hankey MD FRCP FRACP

Consultant Neurologist, Royal Perth Hospital, Perth, Australia

Clinical Professor, School of Medicine and Pharmacology,
University of Western Australia, Perth, Australia

ELSEVIER

EDINBURGH   LONDON   NEW YORK   OXFORD   PHILADELPHIA
ST LOUIS   SYDNEY   TORONTO   2006

THE LANCET

An imprint of Elsevier Limited

First published 2006
© 2006, Elsevier Ltd

No part of this publication may be reproduced, stored in a retrieval system, or transmitted in any form or by any means, electronic, mechanical, photocopying, recording or otherwise, without either the prior permission of the publishers or a licence permitting restricted copying in the United Kingdom issued by the Copyright Licensing Agency, 90 Tottenham Court Road, London W1T 4LP. Permissions may be sought directly from Elsevier's Health Sciences Rights Department in Philadelphia, USA: (+1) 215 239 3804, fax: (+1) 215 239 3805, e-mail: healthpermissions@elsevier.com. You may also complete your request on-line via the Elsevier Science homepage (http://www.elsevier.com), by selecting 'Customer Support' and then 'Obtaining Permissions'.

Main edition	ISBN-13: 978-0-08-044650-9
	ISBN-10: 0-08-044650-7
International edition	EAN: 978-0-08-045038-4
	ISBN: 0-08-045038-5

British Library Cataloguing in Publication Data
A catalogue record for this book is available from the British Library.

Library of Congress Cataloging in Publication Data
A catalog record for this book is available from the Library of Congress.

Note

Knowledge and best practice in this field are constantly changing. As new research and experience broaden our knowledge, changes in practice, treatment and drug therapy may become necessary or appropriate. Readers are advised to check the most current information provided (i) on procedures featured or (ii) by the manufacturer of each product to be administered, to verify the recommended dose or formula, the method and duration of administration, and contraindications. It is the responsibility of the practitioner, relying on their own experience and knowledge of the patient, to make diagnoses, to determine dosages and the best treatment for each individual patient, and to take all appropriate safety precautions. To the fullest extent of the law, neither the Publisher nor the Editor assumes any liability for any injury and/or damage to persons or property arising out of or related to any use of the material contained in this book.   *The Publisher*

ELSEVIER   your source for books, journals and multimedia in the health sciences

www.elsevierhealth.com

The publisher's policy is to use paper manufactured from sustainable forests

Printed in Spain

CONTENTS

Alan J. Carson MB CHB MPHIL MD MRCPSYCH
Consultant Neuropsychiatrist and Part time Senior Lecturer, Department of
Clinical Neurosciences, Western General Hospital, Edinburgh, UK

Brian R. Chambers MBBS MD FRACP
Head of Outpatient Stroke Services, Austin Health, Melbourne, Australia
Associate Director, National Stroke Research Institute, Melbourne, Australia
Principal Fellow, Department of Medicine, University of Melbourne,
Australia

Andrew M. Chancellor MD FRACP
Neurologist, Tauranga Hospital, Tauranga, New Zealand

Helen M. Dewey MBBS PhD FRACP FAFRM(RACP)
Head of Inpatient Stroke Services, Austin Health, Melbourne, Australia
Senior Research Fellow, National Stroke Research Institute, Melbourne,
Australia
Senior Lecturer, Department of Medicine, University of Melbourne,
Australia

David W. Dodick MD
Professor of Neurology, Mayo Clinic, Scottsdale, Arizona, USA

Michael Donaghy DPhil FRCP
Reader in Clinical Neurology, University of Oxford, UK
Consultant Neurologist, The Radcliffe Infirmary, Oxford, UK
Honorary Civilian Consultant Neurologist to the Army, UK

Geoffrey A. Donnan MBBS MD FRACP FRCP
Professor of Neurology, University of Melbourne, Australia
Director, National Stroke Research Institute, Melbourne, Australia

Jeremy Farrar BSc MBBS FRCP DPhil OBE
Director, Oxford University Clinical Research Unit, Hospital of Tropical
Diseases, Ho Chi Minh, Vietnam
Honorary Consultant, John Radcliffe Hospital, Oxford University, UK

Clare J. Fowler FRCP
Professor of Uro-Neurology, Institute of Neuroloy, University College, London, and National Hospital for Neurology and Neurosurgery, London, UK

Geraint Fuller MD FRCP
Consultant Neurologist, Gloucestershire Royal Infirmary, Gloucester, UK

Victor S. C. Fung PhD FRACP
Director, Movement Disorder Unit, Westmead Hospital, Sydney, Australia

Lionel Ginsberg BSc MBBS PhD FRCP
Consultant Neurologist, Royal Free Hospital, London, UK

Robin Grant MBChB MD
Consultant Neurologist, Western General Hospital, Edinburgh, UK
Senior Lecturer in Neurology, University of Edinburgh, UK

David Hilton-Jones MD FRCP FRCPE
Consultant Neurologist, The Radcliffe Infirmary, Oxford, UK

Nicholas Hirsch MBBS FRCA FRCP
Consultant Neuroanaesthetist, Harris Neuromedical Intensive Care Unit, National Hospital for Neurology and Neurosurgery, London, UK

Harry K. McNaughton PhD FRACP FAFRM
Rehabilitation Physician, Wellington Hospital, New Zealand

John Morris DM (Oxon) FRCP FRACP
Head, Department of Neurology, Westmead Hospital, Sydney, Australia

David Neary MD FRCP
Professor of Neurology, Greater Manchester Neuroscience Centre, Hope Hospital, Salford, UK

Jackie Palace BM DM MD FRCP
Consultant Neurologist, The Radcliffe Infirmary, Oxford, UK

Alejandro A. Rabinstein MD
Assistant Professor of Neurology, University of Miami School of Medicine, USA

Paul Reading MA MB BChir PhD FRCP
Consultant Neurologist, Department of Neurology, The James Cook University Hospital, Middlesbrough, UK

John Scadding MD FRCP
Consultant Neurologist, National Hospital for Neurology and
Neurosurgery, London, UK

Michael Sharpe MA MD FRCP FRCPsych
Professor of Psychological Medicine and Symptoms Research, University
of Edinburgh, UK

Simon Shorvon MA MD FRCP
Professor of Clinical Neurology, Institute of Neurology, University College
London, UK

Jon Stone MB ChB MRCP
Consultant Neurologist, Department of Clinical Neurosciences, Western
General Hospital, Edinburgh, UK

Eelco F. M. Wijdicks MD PHD FACP
Professor of Neurology, Mayo Clinic, Saint Mary's Hospital, Rochester,
Minnesota, USA

Adam Zeman MA BM BCh MRCP DM
Professor of Cognitive and Behavioural Neurology, Peninsula Medical
School, Royal Devon and Exeter Hospital, Exeter, UK

FOREWORD

Traditionally, clinical neurology focused on the diagnosis of neurological conditions and relevant clinico-anatomical-pathological correlation. Treatments were sparse, and their effectiveness and safety were evaluated in small case series compared with non-treated historical and literature controls. Flawed conclusions arose from systematic and random errors, and polarised views about treatments prevailed with passion.

More recently, neurological diagnosis has been enhanced by molecular genetic and neuroimaging techniques, treatments have been developed from enhanced understanding of the mechanisms of neurological diseases, and the effectiveness and safety of treatments have been evaluated by more rigorous methods, such as systematic reviews of randomised controlled trials, which minimise systematic and random errors. Treatments can now be judged scientifically.

However, best evidence remains to be translated optimally into best practice, arguably because best evidence is not available for practising clinicians in an easily accessible, clinically relevant and digestible format.

The Lancet Handbook of Treatment in Neurology aims to meet this need. It is a small yet comprehensive work dedicated to the treatment of common, and rare but treatable, neurological conditions. It is written by a team of 'World Cup All-Stars' from around the globe, that has been assembled and directed by its 'captain', Professor Charles Warlow, and 'Board of Management', The Lancet. The content is 'living' (i.e. real-life and relevant to everyday clinical practice) and the style is consistent. The authors assume that the correct diagnosis of each neurological condition has been made, and introduce their chapters with a brief description of the definition, epidemiology, pathology and aetiology where relevant to the treatment of the condition. What follows is an honest and succinct description of the natural (untreated) history of each condition, the favourable and unfavourable effects of available treatments, and how to monitor the treatment effects. The chapters provide a no-nonsense, 'bottom line' guide to appropriate treatment, which is based on the best evidence available, where it exists,

1 MIGRAINE AND OTHER PRIMARY HEADACHE SYNDROMES

David W. Dodick

Headache is the most common neurological symptom encountered in primary care, and also in general neurological practice. In most cases there is no serious underlying cause and the patient will have one of the primary headache syndromes which will be discussed in this chapter.

Migraine

Definition

- Migraine is a familial paroxysmal neurological disorder characterised by spontaneous or triggered attacks of headache that are variably associated with:
  - autonomic disturbance (nausea, pallor)
  - heightened sensitivity to external stimuli (light, noise, odour)
  - neurological symptoms (scotoma, paraesthesiae, dizziness) and less often signs (hemiparesis, aphasia)
  - alteration in mood (anxiety, depression).
- The attacks usually last 4–72 hours but they are often shorter in children (1–2 hours), and may last longer in some adults.
- The frequency of attacks is highly variable. Some individuals have only a few attacks during their lifetime, up to 25% suffer with one attack every week, while some may develop chronic migraine where headache occurs on more days than not.

Prevalence

- Migraine prevalence is similar in developed countries:
  - 18% of women and 6% of men in the USA have had had at least one migraine attack in the previous year. This amounts to more than 28 million sufferers, or one for every four households.
- Migraine prevalence varies by age, sex, ethnic origin and income:
  - before puberty, migraine prevalence is about 4%, after puberty prevalence increases, more rapidly in girls than boys
  - prevalence increases until about the age of 40 years, then declines
  - prevalence is lowest in Asian-Americans, intermediate in African-Americans, and highest in whites
  - migraine prevalence decreases as household income increases.
- Migraine greatly affects quality of life. The World Health Organisation ranks migraine among the world's 20 most disabling medical illnesses.

Types of migraine

- *Migraine with aura* consists of focal neurological symptoms that precede, accompany or (rarely) follow the headache:
  - the aura usually develops over 5–20 minutes, lasts for less than 60 minutes, and may include visual, sensory, motor, language or brainstem dysfunction
  - visual aura is the most common type of aura (90%) and most patients with sensory or motor aura also have visual aura
  - paraesthesiae are often cheiro-oral, where numbness starts in the hand, migrates up the arm and involves the face, lips and tongue
  - weakness is rare, occurs in association with sensory and visual symptoms, and is unilateral.
- *Migraine aura without headache* may occur at any age, but is more common in middle or older age, and there is not always a prior history of migraine with or without aura. These episodes are distinguished from transient ischaemic attacks by their gradual intensification, spread from one body part to another, and their recurrent and stereotyped nature.
- *Basilar migraine* manifests with brainstem symptoms such as ataxia, vertigo, tinnitus, diplopia, nausea and vomiting, nystagmus, dysarthria, bilateral paraesthesia, or a change in level of consciousness and cognition.
- *Hemiplegic migraine* can be sporadic or familial; the attacks are frequently precipitated by minor head injury.
- *Ophthalmoplegic migraine* is now felt to represent an idiopathic inflammatory neuritis.

Investigations

Investigations are generally not necessary in patients who meet the diagnostic criteria for migraine and who have a normal neurological examination. Screening blood tests and a baseline electrocardiogram (ECG) may be required prior to starting drug therapy, depending on the medications to be prescribed. For those who present with a first-time aura, or complex aura with motor, sensory or brainstem symptoms, brain magnetic resonance imaging (MRI) may be warranted.

The clinician must be alert to the fact that migraine may be the presenting manifestation of cerebral autosomal dominant arteriopathy with subcortical ischaemic stroke and leukoencephalopathy (CADASIL) and mitochondrial encephalopathy with lactic acidosis and stroke-like episodes (MELAS).

Box 1.1   International Headache Society criteria for migraine without aura

A. At least five attacks fulfilling criteria B–D.

B. Headache attacks lasting 4–72 hours (untreated or unsuccessfully treated).

C. Headache has at least *two* of the following characteristics:
   – unilateral location
   – pulsating quality
   – moderate or severe pain intensity
   – aggravation by or causing avoidance of routine physical activity (e.g. walking or climbing stairs).

D. During headache at least one of the following:
   – nausea *or* vomiting
   – photophobia *and* phonophobia.

E. Not attributed to another disorder.

A brief validated screening instrument has a 93% positive predictive value (2/3 questions answered yes) and a 98% positive predictive value (3/3 questions answered yes) for the diagnosis of migraine. This can be remembered by the acronym **PIN** ('pin the diagnosis of migraine'):
– Does light bother you a lot more than when you don't have headaches? (**P**hotophobia)
– Do your headaches limit your ability to work, study or do what you need to do for at least one day? (**I**mpairment)
– Do you feel nauseated or sick to your stomach? (**N**ausea)

Treatment for the attacks (Table 1.1)

- Non-specific drugs such as analgesics, non-steroidal anti-inflammatory drugs (NSAIDs) and opioids may control the pain of migraine.
- Specific drugs, such as the triptans and ergots, are effective for the treatment of migraine headache attacks but are not useful for other pain disorders.
- Triptans have largely usurped the role of ergotamine in clinical practice and are first-line treatment in patients with migraine headache of any severity for whom non-specific drugs have failed.
- By the time patients consult a physician for migraine, the attacks are almost always moderate or severe and the patients have already tried over-the-counter analgesics and NSAIDs.
- Developing an acute treatment strategy for an individual patient depends on several factors, including:
  - What percentage of headaches progress to moderate or severe pain if left untreated? If all, then:
  - Does the patient take acute therapy while the pain is still mild? If not, the patient should be encouraged to do so. If so, then:
  - What percentage of headaches respond to non-specific therapies if taken while the pain is still mild? If none, then:
  - The clinician should use a specific migraine drug while the pain is mild. This applies to patients who experience ≤ 4 attacks per month and can distinguish between tension-type and migraine headaches.
  - For patients with more frequent attacks of migraine headache, a preventive drug should also be started (see below), otherwise there is a risk of developing medication-overuse headache.
- Triptans are usually not recommended during the aura phase of an attack, nor are they used in patients with complex auras (sensory, motor, speech). They are contraindicated in hemiplegic migraine, and should be avoided in patients with coronary heart disease, previous stroke or uncontrolled hypertension.
- For those patients with severe nausea and vomiting as frequent features of an attack, especially when these symptoms occur early or during the premonitory phase:
  - a nasal spray or injectable formulation of a triptan, or dihydroergotamine should be considered.
  - antiemetics may also provide relief of nausea and headache: metoclopramide (10–20 mg, oral) or prochlorperazine (10–25 mg, oral, suppository).

Table 1.1 Drugs for the treatment of an acute migraine attack

Drug	Efficacy*	Adverse effects*	Relative contraindications
Acetaminophen (paracetamol)	2+	1+	Liver disease
Aspirin	2+	1+	Kidney disease, peptic ulcer, gastritis, age < 15 years
Butalbital (butobarbitone), caffeine and analgesics combined (Fioricet, Fiorinol)	2+	3+	Use of other sedatives, history of medication overuse
Caffeine	2+	1+	Sensitivity to caffeine
Isometheptene	2+	1+	Uncontrolled hypertension, coronary heart disease, peripheral vascular disease
Opioids	2+	4+	Drug or substance abuse
Non-steroidal anti-inflammatory drugs	2+	1+	Kidney disease, peptic ulcer, gastritis
Dihydroergotamine:			Uncontrolled hypertension, coronary heart disease, peripheral vascular disease
iv, im or sc	4+	2+	
intranasal	3+	1+	
Ergotamine:			Prominent nausea or vomiting, uncontrolled hypertension, coronary heart disease, peripheral vascular disease
tablets	2+	2+	
suppositories	2+	3+	
Triptans			Uncontrolled hypertension, coronary heart disease, peripheral vascular disease
Almotriptan: tablets	3+	+/–	
Eletriptan: tablets	3+	1+	
Frovatriptan: tablets	2+	1	
Naratriptan: tablets	2+	+/–	
Rizatriptan: tablets	3+	1+	
Zolmitriptran: tablets, intranasal	3+	1+	
Sumatriptan:			
sc	4+	2+	
intranasal	3+	1+	
tablets	3+	1+	

*Ratings are on a scale from 1+ (lowest) to 4+ (highest) based on response rates and consistency of response in double-blind placebo-controlled trials and clinical experience.

- A patient should not be considered a triptan non-responder until every triptan (including nasal and injectable formulations) has been tried at a stage of the attack when the pain is mild, and for at least three attacks.
- Opioids should be avoided unless absolutely necessary because of inadequate efficacy and risk of habituation, medication-overuse headache, and development of resistance to other acute headache medications.
- For those patients with a suboptimal response to a single drug, a combination of an analgesic or NSAID, triptan and antiemetic may be useful.
- In patients with status migrainosus, or prolonged migraine attacks not responsive to usual therapy, parenteral therapy is often required and a variety of options is available (Box 1.2).
- Pregnancy:
  - small doses of caffeine (< 300 mg) and acetaminophen (paracetamol) are safe after the first trimester
  - although there are no good studies, NSAIDs, including diclofenac, flurbiprofen, ibuprofen, ketoprofen, naproxen, piroxicam and indomethacin, appear to pose minimal risk to the fetus

---

Box 1.2   Treatment protocols for refractory migraine

- Prochlorperazine 10 mg iv over 2 minutes (may repeat in 30 minutes), or 10 mg iv + dihydroergotamine 0.5–1.0 mg iv over 10 minutes (may repeat in 60 minutes).
- Metoclopramide 10–20 mg iv, may repeat for up to 3 doses (30–60 mg cumulative maximum) over 2 hours, or 10 mg iv followed in 15 minutes by dihydroergotamine 0.5–1.0 mg iv.
- Droperidol 0.625 mg every 10 minutes (dose titration in this fashion may decrease the dose necessary for headache relief while minimising adverse effects). Average effective dose 3.15 mg.

Note: For all dopamine antagonists, diphenhydramine 25–50 mg iv or benztropine 1 mg iv may be given if extrapyramidal adverse effects (dystonia, akathisia) develop.

- Divalporex sodium (valproate) 500 mg iv in 100 ml normal saline over 15 minutes.
- Magnesium sulphate 1.0 g iv over 15 minutes.
- Dexamethasone 8–20 mg iv over 5–10 minutes, or hydrocortisone 100–250 mg iv over 10 minutes, every 8–12 hours for 24 hours.
- Ketorolac, 30–60 mg iv or im.

- after the first trimester, pyridoxine, dimenhydrinate, diphenhydramine, codeine, prochlorperazine, promethazine, metoclopramide and prednisolone are generally considered safe
- NSAIDs, meperidine and morphine should all be avoided in the third trimester
- aspirin, ergotamine and dihydroergotamine should be avoided
- there is no evidence of any increased risk of triptans to mother or fetus during pregnancy, but their use is generally discouraged.

Preventive treatment

Preventive drugs reduce attack frequency, duration or severity and are indicated when:
- migraine substantially interferes with the patient's daily routine, despite treatment of acute attacks
- there is failure of, contraindication to, overuse of, or troublesome adverse effects from acute drugs
- headaches are frequent (> 1 per week)
- there are special circumstances such as hemiplegic migraine, basilar-type migraine, or attacks associated with disorders such as CADASIL.

■ The preventive drugs with the best documented effectiveness are the beta-blockers (all except those with intrinsic sympathomimetic activity), valproate and topiramate (Table 1.2). The choice for a given patient is based on effectiveness, potential adverse effects, coexistent and comorbid conditions, and patient preference which is often based on the likely adverse effects. For example, a patient with coexisting hypertension may be started on a beta-blocker whereas a patient with depression and insomnia may be tried first on a tricyclic antidepressant. Drugs which have the potential for weight gain (tricyclics, valproate) should be avoided in an overweight patient or in those who would be adversely affected by weight gain (diabetes mellitus, hypertension, arthritis).

■ Every drug should be started at a low dose and increased slowly until satisfactory control is achieved, the maximum dose is reached, or dose-limiting adverse effects occur. A full therapeutic trial can take 2–6 months. It is important to remember that the efficacy of preventive drugs may increase over time. Therefore, when a partial response is seen at 1 or 2 months, patience is recommended as efficacy can increase over the ensuing several months.

■ Acute headache drugs should not be overused because of the prevailing belief that their overuse neutralises the effect of preventive medications.

Table 1.2	Preventive treatments in migraine		
Drug class	**Efficacy***	**Adverse effects***	**Relative contraindications**
Beta-blockers	4+	2+	Asthma, depression, cardiac failure, Raynaud's, heart block
Antiserotonin:			
Pizotifen	3+	2+	Weight gain
Methysergide	4+	4+	Angina, peripheral vascular disease
Calcium channel blockers:			
Verapamil	2+	1+	Constipation, hypotension, parkinsonism
Flunarizine	4+	2+	
Antidepressants:			
Tricyclics	3+	2+	Mania, urinary retention, arrhythmia
SSRIs	2+	1+	Mania
Antiepileptic drugs:			
Valproate	4+	2+	Liver disease, bleeding disorders
Gabapentin	2+	2+	Previous sensitivity
Topiramate	4+	2+	Kidney stones

SSRI, selective serotonin reuptake inhibitor.
*Ratings are on a scale from 1+ (lowest) to 4+ (highest).

- If headaches are well controlled for a period of 6 months, preventive treatment can be tapered and discontinued because periods of remission can occur.

Pre-emptive preventive therapy

This is used when there are predictable triggers:
- Menstrually associated migraine must be elicited by careful questioning because it is frequently overlooked, and it is often managed differently. NSAIDs (bd), oestradiol patch (100 µg/day) or a triptan (often bd) beginning 2 days prior to menstruation and continuing for several days, or for the duration of menses, are effective in this setting.
- High-altitude headache may be prevented with methazolamide (acetazolamide).

Pregnancy and preventive therapy

- In women of child-bearing age and potential, adequate contraception should be used in those started on preventive drugs.
- In general, preventive migraine medications should be avoided in pregnant women and in those attempting to conceive. This is especially true for valproate and ergotamine.
- Beta-blockers have been associated with small for gestational age infants, and tricyclic antidepressants may be associated with an increase in the rate of spontaneous abortion.
- Non-pharmacological techniques should be employed whenever possible (see below).
- During the post-partum period, antihistamines, ergotamine, bromo-criptine and tricyclics should be avoided. Caution is recommended with triptans, benzodiazepines, antidepressants and neuroleptics.

Non-pharmacological treatments

- Patients should be encouraged to keep a headache diary to document headache frequency and identify any potential triggers that have not already been identified.
- Behavioural and psychological interventions include relaxation training, thermal biofeedback combined with relaxation training, electromyography biofeedback, and cognitive–behavioural treatments. These techniques can augment the preventive effect of drugs, and may be particularly useful in patients with anxiety and depression, when stress is a particularly robust trigger, or for pregnant women where medications are avoided as much as possible.

Chronic daily headache

The term 'chronic daily headache' refers to a group of primary and secondary disorders characterised by very frequent headaches ($\geq$ 15 days per month).

Secondary chronic daily headache has an identifiable underlying cause such as acute headache medication overuse, head trauma and disorders of intracranial pressure.

Primary chronic daily headache is subdivided into long- and short-duration disorders, based on whether each headache episode lasts more or less than 4 hours.

- When headache lasts less than 4 hours, the differential diagnosis includes cluster headache, paroxysmal hemicrania, primary stabbing headache, hypnic headache and SUNCT (see below).
- When headache lasts longer than 4 hours, the major primary disorders include transformed migraine (Box 1.3), hemicrania continua, chronic tension-type headache and new daily persistent headache.
  - Long-duration chronic daily headache is a significant public health concern with a worldwide prevalence of 3–5%.
  - Transformed migraine accounts for 50% of patients with chronic daily headache, but up to 80% of those who present to the subspecialty of headache and neurological practice.
  - Most patients with transformed migraine overuse acute headache medications. However, not all of them suffer from medication-overuse headache (Box 1.4) and frequent headaches may persist even after withdrawal.

Management

The objectives are to decrease the frequency, severity and duration of the headaches. Since most chronic daily headache patients seen in a headache clinic will be overusing acute headache medications, a major component of the treatment plan is acute medication withdrawal. During withdrawal of acute medications, a transitional or bridge strategy is required and, once the medications have been effectively withdrawn, patients need a new acute treatment plan. Many authorities advocate the use of preventive medications

---

Box 1.3   Silberstein–Lipton criteria for transformed migraine

- Daily or almost daily (> 15 days/month) head pain for > 1 month.
- Average headache duration of > 4 hour/day (if untreated).
- At least one of the following:
  - history of episodic migraine meeting International Headache Society criteria
  - history of increasing headache frequency with decreasing severity of migrainous features over at least 3 months
  - headache at some time meets International Headache Society criteria for migraine, other than duration.
- Does not meet criteria for new daily persistent headache, or hemicrania continua.
- Not attributed to another disorder.

Box 1.4   Diagnostic criteria for medication-overuse headache

A. Headache present on > 15 days/month fulfilling criteria C and D.

B. Regular overuse of a medication for > 3 months:
   - ergotamine, triptans, opioids and combination analgesics ≥ 10 days/month
   - simple analgesics ≥ 15 days/month
   - total exposure of all acute medications ≥ 7 days/month.

C. Headache has developed or markedly worsened during medication overuse.

D. Headache resolves or reverts to its previous pattern within 2 months of discontinuation of overused medication.

---

from the outset since these may ameliorate withdrawal symptoms, reduce headache frequency during and after the withdrawal phase, and minimise the risk of relapse. Many patients, but certainly not all, improve or revert to an episodic pattern of headache after overused acute medications have been withdrawn.

Box 1.5 outlines the management of transformed migraine with medication overuse.

- Non-pharmacological measures are important: patients should be encouraged to eat, sleep and exercise in a regular pattern, and caffeine consumption should be limited or eliminated.
- Any comorbid depression and anxiety must be treated.
- Relaxation techniques and biofeedback may be very helpful, and certainly their benign adverse effect profile is appealing.
- Patients overusing acute medications need education that this behaviour may reduce or completely prevent the efficacy of preventive medications, and that during the withdrawal period the headaches may get worse for 1–4 weeks before subsequently improving. It must also be emphasised that headaches will continue to occur frequently, if not daily, so long as the overuse of acute headache medications continues.
- Withdrawal symptoms, including severe headaches, nausea, vomiting, agitation, restlessness, sweating and insomnia may occur. These typically last 2–10 days, although they may persist for 2–4 weeks. In most patients there is significant headache improvement by 4–8 weeks.
- The withdrawal of overused acute medications can be managed on an outpatient basis in most patients.
- If outpatient treatment fails, is not safe due to concern for a barbiturate or opioid withdrawal syndrome, or if there is significant medical or psychiatric comorbidity, inpatient treatment may be needed.

Box 1.5   Treatment of transformed migraine with medication overuse

Outpatient protocols
- Education, support and close follow-up for 8–12 weeks.
- Encourage lifestyle modification (smoking, exercise, meals, sleep, caffeine).
- Biobehavioural therapy (relaxation therapy, biofeedback).
- Withdrawal of overused medications:
  - analgesics, ergotamine or triptans – may be abrupt, or rapid taper over 1–2 weeks
  - butalbital (butobarbitone) overuse, taper over 2–4 weeks; if concern for withdrawal syndrome, provide tapering course of phenobarbital 30 mg bd for 2 weeks followed by 15 mg bd for 2 weeks
  - opioid overuse, taper over 2–4 weeks; if concern for withdrawal syndrome, use clonidine patch for 2–4 weeks.
- Transitional strategies for relief of withdrawal headaches (not to exceed 10 treatment days per month):
  - prednisolone 100 mg/day for 5 days
  - NSAIDs (naproxen sodium 550 mg, ketoprofen 50–100 mg, ibuprofen 400–800 mg)
  - antiemetics (metoclopramide, prochlorperazine, domperidone)
  - dihydroergotamine 1 mg sc or im
  - preventive drug therapy (Table 1.3).

Inpatient protocols
- Intravenous infusions every 8 hours for 2–4 days:
  - dihydroergotamine 0.5–1.0 mg + metaclopramide 10–20 mg or prochlorperazine 10 mg
  - or sodium valproate 6.4 mg/kg
  - or methylprednisolone 250–500 mg every 12 hours
  - or ketorolac 10 mg.
- Initiate preventive therapy (Table 1.3).
- Discontinue overused medication (analgesics, ergotamine, triptan) or begin taper (barbiturates or opioids).

- The 4-year relapse rate is approximately 50%. The vast majority of patients relapse within the first year after withdrawal, and the relapse rate is higher in those overusing analgesics compared with those overusing triptans.
- Preventive therapy for patients with transformed migraine, even in those overusing acute medications, should generally be started immediately, and not delayed until acute medications are withdrawn (Table 1.3).

Table 1.3   Preventive medications for transformed migraine (± acute headache medication overuse)*

Medication class	Drug	Starting daily dose	Target daily dose	Titration period	Common adverse effects
Antidepressant	Amitriptyline	10 mg	50–100 mg	1 month	Weight gain, dry mouth, constipation, palpitations, drowsiness, dizziness, fatigue
	Fluoxetine	20 mg	20–60 mg	1 month	Anorexia, insomnia, anxiety, tremor, asthenia, dizziness, somnolence
	Nefazodone	200 mg	200–450 mg	1 month	Asthenia, dizziness, somnolence, blurred vision, nausea, constipation, dry mouth
Antiepileptic drugs	Valproate	250 mg	500–2000 mg	2 weeks	Nausea, somnolence, dizziness, vomiting, tremor, alopecia, weight gain
	Gabapentin	300 mg	900–3600 mg	1 month	Dizziness, somnolence, ataxia, abnormal thinking, peripheral oedema, weight gain, incoordination
	Topiramate	25 mg	100–200 mg	1–2 months	Paraesthesia, difficulty concentrating, word-finding memory, urolithiasis, acute glaucoma
Alpha$_2$-adrenergic agonist	Tizanidine	4 mg	8–20 mg	1 month	Dry mouth, somnolence, asthenia, dizziness, constipation, hypotension, bradycardia
Neurotoxin	Botulinum toxin type A		25–250 units	Injection every 3 months	Weakness, muscle pain, ptosis, bruising

*A long-acting NSAID used for 4–8 weeks may provide useful adjunctive relief of headache and associated symptoms when used in combination with any of the medications listed above.

Preventive medications may minimise withdrawal symptoms as well as reduce headache frequency and relapse rate after drug withdrawal.

Tension-type headache

Tension-type headache is defined by recurrent attacks of mild to moderate intensity headache that last 30 minutes to 1 week untreated. The headaches are frequently bilateral and are often described as a dull pressure or squeezing discomfort. The pain is not throbbing, unilateral or aggravated by physical activity, nor is it associated with photophobia, phonophobia or nausea. These headaches, in other words, are 'featureless'.

Chronic tension-type headache is differentiated from **episodic tension-type headache** by headache on more than 15 days per month for more than 6 consecutive months. About 80% of the general population experience a tension-type headache during their lifetime. By contrast, the prevalence of chronic tension-type headache is much lower at 2–3%. Episodic tension-type headache prevalence appears to peak in the 30s and 40s and declines thereafter, whereas chronic tension-type headache appears to increase with age.

Although tension-type headache is the most common primary headache type in the general population, patients who present in neurological practice rarely have tension-type headache as their only headache type. Because migraine is frequently associated with neck pain and tenderness, may be bilateral, is often associated with stress as a trigger, and depression or anxiety as comorbid disorders, migraine patients are often misdiagnosed as having tension-type headache. In fact only 10% of the headaches that migraine sufferers experience meet the criteria for tension-type headache, and even many of these phenotypic tension-type headaches respond to triptans and are felt to be biologically similar to migraine ('mild migraine').

Treatment

- Non-pharmacological therapy:
  - physical exercise
  - relaxation therapy
  - cognitive therapy
  - biofeedback
  - physical therapy (hot/cold packs, massage).
- Oral pharmacological therapy for symptomatic relief:
  - aspirin 500–1000 mg
  - acetaminophen (paracetamol) 500–1000 mg

- ibuprofen 200–400 mg
- naprosyn 275–550 mg
- ketoprofen 25–50 mg
- aspirin + acetamiophen (paracetamol) + caffeine.
■ Prophylaxis:
- amitriptyline 10–100 mg/day.

Trigeminal–autonomic cephalalgias

Trigeminal–autonomic cephalalgias are a group of primary headache syndromes manifested by pain in the distribution of the trigeminal nerve along with one or more autonomic signs including lacrimation, conjunctival injection, nasal congestion, rhinorrhoea, ptosis, meiosis, facial pallor or sweating, and periorbital oedema. With the exception of hemicrania continua, these disorders are characterised by discrete, stereotyped and relatively short-lasting (seconds to 3 hours) episodes of severe unilateral pain that is often confined to or maximal in the orbital/periorbital region. The attacks are separated by pain-free intervals, but often recur on a daily basis either continuously (chronic) or for a defined period of time (episodic) with intervening periods of remission. They are differentiated from each other on the basis of the duration of the individual attacks, the daily frequency of attacks and the response to medication (Table 1.4). These disorders are highly disabling and yet eminently treatable, underscoring the importance of an accurate diagnosis.

Structural lesions may mimic the trigeminal–autonomic cephalalgias and these should be considered at presentation. Clues include the absence of periodicity, a low-grade background headache that does not subside between attacks, and an inadequate or incomplete response to therapy. It is prudent to obtain an MRI scan on all patients suspected of having a trigeminal–autonomic cephalalgia at presentation.

CLUSTER HEADACHE

■ Cluster headache is an excruciatingly severe unilateral headache that is maximal in the orbital–temporal region and is associated with cranial autonomic features such as ipsilateral lacrimation, ptosis, rhinorrhoea and conjunctival injection. The attacks often occur with a stereotyped periodicity (same time of day or night), nocturnal predilection (awaken patient from sleep) and last on average 60 minutes (range 30–180 minutes). Patients may experience 1–8 attacks per day. The period during which recurrent attacks occur, typically weeks yet at times months or years, is referred to as the 'cluster period'. Remissions may last from months to years.

■ Cluster headache is uncommon, with a prevalence of 0.4%, and the male/female ratio is about 4:1 (cluster headache and SUNCT are the only primary headache disorders more common in males).

■ The acute and preventive treatment of cluster headache is outlined in Tables 1.5 and 1.6.
  – Since the pain intensity peaks within 5–10 minutes and lasts for only 30–180 minutes, acute treatments are most effective when delivered intranasally or parenterally.
  – Because the attacks occur daily, and sometimes many times every day for weeks or months, transitional and/or preventive treatment is initiated in all patients.
  – Transitional strategies are designed to rapidly suppress or reduce the frequency and severity of attacks during the period of time it takes for the effect of the preventive medication to become evident. Since the duration of the cluster periods is usually predictable for an individual patient based on prior experience, these medications are usually used for the duration of the cluster period plus 2 weeks.

Table 1.4   Differentiating features of the trigeminal–autonomic cephalalgias

Feature	Cluster headache	Paroxysmal hemicrania	SUNCT
Sex ratio (M:F)	4:1	1:3	2:1
Attack duration (range)	60 minutes (30–180 minutes)	20 minutes (2–45 minutes)	40 seconds (5–200 seconds)
Attack frequency	1–8/day (typically 1–3/day)	1–20/day (typically 5–10/day)	1/day to 30/hour (typically > 10/day)
Indomethacin response (first-line treatment)	Verapamil	Indomethacin	Tamotrigine

SUNCT, short-lasting unilateral neuralgiform pain with conjunctival injection and tearing.

Trigeminal neuralgia, see Chapter 7.

Table 1.5	Drugs used as acute treatment for cluster headache				
Drug	**Standard dose**	**Route***	**Contraindications**	**Remarks**
Oxygen	100%, 7–10 l/min for 10–15 minutes	Nasal	None	Major draw back: inconvenience
Sumatriptan	6 mg 20 mg	sc Intranasal	Cardiovascular disease, uncontrolled hypertension, pregnancy	Avoid in patients with multiple daily attacks
Dihydro-ergotamine mesylate	0.5–1 mg 0.5–1 mg 2 mg	iv im Intranasal	Peripheral vascular disease, cardio-vascular disease, uncontrolled hypertension, pregnancy	Fewer adverse effects than ergotamine
Zolmitriptan	5 mg, 10 mg 5 mg	Oral Intranasal	Same as sumatriptan	Same as sumatriptan
Somatostatin	100 μg	sc	Hypersensitivity to somatostatin	–
*Route of administration.				

- In patients with chronic cluster headache where there are no remissions, preventive medications (often a combination of drugs) are used indefinitely, or until a remission of at least 3 months has been achieved.
- In patients with chronic cluster headache lasting for more than 2 years that has failed to respond to maximal medical therapy (combinations of up to three preventive drugs), surgery is a last resort (Box 1.6).

PAROXYSMAL HEMICRANIA AND HEMICRANIA CONTINUA

Paroxysmal hemicrania is similar to cluster headache, and the differentiating features are outlined in Table 1.4.

Hemicrania continua is characterised by a headache that is unilateral, continuous and moderately severe. The continuous background pain is punctuated by severe exacerbations that can last from hours to days, cranial

Table 1.6   Prevention of cluster headache

Intervention	Standard dose	Contraindications	Adverse effects	Remarks
Transitional				
Prednisolone	40–60 mg/day initially, oral, taper by 10 mg every 3 days	Poorly controlled diabetes mellitus, active peptic ulcer, osteoporosis	Hyperglycaemia, insomnia, restlessness, personality changes, hyponatraemia, osteoporosis, Cushing's syndrome, cataract, glaucoma, oedema, myopathy, peptic ulcer, hypertension, hip necrosis	Long-term use is not warranted
Ergotamine	1–2 mg, oral or rectal, once or twice daily	Vascular disease, uncontrolled hypertension, decreased liver or kidney function, pregnancy	Nausea, vomiting, paraesthesias, cold hands and feet, claudication, ergotism	Long-term use is not recommended
Occipital nerve block	3–5 ml 0.5% bupivicaine + 10–20 mg methylprenisolone	Hypersensitivity to any of the ingredients	Numbness posterior scalp, haematoma	May provide effective relief for 1–2 weeks
Maintenance				
Verapamil	120–720 mg/day in three divided doses	Heart block, heart failure	Constipation, oedema, hypotension, dizziness, nausea, fatigue, paraesthesiae	Medication of choice for episodic cluster headache

	Dose	Contraindications	Side effects	Comments
Methysergide	2–6 mg/day up to 12 mg, in three divided doses	Vascular disease	Muscle cramps, cold extremities, nausea, diarrhoea, pleuropulmonary and retroperitoneal fibrosis	Physicians Desk Reference advises that therapy be interrupted every 4–6 months
Lithium carbonate	300 mg, oral, 2 or 3 times daily	Vascular disease, kidney dysfunction, pregnancy	Nausea, weakness, tremor, polydipsia, polyuria, diarrhoea, myxoedema, arrhythmias, lethargy, blurred vision, slurred speech, extrapyramidal signs	Serum concentration and thyroid and kidney function must be monitored during long-term treatment. Major drug interactions: diuretics and NSAIDs
Valproate	500–2000 mg/day, may be given as 1 dose sustained release, or bd	Pregnancy, liver and pancreatic disease	Nausea, tremor, weight gain, lethargy, alopecia, occasionally abnormal liver function, pancreatitis	Periodic monitoring of liver function if long-term treatment
Topiramate	50–200 mg/day, up to 200 mg as a single dose, or in two divided doses	Renal calculi, pregnancy	Paraesthesiae, somnolence, cognitive symptoms, dizziness, ataxia. Patients must be aware of rare adverse effect of acute angle closure glaucoma. Renal calculi occurs in 1%	Preliminary open-label data
Gabapentin	900–3600 mg/day, oral, in 3 divided doses	Hypersensitivity to the drug	Peripheral oedema, dizziness, somnolence	Open-label data

---

Box 1.6 Surgical treatment for cluster headache

- Procedures directed toward the sensory trigeminal nerve:
  - radiofrequency trigeminal rhizotomy
  - retrogasserian glycerol injection
  - alcohol injection into gasserian ganglion
  - alcohol injection into supraorbital and intraorbital nerves
  - trigeminal nerve root section
  - gamma-knife surgery of root exit zone of trigeminal nerve
  - avulsion of intraorbital, supraorbital and supratrochlear nerves
  - microvascular decompression of trigeminal nerve root, or of nervus intermedius (parasympathetic fibres of 7th cranial nerve)
  - occipital nerve stimulation.
- Procedures directed towards the autonomic pathways:
  - section of greater superficial petrosal nerve
  - section of intermediate nerve
  - section or cocainisation of sphenopalatine ganglion.
- Hypothalamic deep brain stimulation.

---

autonomic symptoms, ice-pick pains and symptoms that are commonly associated with migraine (photophobia, phonophobia, nausea). It is therefore easily mistaken for migraine or chronic migraine. Thus in patients with a continuous unilateral headache, if not contraindicated it is always worth a brief (3–7 days) trial of indomethacin with up to 300 mg/day if necessary.

- Indomethacin is not only the treatment of choice for paroxysmal hemicranias and hemicrania continua, but a response to this drug is an obligatory diagnostic criterion.
- Treatment is usually initiated at 25 mg tds, oral, with meals.
- Most patients have complete headache relief within 24 hours, frequently within 8 hours.
- If headache relief is not obtained within 48 hours, the dose should be increased to 50 mg tds.
- Treatment failure should be considered only if a patient does not respond to 300 mg/day.
- After an effective dose has been established for several weeks, it should be decreased gradually to ascertain the lowest effective dose. Maintenance doses between 25 and 100 mg/day are usually adequate to suppress the headache.
- Occasionally, dose adjustments are necessary to treat the fluctuations in headache severity that occur in these disorders.

- Because nocturnal attacks or exacerbations may occur, a bedtime dose of sustained-release indomethacin may be useful.
- Some patients are so exquisitely sensitive to indomethacin that skipping even one dose allows the headache to recur.
- Although long-term, indefinite treatment is often required, a periodic attempt to withdraw the medication is important because long-term remissions have been described.
- If the headache is refractory to indomethacin, the diagnosis should be reconsidered, even though some apparently typical cases have been described where the headache was unresponsive to indomethacin. Patients who require a continuous high dose of indomethacin and those who require increasing doses after an initial response to a lower dose may have an underlying structural lesion and need careful evaluation for parasellar, pituitary and posterior fossa lesions.
- In patients who fail to respond to or tolerate indomethacin, several drugs have been reported as effective, including other NSAIDs, dihydroergotamine, methysergide, corticosteroids, acetaminophen with caffeine, lamotrigine, gabapentin and lithium carbonate.

SUNCT SYNDROME

SUNCT (short-lasting unilateral neuralgiform pain with conjunctival injection and tearing) is a rare primary headache disorder that is more common in males (2:1) and usually begins between the age of 40 and 70 years. The individual attacks of pain are very brief, lasting less than 40 seconds on average (range 5–200 seconds). The pain is moderate or severe, exclusively unilateral, maximal in the orbital, periorbital or frontal location, and often described as an electric-shock or a stabbing, piercing or burning pain. The pain peaks and resolves abruptly. Most patients are completely pain-free between attacks, although some report a persistent dull discomfort. The attack frequency between and among individual sufferers varies considerably, occurring as infrequently as once a day to more than 30 attacks an hour. Unlike cluster headache, nocturnal attacks are seldom reported. The cranial autonomic symptoms occur in synchrony with the pain.

SUNCT can be differentiated from paroxysmal hemicrania by the brevity of the attacks (seconds) and lack of response to indomethacin. Unlike SUNCT, the pain associated with primary stabbing headache (previously 'ice-pick headache') lasts only 1–3 seconds and the stabs of pain are not usually confined to the orbital/periorbital region, occur on both sides of the head, and are not associated with cranial autonomic symptoms.

Because of the considerable overlap in the clinical phenotype, differentiating SUNCT from trigeminal neuralgia can be very challenging. Both are characterised by frequent unilateral stabbing or electric-like shocks of pain of brief duration that are associated with trigger zones in the face, and both occur in middle or older age. However, unlike SUNCT, the pain of trigeminal neuralgia is rarely confined to the ophthalmic division of the trigeminal nerve or accompanied by cranial autonomic features (see Chapter 7).

Treatment

■ Unlike other trigeminal–autonomic cephalalgias, patients with SUNCT do not respond to indomethacin, nor do they respond to medications typically effective for patients with cluster headache.

■ Lamotrigine 100–200 mg/day has been reported to be highly effective in several patients and is widely considered to be the treatment of first choice.

■ Gabapentin, topiramate and carbamazepine have also been reported to be effective.

■ It has been recently demonstrated that intravenous lidocaine (lignocaine) can completely suppress attacks of SUNCT, so this should be considered in patients where continuous suppression of attacks is needed for a short period of time. For example, in patients with dozens or more than 100 attacks per day, respite from pain may be needed until effective preventive medication can be established.

Hypnic headache

Hypnic headache is a rare syndrome that has been called 'alarm-clock headache' because it occurs exclusively during sleep and often at the same time each night. The mean age of onset is 62 years (range 26–84 years). The pain is bilateral in about two-thirds of cases, and mild to moderate; although severe pain is reported by about 20% of patients. The attacks usually last from 15 to 180 minutes. Patients often need to get out of bed to relieve the pain. Spontaneous remission is rare.

The older age of onset, absence of cranial autonomic features such as lacrimation and rhinorrhoea, lack of remission periods, the mild to moderate nature of the pain, and the often bilateral location of the pain, should allow this disorder to be differentiated from cluster headache, which can also awaken patients predictably at the same time each night.

New-onset nocturnal headache in the elderly should raise concern about causes such as raised intracranial pressure, giant cell arteritis, obstructive sleep apnoea, nocturnal hypertension, glaucoma, medication-overuse headache and nocturnal hypoglycaemia.

Treatment

- Aspirin has been demonstrated to provide acute relief of hypnic headache attacks.
- For prevention, lithium has been used most frequently and has also showed the best overall efficacy (300–600 mg/day, oral, in 2–3 divided doses). Sustained-release lithium carbonate at a dose of 300–450 mg/day may be effective (see also Chapter 13).
- Indomethacin (25–75 mg at bedtime), flunarizine (10 mg qds) and caffeine (coffee or 60–200 mg at bedtime) have also been reported to be effective.

Atypical facial pain

'Atypical facial pain' has become an umbrella term for facial pain of indeterminate origin. Historically, pain not clearly identifiable as one of the typical, well-defined neuralgic syndromes, was assumed to be of psychogenic origin. In contrast to the highly stereotyped and distinguishing features of neuralgic pain (e.g. trigeminal neuralgia), this syndrome is characterised by:

- Constant poorly localised pain, described as deep and aching, boring, burning or throbbing.
- No trigger zones or cutaneous triggers (e.g. teeth-brushing, touching the face).
- Areas of localised tenderness with spread of pain to other areas of the face, head or neck.
- Greater prevalence in women and younger or middle-aged groups.
- Lack of response to antiepileptic drugs or ablative lesions of the trigeminal nerve.

In most cases the pain is organic even if a demonstrable cause is not readily identified. If the cause is not clear from the history and examination, a careful evaluation of the skull, brain, cervical spine, cerebrospinal fluid (CSF), and of dental, nasal, eye, throat, sinus, ear and chest structures is necessary. The diagnosis of facial pain of unknown origin (atypical facial pain) can only be made after excluding:

- nasopharyngeal carcinoma
- lung carcinoma (invasion/compression of the ipsilateral vagus nerve)

- mandibular or maxillary bone cavities, postsurgical (root canal) microabscesses, cracked tooth syndrome
- sinusitis (including ethmoidal and sphenoidal)
- carotid dissection
- vascular (discrete episodes of throbbing pain) or autonomic features (tearing, rhinorrhoea) suggestive of migraine or cluster headache
- post-traumatic or postsurgical pain (sinus procedures, dental extractions)
- posterior fossa tumours.

If no obvious underlying cause is uncovered, the mainstay of therapy usually involves biofeedback and relaxation therapy. Biobehavioural techniques may be particularly useful in patients with comorbid anxiety or depression. Since depression is common in this group of patients, tricyclic antidepressants are often useful to ameliorate the pain as well as to treat any underlying depression.

Thunderclap headache

- 'Thunderclap headache' refers to an excruciating headache of instantaneous onset – as sudden and as unexpected as a clap of thunder. The term was first used to describe this type of headache as a presentation of an unruptured cerebral aneurysm, but there are a number of other causes (Box 1.7).
- Primary thunderclap headache is self-limited and treatment is supportive by providing analgesia if the headache persists.
- For all new presentations of exertional or sexual headache, appropriate imaging should be performed to search for subarachnoid haemorrhage or an intracranial lesion.

Box 1.7   Causes of thunderclap headache

Primary causes
- Primary thunderclap headache.
- Primary cough headache.
- Primary exertional headache.
- Primary sexual headache.

Secondary causes
- Subarachnoid haemorrhage.
- Intracranial venous thrombosis.
- Carotid/vertebral dissection.
- Pituitary apoplexy.
- Spontaneous CSF leak.
- Retroclival haematoma.
- Hypertensive crisis.
- Unruptured intracranial aneurysm.

- Various posterior fossa abnormalities have been described in patients who have cough headache, the Arnold–Chiari type I malformation being the most common.
- For cough headache (often occurs with a variety of activities that produce a valsalva manoeuvre, e.g. laugh, strain, cry, bend, sneeze), if it is persistent, indomethacin 2–3 times daily (25–150 mg in total, oral) with meals is often very helpful.
- For those with recurrent primary exertional or sexual headache, a 25–75 mg oral dose of indomethacin 1–2 hours prior to the activity is usually effective.

Primary stabbing headache (ice-pick headache)

- Primary stabbing headache (ice-pick headache) is a benign, common but unusual disorder characterised by ultrashort (1–2 seconds) attacks of stabbing pain, unilateral or bilateral, varying from one part of the head to another.
- The treatment of choice is indomethacin in 2–3 divided doses in a total daily dose of 25–200 mg oral.
- Treatment is often not necessary, however, unless attacks of pain occur repeatedly on a near-daily basis.
- Once remission occurs, indomethacin can be discontinued.

Intracranial hypotension

Low CSF pressure, usually due to a leak through the spinal dura, causes low intracranial pressure and the striking clinical feature of orthostatic headache (i.e. rapid resolution with lying down) with, in severe cases, neck pain, nausea, vomiting, diplopia, blurred vision and distorted hearing. Intracranial hypotension results in mechanical distortion of intracranial contents. The CSF leak may be:
- spontaneous
- due to dural connective tissue weakness, as in Marfan's syndrome
- iatrogenic, most commonly following diagnostic lumbar puncture but also spinal surgery, spinal anaesthesia or epidural anaesthesia.

Prevention at diagnostic lumbar puncture

- Smallest needle size compatible with pressure measurement and removal of CSF.

Table 2.1   Classification of seizure type

Seizure type	Description
Generalised seizures	
Tonic–clonic seizures	Occur mainly in idiopathic generalised epilepsy. Also in acute symptomatic epilepsy due to metabolic/toxic/anoxic causes
Absence seizures	Occur only in idiopathic generalised epilepsy
Myoclonic seizures	See Box 2.3
Tonic seizures, atonic seizures	Only in severe epilepsy syndromes (e.g. Lennox–Gastaut syndrome)
Clonic seizures	Only in infants
Partial seizures	
Partial seizures Secondarily generalised seizures	Occur in many forms of symptomatic and cryptogenic epilepsy

- About 40% of patients who develop epilepsy do so below 16 years of age and about 20% over the age of 65 years.
- The cumulative incidence of epilepsy – the risk of an individual having a seizure in their lifetime – is about 4%.
- Isolated (first and only) seizures (20/100,000/year) and febrile seizures (50/100,000/year) are not usually included in epilepsy statistics.
- In a population of one million, there are about 5000 with active epilepsy on treatment and about 15,000 with a history of epilepsy in remission.
- The standardised mortality is 2–3 times higher in patients with epilepsy than the background population. In newly diagnosed epilepsy this excess mortality is due largely to the underlying cause of the epilepsy. In chronic epilepsy the excess mortality is largely due to death in epileptic seizures (sudden unexpected death in epilepsy (SUDEP), accidents, etc.) – about one death per 2500 patients per year in mild epilepsy, to one per 100 patients per year amongst those with severe and intractable epilepsy.

Prognosis

- In about 60% of those developing seizures, initial therapy is completely effective, and the mean duration of active epilepsy is short (< 5 years) in about 50%.
- In the other 40%, seizures persist in spite of initial therapy, and alternative therapies are needed.

- In about 20%, seizures remain uncontrolled for long periods of time, in spite of drug therapy.
- About 15% of those on treatment have more than 50 seizures per year, 25% between 10 and 50 per year, and 60% less than 10 seizures a year.

Learning and other disabilities

- About one-third to one-half of children, and about one-fifth of adults, with epilepsy have, in addition, learning disability.
- Similarly, epilepsy occurs in about 20% of those with learning disability.
- 18% of adults with newly diagnosed epilepsy have cognitive disabilities, 6% have motor disabilities and 6% severe psychiatric disorders.
- About one in 15 patients with epilepsy is dependent on others for daily living because of epilepsy and the associated handicaps – amongst neurological diseases, only stroke and dementia have a greater impact.
- Stigmatisation of patients with epilepsy is common, and social attitude change would alleviate many of the problems encountered by patients with epilepsy – this is as important as any medical therapy.

CHOICE OF DRUGS FOR DIFFERENT SEIZURE TYPES

The approach to drug treatment of epilepsy broadly depends upon:
- seizure type
- stage (newly diagnosed, chronic epilepsy, epilepsy in remission)
- epilepsy syndrome
- special patient groups.

Table 2.1 is a summary of the International League against Epilepsy classification of seizure type, Table 2.2 lists the effective drugs in these different seizure types and Table 2.3 shows the licensed drugs in Europe (the licensed indications for individual drugs vary in different countries) There is considerable off-label use of drugs.

The choice of drug depends on various factors, and as far as possible drug treatment should be tailored individually:
- People differ in their willingness to risk adverse effects, or to try new therapy.
- Patients' preferences depend on their age, gender and comorbidity, comedication, drug formulation and dosing frequencies, and other factors such as risks in pregnancy and a whole range of social aspects.
- The pattern of drug usage varies widely between countries, reflecting differences in medical systems, cost, marketing pressures and medical preferences.

Table 2.2   Choice of antiepileptic drugs in different seizure types

Effective drugs

	Seizure type						
	Partial	Secondarily generalised tonic–clonic	Generalised tonic–clonic	Absence	Myoclonic	Atypical absence	Tonic and atonic
Clobazam	●	●	●	●	●	●	●
Clonazepam	●	●	●	●	●	●	●
Carbamazepine	●	●	●				
Ethosuximide				●			
Gabapentin	●	●					
Lamotrigine	●	●	●	●	●	●	●
Levetiracetam	●	●	●	●	●	●	●
Oxcarbazepine	●	●	●				
Phenobarbital	●	●	●	●	●	●	●
Phenytoin	●	●	●			●	●
Piracetam					●		
Pregabalin	●	●					
Primidone	●	●	●			●	●
Tiagabine	●	●	●				
Topiramate	●	●	●			●	●
Valproate	●	●	●	●	●	●	●
Zonisamide	●	●	●	●	●	●	●

This list shows seizure types that have been shown in studies (often non-randomised) to respond, but in many countries licensing is more restricted. See Table 2.3.

- Some drugs worsen certain seizure types (e.g. the frequent worsening of absence seizures by carbamazepine, gabapentin, oxcarbazepine and tiagabine).

Initial antiepileptic drug choice in drug-naive patients (Box 2.1)

In partial seizures and secondarily generalised seizures

- Carbamazepine (in most countries in Europe).
- Valproate, phenytoin (in the USA) or lamotrigine are commonly used alternatives.
- In some countries in the developing world, phenobarbital.
- There are a few controlled studies comparing these drugs and no differences in efficacy have been found.

In generalised tonic–clonic seizures

- Valproate.
- Carbamazepine, lamotrigine or phenytoin are commonly used alternatives.
- In some countries, in the developing world, phenobarbital.
- There are a few controlled studies comparing these drugs and no differences in efficacy have been found.

In myoclonus

- Valproate.
- Alternatives are clonazepam, lamotrigine (sometimes worsens myoclonus).

In absence seizures

- Valproate or ethosuximide.

Choice of antiepileptic drugs in established active epilepsy (i.e. when seizures continue despite initial drug therapy)

- Depends on seizure type (see Tables 2.2 and 2.3).
- Most randomised trials have been in patients with uncontrolled chronic partial (and secondarily generalised) epilepsies; they have almost uniformly failed to show significant differences between antiepileptic drug efficacy. Similarly, as monotherapy in early epilepsy, topiramate,

Table 2.3　Licensed indications for antiepileptic drugs in Europe

	Licensed indications	Monotherapy	Age
Carbamazepine, phenytoin, phenobarbital, valproate	No restrictions	Yes	Any age
Clobazam	Adjunctive therapy for epilepsy (no restrictions by seizure type)	Not licensed for monotherapy	≥ 3 years (can be used in children over 6 months in exceptional circumstances)
Gabapentin	Adjunctive second-line therapy in partial and secondarily generalised tonic–clonic seizures	Not licensed for monotherapy	≥ 6 years
Lamotrigine	Partial and tonic–clonic seizures (primary or secondarily generalised) and Lennox–Gastaut syndrome	Yes	≥ 2 years; ≥ 12 years in monotherapy
Levetiracetam	Adjunctive therapy in partial and secondarily generalised tonic–clonic seizures	Not licensed for monotherapy	≥ 16 years
Oxcarbazepine	Partial and tonic–clonic seizures (primary or secondarily generalised)	Yes	≥ 6 years
Pregabalin	Adjunctive therapy in partial and secondarily generalised tonic–clonic seizures	Not licensed for monotherapy	≥ 16 years
Tiagabine	Adjunctive second-line therapy in partial and secondarily generalised tonic–clonic seizures	Not licensed for monotherapy	≥ 12 years

Continued

Table 2.3	Continued		
	Licensed indications	**Monotherapy**	**Age**
Topiramate	Partial and tonic–clonic seizures (primary or secondarily generalised) and Lennox–Gastaut syndrome	Yes	≥ 2 years; ≥ 6 years in monotherapy
Zonisamide	Adjunctive therapy in partial seizures with or without secondary generalisation	Not licensed for monotherapy	≥ 18 years

valproate, carbamazepine, phenytoin and lamotrigine have all been shown to be equally effective in comparative randomised trials.

- Adverse effect profiles differ and must be taken into account.
- Patient preference is often dictated by differing adverse effect profiles. Where possible, treatment should be tailored to individual patient needs.
- Drug choice may differ in special patient groups (e.g. pregnancy, elderly) – see below.
- Fashion and pharmaceutical company marketing play a large part in prescribing patterns.

PRINCIPLES OF TREATMENT
Newly diagnosed patients

- The decision to treat depends essentially on a balance between the benefits and drawbacks of therapy, and any treatment should be tailored to the requirements of the individual patient.
- The physician should explain the relative advantages and disadvantages of therapy, although the final decision must be left to the patient.
- Individuals differ greatly in their views about epilepsy and its treatment. For some, seizure control is paramount (e.g. for driving or employment). Others have concerns about the concept of long-term medication or specific adverse effects and would prefer to risk an occasional seizure.

Factors influencing the decision to treat

- *Diagnosis*: it is essential to establish a firm diagnosis of epilepsy before therapy is started. There is almost no place for a 'trial of treatment' to clarify the diagnosis because it seldom does.

Box 2.1   Protocol for the treatment in drug-naive patients

The aim of initial treatment is, in the vast majority of cases, complete control of seizures without adverse effects.

Establish diagnosis unequivocally and classify seizure type/syndrome/aetiology.

Identify and counsel about any precipitating factors.

Decide on the need for antiepileptic drug therapy.

Counsel the patient.

Baseline haematological and biochemical investigations.

Start monotherapy with the first-choice drug, initially at low dose, titrating up slowly to a low maintenance dose (see Tables 2.4 and 2.5). Emergency drug loading is seldom necessary except where status epilepticus threatens. In new patients low drug doses will usually suffice.

If seizures continue, titrate the dose upwards to higher maintenance dose levels, guided, where appropriate, by serum level monitoring.

In about 60% of patients, these simple steps will result in complete seizure control. In remaining patients:

Alternative monotherapy should be tried with another appropriate first-choice antiepileptic drug. The second drug should be introduced incrementally at suitable dose intervals, and the first drug then withdrawn in slow decremental steps (see Table 2.4). The second drug should first be titrated to low maintenance doses and then, if seizures continue, the dose increased incrementally to maximal doses.

If seizures continue, or recur after initial therapy with 2–3 drugs tried in monotherapy as above, the diagnosis should be reassessed. It is not uncommon in this situation to find that the attacks do not have an epileptic basis.

Alternative monotherapies or polytherapy should be considered.

The patient should be referred for specialist advice.

- *The risk of seizure recurrence* is obviously a key factor:
  - overall the risk after an isolated first seizure is 50–80%
  - the risk is high initially and then falls over time (about 45% in the initial 6 months, 30% in the next 6 months, 15% in the second year)
  - the risk is greater in those with structural brain disease, and less in acute symptomatic seizures provoked by metabolic or drug/toxin exposure
  - different epilepsy syndromes have different recurrence risks, as do different seizure types
  - the risk of recurrence of 'idiopathic' or 'cryptogenic' tonic–clonic seizures is approximately 50%
  - the risk is greater in those under the age of 16 or over the age of 60 years.
- *The type, timing and frequency of seizures* – some types of epileptic seizure have minimal impact on quality of life (e.g. simple partial seizures, absences, sleep attacks). The benefits of treating such seizures, even if happening frequently, can be outweighed by the disadvantages.
- *Reflex seizures and acute symptomatic seizures* – occasionally seizures occur only in specific circumstances (e.g. photosensitivity, fatigue, alcohol) and avoiding these may avoid the need for drug therapy.
- *The risks of therapy (adverse effects) and of epilepsy (morbidity and mortality).*

There can be no absolute rules about when to start therapy and when not to do so. In general terms, if there is a risk of recurrence of convulsive seizures, or seizures with risk of injury or death, treatment is indicated. In other circumstances, however, the requirement to initiate therapy can be quite individual. Where seizures are infrequent and minor, where non-convulsive seizures occur exclusively at night, or for the benign syndromes of childhood epilepsy, treatment is often not indicated at all, even in established cases. In all situations, the patient should be given advice based on the best available data and be allowed to make the final decision. A protocol for treatment is shown in Box 2.1.

Patients with established active epilepsy

The goal of drug therapy in most newly diagnosed cases is complete seizure control. This is obtained in about 60–70% of patients in the longer term, which means that about 30–40% of cases have continuing seizures. The treatment of this 'chronic active' epilepsy is more complex and more difficult than that of a drug-naive case. Different issues are raised, and the perspectives of therapy are different. There remain a number of patients – perhaps 10% of all those developing epilepsy – whose seizures persist and are disabling. The epilepsy often coexists with learning disability, psychosocial problems or other neurological handicaps, and these factors complicate medical therapy further. Patient choice is as important as in newly diagnosed epilepsy, but the aims of treatment may be modified, accepting the limits of therapy in some patients, in whom treatment should be a balance between seizure suppression and minimising adverse effects. The patient must be thoroughly assessed and a treatment plan formulated.

- Assessment:
  - Review the diagnosis of epilepsy.
  - Establish the cause.
  - Classify seizure type.
  - Review of previous treatment history is an absolutely essential step, which is often omitted. The response to a drug is, generally speaking, relatively consistent over time. Find out which drugs have been tried previously, what the response was (effectiveness/adverse effects), what the maximum dose was, and why the drug was withdrawn.
  - Review compliance.
- Treatment plan:
  - A treatment plan should be formed on the basis of the assessment.
  - It consists of a stepwise series of treatment trials, each available antiepileptic in turn, in a reasonable dose, singly or as two-drug therapy (or, more rarely, three-drug combinations) if the previous trial fails to meet the targeted level of seizure control.
  - There is often inertia in much of the treatment of chronic epilepsy but this should be resisted, and an active and logical approach to therapy can prove very successful.
- Choice of drug to introduce or retain – generally these are drugs that are appropriate for the seizure type and which have either not been previously used in optimal doses or which have been used and did prove helpful.
- Choice of drug to withdraw – these should be drugs that have been given an adequate trial at optimal doses and which were either ineffective or caused unacceptable adverse effects.
- Duration of any treatment trial depends on the baseline seizure rate.
- Drug withdrawal:
  - sudden reduction in dose can result in a severe worsening of seizures or in status epilepticus, even if the withdrawn drug was apparently not contributing much to seizure control
  - drug doses should be reduced in a stepped fashion (see Table 2.4)
  - only one drug should be withdrawn at a time

Table 2.4   Usual dosing regimens and fastest routine incremental and decremental rates in adults

Drug	Initial dose (mg/day)	Drug initiation: usual dose increment (mg/day) stepped up every 2 weeks	Usual maintenance dose for mono-therapy (mg/day)	Usual maximum dose (mg/day)	Dosing intervals (per day)	Drug reduction/withdrawal: usual dose decrement (mg/day) stepped down every 4 weeks
Carbamazepine	100	100–200	400–1600	2000	2–3	200
Clobazam	10	10	10–30	30	1–2	10
Clonazepam	0.25	0.25–0.5	0.5–4	4	1–2	1
Ethosuximide	250	250	750–1500	1500	2–3	250
Gabapentin	300–400	300–400	900–2400	3200	2–3	300
Lamotrigine	12.5–25	25–100	100–200	600	2	100
Levetiracetam	125–250	250–500	500–1500	4000	1–2	250
Oxcarbazepine	600	300	600–2400	3000	2	300
Phenobarbital	30	30–60	60–120	180	1–2	30
Phenytoin	200	25–100	200–300	450	1–2	50
Pregabalin	150	50–100	150–600	600	2	150
Primidone	62.5–125	125–250	250–750	1500	2	125
Tiagabine	4–5	4–15	15–30	56–60	2–3	5
Topiramate	25–50	50–100	100–300	600	2	50
Valproate	200–500	200–500	600–1500	3000	2–3	200
Zonisamide	100	100	200–400	600	1–2	100

The incremental and decremental rates are the fastest that should be attempted in routine clinical situations. Often slower rates are advisable. Comedication with other antiepileptic drugs can affect the dose of carbamazepine, ethosuximide, lamotrigine, oxcarbazepine, phenobarbital, phenytoin, primidone, tiagabine, topiramate, valproate and zonisamide.

- if the withdrawal period is likely to be difficult, the dangers can be reduced by covering the withdrawal with a benzodiazepine (usually clobazam 10 mg/day).
■ Drug addition:
  - new drugs added to a regimen should usually be introduced slowly (see Table 2.4), as this results in better tolerability
  - it is usual to aim initially for a low maintenance dose, but in severe epilepsy higher doses are often required.
■ Concomitant medication – changing the dose of one antiepileptic (either incremental or decremental) can influence the serum levels of other drugs, contributing to changing adverse effects or effectiveness.
■ Drug therapy will fail in about 10–20% of patients, when the epilepsy can then be categorised as 'intractable' and the goal of therapy changes to defining the best compromise between inadequate seizure control and drug-induced adverse effects.
■ Counselling should be offered to patients with chronic epilepsy and this is needed on a wide range of topics.
■ Single-drug therapy will provide optimal seizure control in about 70–80% of all patients with epilepsy, and should be chosen whenever possible. The advantages of monotherapy are:
  - better tolerability and fewer adverse effects
  - simpler and less intrusive regimens
  - better compliance
  - avoidance of pharmacokinetic and pharmacodynamic interactions.
■ Combination therapy is needed in about 20–30% of all those developing epilepsy, and in a higher proportion of those with epilepsy which has remained uncontrolled in spite of initial monotherapy (chronic active epilepsy).

Patients with epilepsy in remission

Epilepsy can be said to be in remission when seizures have not occurred over long time periods (conventionally 2 or 5 years). The clinical management of ongoing therapy is generally straightforward:
■ In most cases, appropriate management can be provided at primary care level, with occasional specialist visits.
■ Seizure type, epilepsy syndrome, aetiology, investigations and previous treatment should be recorded.
■ Annual haematological and biochemical checks are recommended in asymptomatic individuals.

- Inquiry should be made of long-term adverse effects (e.g. bone disease in postmenopausal women).
- Counselling about issues such as pregnancy should be offered where appropriate.

Discontinuation of drug therapy

It is often difficult to decide when (if ever) to stop drug treatment. The decision should be made by a specialist who is able to provide an estimate of the risk of reactivation of the epilepsy (see Box 2.2).

Box 2.2   Calculation of the risk of a recurrent seizure following continued treatment or slow withdrawal of antiepileptic drugs when a patient has been in remission and seizure-free for more than 2 years while on treatment

	Factor value to be added to score
1. Starting score for all patients	175
Age > 16 years	45
Taking more than one antiepileptic drug	50
Seizures occurring after the start of treatment	35
History of any tonic–clonic seizure (generalised or partial in onset)	35
History of myoclonic seizures	50
EEG while in remission:	
not done	15
abnormal	20
Duration of seizure-free period (years), D	$200/D$
2. Total score	T
3. Exponentiate $T/100$ ($Z = \exp(T/100)$)	Z

Probability of seizure recurrence	By 1 year	By 2 years
On continued treatment	$1 - 0.89Z$	$1 - 0.79Z$
On slow withdrawal of treatment	$1 - 0.69Z$	$1 - 0.60Z$

From: Chadwick D. Management of epilepsy in remission. In: The treatment of epilepsy (eds Shorvon SD, Perucca E, Fish DR, Dodson E). Blackwell, Oxford, 2004, pp. 174–179.

About 40% of patients who stop treatment will have further seizures on drug reduction over the next 2 years (compared with 20% of patients who continue treatment). The factors influencing the risk of recurrence include:

■ Duration of remission – the longer the patient is seizure-free prior to drug reduction, the less the chance of relapse. The overall risk of relapse after drug withdrawal, for instance after a seizure-free period of 5 years, is < 10%.
■ Duration of active epilepsy – the shorter the duration of epilepsy, the less the risk of relapse.
■ Type and severity of epilepsy – symptomatic epilepsy, secondarily generalised or myoclonic seizures, neurological deficit or learning disability greatly lessen the chance of remission.
■ Electroencephalographic (EEG) abnormality – the persistence of spike wave in idiopathic generalised epilepsy indicates a higher chance of relapse. Other EEG abnormalities have no great prognostic utility.
■ Seizure syndrome – prognosis varies in different syndromes.

How to withdraw therapy – the importance of slow reduction

Half of patients who experience seizure recurrence on withdrawal do so during the reduction phase, and 25% do so in the first 6 months after withdrawal. To maximise success:

■ one drug should be discontinued at a time
■ withdrawal should be slow (see Table 2.4)
■ the patient should be counselled fully (there is no guarantee that treatment withdrawal will be successful, and if seizures do recur, there is no guarantee that a return to therapy will ensure future remission)
■ an estimate of the risks of recurrence on withdrawal and of further recurrence on return to therapy should be given (see Box 2.2)
■ driving should be avoided during the withdrawal phase
■ if relapse on drug withdrawal does occur, about 10% of patients will not regain seizure control when the drugs are replaced.

TREATMENT OF THE COMMON EPILEPSY SYNDROMES
(Table 2.5)

Febrile seizures
Emergency treatment

■ Preventing seizures becoming prolonged is the aim of therapy. The majority (90%) of seizures are self-limiting, but if a seizure continues for 5–10 minutes emergency therapy is needed.

Table 2.5   The antiepileptic drugs

Carbamazepine

Primary indications	Partial and generalised seizures (excluding absence and myoclonus). Also childhood epilepsy syndromes. Adults and children
Usual preparations	Tablets: 100, 200, 400 mg Chewtabs: 100, 200 mg Slow-release formulations: 200, 400 mg Liquid: 100 mg/5ml; suppositories: 125, 250 mg
Usual dosage – adults	Initial: 100 mg at night Maintenance: 400–1600 mg/day (maximum 2400 mg) (Slow-release formulation, higher dosage)
Usual dosage – children	< 1 year: 100–200 mg/day 1–5 years: 200–400 mg/day 5–10 years: 400–600 mg/day 10–15 years: 600–1000 mg/day (Slow-release formulation, higher dosage)
Dosing intervals	2–3 times/day (2–4 times/day at higher doses or in children)
Common/important adverse effects	Drowsiness, fatigue, dizziness, ataxia, diplopia, blurred vision, sedation, headache, insomnia, gastrointestinal disturbance, tremor, weight gain, impotence, effects on behaviour and mood, hepatic disturbance, rash and other skin reactions, marrow dyscrasia, leukopenia, hyponatraemia, water retention, endocrine effects
Major mechanism of action	Inhibition of voltage-dependent sodium conductance. Also action on monoamine, acetylcholine and NMDA receptors

Clobazam

Primary indications	Partial and generalised seizures. Also for intermittent therapy, one-off prophylactic therapy. Adults and children
Usual preparations	Tablet, capsule: 10 mg
Usual dosage – adults	10–20 mg/day, higher doses can be used.
Usual dosage – children	3–12 years: 5–10 mg/day

Continued

Table 2.5   *Continued*

Clobazam – *continued*

Dosing intervals	1–2 times/day
Common/important adverse effects	Sedation, dizziness, weakness, blurred vision, restlessness, ataxia, aggressiveness, behavioural disturbance, withdrawal symptoms
Major mechanism of action	GABA$_A$ receptor agonist

Clonazepam

Primary indications	Partial and generalised seizures (including absence and myoclonus). Also Lennox–Gastaut syndrome, neonatal seizures, infantile spasms and status epilepticus. Adults and children
Usual preparations	Tablets: 0.5, 1, 2 mg Liquid: 1 mg in 1 ml diluent
Usual dosage – adults	Initial: 0.25 mg at night Maintenance: 0.5–4 mg/day
Usual dosage – children	< 1 year: 1 mg/day 1–5 years: 1–2 mg/day 5–12 years: 1–3 mg/day
Dosing intervals	1–2 times/day
Common/important adverse effects	Sedation (common and may be severe), cognitive effects, ataxia, hyperactivity, restlessness, aggressiveness, hypersalivation, tone changes, withdrawal symptoms
Major mechanism of action	GABA$_A$ receptor agonist

Ethosuxamide

Primary indications	Generalised absence seizures. Adults and children
Usual preparations	Capsules: 250 mg Syrup: 250 mg/5 ml
Usual dosage – adults	Initial: 250 mg Maintenance: 750–2000 mg/day

Continued

Table 2.5   Continued

Usual dosage – children	Initial: 10–15 mg/kg/day Maintenance: 20–40 mg/kg/day
Dosing intervals	2–3 times/day
Common/important adverse effects	Gastrointestinal symptoms, drowsiness, ataxia, diplopia, headache, dizziness, hiccups, sedation, behavioural disturbances, acute psychotic reactions, extrapyramidal symptoms, blood dyscrasia, rash, lupus-like syndrome, severe idiosyncratic reactions
Major mechanism of action	Effects on calcium T-channel conductance

Gabapentin

Primary indications	Partial or secondarily generalised epilepsy. Adults and children (over age of 3–6 years)
Usual preparations	Capsules: 100, 300, 400 mg
Usual dosage – adults	Initial: 300 mg/day Maintenance: 900–3600 mg/day
Dosing intervals	2–3 times/day
Common/important adverse effects	Drowsiness, dizziness, seizure exacerbation, ataxia, headache, tremor, diplopia, nausea, vomiting, rhinitis
Major mechanism of action	Not known

Lamotrigine

Primary indications	Partial and generalised epilepsy. Also Lennox–Gastaut syndrome and other generalised epilepsy syndromes. Adults and children over 2 years of age
Usual preparations	Tablets: 25, 50, 100, 200 mg Chewtabs: 5, 25, 100 mg
Usual dosage – adults	Initial: 12.5–25 mg/day Maintenance: 200–600 mg/day But varies with comedication and with enzyme-inducing drugs
Usual dosage – children	Depends on comedication

Continued

Table 2.5   *Continued*

Lamotrigine – *continued*

Dosing intervals	2 times/day
Common/important adverse effects	Rash (sometimes severe), headache, blood dyscrasia, ataxia, asthenia, diplopia, nausea, vomiting, dizziness, somnolence, insomnia, depression, psychosis, tremor, hypersensitivity reactions
Major mechanism of action	Inhibition of voltage-dependent sodium conductance

Levetiracetam

Primary indications	Partial seizures with or without secondarily generalised seizures. Adults only
Usual preparations	Tablets: 250, 500, 750, 1000 mg
Usual dosage – adults	Initial: 125–250 mg/day Maintenance: 750–4000 mg/day
Dosing intervals	1–2 times/day
Common/important adverse effects	Somnolence, asthenia, infection, dizziness, headache, irritability, aggression, behavioural and mood change
Major mechanism of action	Action via binding to SV2A synaptic vesicle protein

Oxcarbazepine

Primary indications	Partial and secondarily generalised seizures. Adults and children
Usual preparations	Tablets: 150, 300, 600 mg
Usual dosage – adults	Initial: 600 mg/day Maintenance: 900–2400 mg/day
Usual dosage – children	Initial: 8–10 mg/kg per day Maintenance: 30 mg/kg (maximum 46 mg/kg)
Dosing intervals	2 times/day
Common/important adverse effects	Somnolence, headache, dizziness, diplopia, ataxia, rash, hyponatraemia, weight gain, alopecia, nausea, gastrointestinal disturbance

Continued

Table 2.5   Continued

Major mechanism of action	Inhibition of voltage-dependent sodium conductance. Also affects on potassium conductance, N-type calcium channels, NMDA receptors

Phenobarbital

Primary indications	Partial or generalised seizures (including absence and myoclonus). Status epilepticus. Lennox–Gastaut syndrome. Other childhood epilepsy syndromes. Febrile convulsions. Neonatal seizures
Usual preparations	Tablets: 15, 30, 50, 60, 100 mg Elixir: 15 mg/5 ml Injection: 200 mg/ml
Usual dosage – adults	Initial: 30 mg/day Maintenance: 30–180 mg/day
Usual dosage – children	Neonates: 3–4 mg/day Children: 3–4 mg/day
Dosing intervals	1–2 times/day
Common/important adverse effects	Sedation, ataxia, dizziness, insomnia, hyperkinesis (children), mood changes (especially depression), aggressiveness, cognitive dysfunction, impotence, reduced libido, folate deficiency, vitamin K and vitamin D deficiency, osteomalacia, Dupuytren's contracture, frozen shoulder, connective tissue abnormalities, rash. Risk of dependency. Potential for abuse
Major mechanism of action	Enhances activity of $GABA_A$ receptor. Also depresses glutamate excitability, affects sodium, potassium and calcium conductance

Phenytoin

Primary indications	Partial and primary and secondarily generalised seizures (excluding myoclonus and absence), status epilepticus, childhood epilepsy syndromes
Usual preparations	Capsules: 25, 30, 50, 100, 200 mg Chewtabs: 50 mg Liquid suspension: 30 mg/5 ml, 125 mg/50 ml Injection: 250 mg/5 ml

Continued

Table 2.5 *Continued*

Phenytoin – *continued*

Usual dosage – adults	Initial: 200 mg at night Maintenance: 200–500 mg/day (Higher doses can be used, guided by serum level monitoring)
Usual dosage – children	10 mg/kg/day (Higher doses can be used, guided by serum level monitoring)
Dosing intervals	1–2 times/day
Common/important adverse effects	Ataxia, dizziness, lethargy, sedation, headache, dyskinesia, acute encephalopathy (phenytoin intoxication), hypersensitivity, rash, fever, blood dyscrasia, gingival hyperplasia, folate deficiency, megaloblastic anaemia, vitamin K deficiency, thyroid dysfunction, decreased immunoglobulins, mood change, depression, coarsened facies, hirsutism, peripheral neuropathy, osteomalacia, hypocalcaemia, hormonal dysfunction, loss of libido, connective tissue alterations, pseudolymphoma, hepatitis, vasculitis, myopathy, coagulation defects, bone marrow hypoplasia
Major mechanism of action	Inhibition of voltage-dependent sodium channels

Pregabalin

Primary indications	Partial seizures with or without secondary generalisation. Adults only
Usual preparations	Capsules: 25, 50, 75, 150, 300 mg
Usual dosage – adults	Initial: 150 mg/day Maintenance: 150–600 mg/day
Dosing intervals	2 times/day
Common/important adverse effects	Somnolence, dizziness, ataxia
Major mechanism of action	Binds to voltage-gated calcium channel. Also reduces release of glutamate and other neurotransmitters

Continued

Table 2.5 Continued

Primidone

Primary indications	Partial and primary and secondarily generalised seizures. Adults and children
Usual preparations	Tablet: 250 mg
Usual dosage – adults	Initial: 62.5–125 mg/day
Usual dosage – children	Maintenance: 250–1500 mg/day
Dosing intervals	2 times/day
Common/important adverse effects	As for phenobarbital. Also, dizziness, nausea on initiation of therapy
Major mechanism of action	As for phenobarbital

Tiagabine

Primary indications	Partial and secondarily generalised seizures. Patients ≥ 12 years of age only
Usual preparations	Tablets: 5, 10, 15 mg
Usual dosage – adults	Initial: 15 mg/day Maintenance: 30–45 mg/day
Dosing intervals	2–3 times/day
Common/important adverse effects	Dizziness, tiredness, nervousness, tremor, diarrhoea, nausea, headache, confusion, psychosis, flu-like symptoms, ataxia, depression, word-finding difficulties
Major mechanism of action	Inhibits GABA reuptake

Topiramate

Primary indications	Partial and secondarily generalised seizures. Also Lennox–Gastaut syndrome. Idiopathic generalised epilepsy. Adults and children > 2 years old
Usual preparations	Tablets: 25, 50, 100, 200 mg Sprinkle: 15, 25 mg
Usual dosage – adults	Initial: 25–50 mg/day Maintenance: 100–500 mg/day

Continued

Table 2.5   *Continued*

Topiramate – *continued*

Usual dosage – children	Initial: 0.5–1 mg/kg/day Maintenance: 5–9 mg/kg/day
Dosing intervals	2 times/day
Common/important adverse effects	Dizziness, ataxia, headache, paraesthesia, tremor, somnolence, cognitive dysfunction, confusion, agitation, amnesia, depression, emotional lability, nausea, diarrhoea, diplopia, weight loss
Major mechanism of action	Inhibition of voltage-gated sodium channels; potentiation of GABA-mediated inhibition at the $GABA_A$ receptor; reduction of AMPA receptor activity; inhibition of high voltage calcium channels; carbonic anhydrase activity

Valproate

Primary indications	Primary and secondarily generalised seizures (including myoclonus and absence) and partial seizures. Lennox–Gastaut syndrome. Idiopathic generalised epilepsy. Childhood epilepsy syndromes. Febrile convulsions
Usual preparations	Enteric-coated tablets: 200, 500 mg Crushable tablets: 100 mg Capsules: 150, 300, 500 mg Syrup: 200 mg/5 ml Liquid: 200 mg/5 ml Slow-release tablets: 200, 300, 500 mg Divalproex tablets: 125, 300, 500 mg
Usual dosage – adults	Initial: 200–500 mg/day Maintenance: 500–3000 mg/day
Usual dosage – children	Initial: 20 mg/kg/day (children < 20 kg); 40 mg/kg/day (children > 20 kg) Maintenance: 20–30 mg/kg/day (children < 20 kg); 20–40 mg/kg/day (children > 20 kg)
Dosing intervals	2–3 times/day

Continued

Table 2.5   *Continued*

Common/important adverse effects	Nausea, vomiting, hyperammonaemia and other metabolic effects, endocrine effects, severe hepatic toxicity, pancreatitis, drowsiness, cognitive disturbance, aggressiveness, tremor, weakness, encephalopathy, thrombocytopenia, neutropenia, aplastic anaemia, hair thinning and hair loss, weight gain, polycystic ovarian syndrome
Major mechanism of action	Effects on GABA and glutaminergic activity, T-type calcium channels conductance and potassium conductance

Zonisamide

Primary indications	Refractory partial epilepsy and generalised epilepsy (all types). Lennox–Gastaut syndrome. West syndrome. Progressive myoclonic epilepsy. Licensed in Japan and Asia in children and adults. Licensed in the USA only for refractory partial epilepsy in patients ≥ 16 years of age
Usual preparations	Capsules: 100 mg (USA) Tablets: 100 mg (Japan, Korea) Powder: 20% (Japan, Korea)
Usual dosage – adults	200–600 mg/day
Usual dosage – children	Initial: 2–4 mg/kg/day Maintenance: 4–8 mg/kg/day
Dosing intervals	1–2 times/day
Common/important adverse effects	Somnolence, ataxia, dizziness, fatigue, nausea, vomiting, irritability, anorexia, impaired concentration, mental slowing, itching, diplopia, insomnia, abdominal pain, depression, skin rashes, hypersensitivity. Significant risk of renal calculi (in US and European, but not Japanese, studies). Oligohidrosis and risk of heat stroke
Major mechanism of action	Inhibition of voltage-gated sodium channel, T-type calcium currents, benzodiazepine $GABA_A$ receptor excitatory glutaminergic transmission, carbonic anhydrase

- Standard out-of-hospital treatment is diazepam solution by rectal instillation:
  - Stesolid (Diastat) is a convenient ready-made-up proprietary preparation.
  - If there is no rapid effect, the same dose should be repeated (to a maximum of two doses in an out-of-hospital setting).
  - An alternative is intramuscular or buccal midazolam 0.1–0.2 mg/kg.
- In a hospital setting, diazepam is given at a dose of 0.2–0.5 mg/kg iv (not exceeding 2 mg/min) or by rectal administration. A total dose (rectal plus intravenous) of 20–30 mg is often required. An alternative is lorazepam 0.05–0.1 mg/kg iv.
- It is often recommended that the child should be cooled immediately (cold water, cold flannels, tepid sponging, and removing clothes and bedcovers).
- Any underlying cause should be established and treated:
  - blood and urine culture
  - full haematological and biochemical screening
  - cerebrospinal fluid (CSF) examination (to exclude meningitis) and brain computed tomography (CT) in all children < 18 months old at the time of presentation of the first seizure, and in any child with meningism.

Long-term prophylaxis

- Given only to infants < 1 year old who have had episodes lasting 30 minutes or more, or who have had multiple seizures: oral phenobarbital 15 mg/kg/day or oral valproate 20–40 mg/kg/day in two divided doses.

Parental counselling

- A febrile seizure is a profoundly distressing experience.
- Almost all parents, at the time of a first febrile seizure, think their child is about to die.
- Parents should be reassured that the risk of brain damage is extremely small, that febrile seizures are common and harmless, and subsequent epilepsy develops in only a small percentage of cases (2–10% risk of later developing afebrile seizures).
- Information about the management of subsequent seizures and first aid should be given:
  - place child on his/her side
  - do not force anything between the teeth

- emergency therapy (see above)
- call the emergency services or get the child to a medical facility if a seizure lasts more than 5 minutes.

Infantile spasms

These are amongst the most serious and resistant of the epilepsy syndromes. Adrenocorticotrophic hormone (ACTH) is usually the preferred first-line therapy in the USA and Japan, and vigabatrin is preferred in most European countries, Asia and Canada. In other countries, corticosteroids are only prescribed as second line after pyridoxine or high-dose valproate. Pyridoxine 100 mg iv is usually also given in most centres.

- ACTH 40 IU (3–6 IU/kg) daily im for 1–5 months. If seizures relapse either on therapy or after withdrawal, the ACTH should be recommenced immediately and doses of 60–80 IU/day may be needed. Almost all children become cushingoid. Other common adverse effects include infections, increased blood pressure, gastritis and hyperexcitability.
- Vigabatrin is the drug of first choice for infantile spasms in tuberous sclerosis (100–150 mg/kg/day, oral), and in some centres for all forms of infantile spasms. There are no long-term data about toxicity or visual or intellectual function.
- Valproate and clonazepam control 25–30% of cases, but relapse rates are high.
- Carbamazepine can worsen the spasms.
- Ketogenic diet, intravenous immunoglobulin, topiramate, lamotrigine, felbamate and zonisamide have all been reported to help in small open case series.

Lennox–Gastaut syndrome

This syndrome, starting in childhood but often continuing into adult life, is characterised by severe epilepsy, learning disability, other neurological handicaps and characteristic seizure and EEG patterns.

- Complete seizure control is rare; almost all patients require polytherapy.
- A balance has to be set between best seizure control and adverse drug effects. It is important to resist the tendency, in the face of ongoing epilepsy, continually to escalate treatment.
- High-dose polypharmacy may cause drowsiness, which is a potent activator of the atypical absence and tonic seizures, and non-convulsive status epilepticus.

- Valproate is the drug usually given initially, but is prescribed with caution in children below 3 years of age in view of the risk of hepatic failure.
- Lamotrigine is an alternative initial therapy, but caution is needed in view of possible severe hypersensitivity reactions.
- The underlying cause should be treated where possible (often it is not).

Benign partial epilepsy syndromes of childhood

There is a variety of benign syndromes of partial epilepsy at various stages of childhood that have an excellent prognosis. The commonest is benign epilepsy with centrotemporal spikes.

- Treatment is usually straightforward and indeed drug treatment is not necessary at all in many mild cases.
- Carbamazepine and valproate are both highly effective in low-dose monotherapy.
- Withdrawal of medication should be considered after 1–2 years free of attacks, even if the EEG is still abnormal.

Idiopathic generalised epilepsies

These are common and important, and generally easily treated. The seizure types include generalised tonic–clonic, absence and myoclonic seizures.

- For generalised tonic–clonic seizures the drugs most commonly used as first line include valproate, carbamazepine, lamotrigine and phenytoin. There is a clinical suspicion that valproate is the most effective. Other drugs with proven efficacy include topiramate and zonisamide. Anecdotal studies suggest levetiracetam is also highly efficacious.
- For absence seizures, valproate, ethosuximide and lamotrigine are commonly drugs of first choice. The benzodiazepines, phenobarbital and topiramate are reserved for more resistant cases. Anecdotal studies also suggest that levetiracetam is effective.
- Only moderate doses are generally required to control seizures.
- Myoclonic seizures are usually treated first with valproate. Alternatives include topiramate, lamotrigine and benzodiazepines. Anecdotal experience with levetiracetam suggests a strong antimyoclonic effect.
- Tiagabine, vigabatrin, oxcarbazepine, gabapentin and carbamazepine can exacerbate absence or myoclonic seizures.
- Lifestyle manipulation can be very helpful: avoiding sleep deprivation, excessive alcohol intake, stress or (in photosensitive patients) photic stimulation may improve seizure control.

Epilepsies with myoclonic seizures

- Myoclonus occurs in a number of different epilepsy syndromes and clinical settings (Box 2.3):
  - most commonly, myoclonus is part of idiopathic generalised epilepsy (see above), occurring particularly in the juvenile myoclonic epilepsy subgroup
  - myoclonus also occurs in diffuse symptomatic epilepsies, especially those due to anoxia, infection, toxins, drugs or poisoning, and some childhood epilepsy syndromes
  - focal myoclonus can occur in symptomatic occipital and frontocentral epilepsies
  - the progressive myoclonic epilepsies form a distinctive clinical phenotype.

Box 2.3   Epilepsies with myoclonic seizures

- Idiopathic generalised epilepsies and benign myoclonic epilepsy syndromes:
  - juvenile myoclonic epilepsy
  - epilepsy of infancy
  - myoclonic astatic epilepsy
  - eyelid myoclonia with absence
  - benign myoclonic epilepsy of infancy.
- Severe myoclonic epilepsy syndromes of childhood:
  - Dravet syndrome
  - myoclonic encephalopathies.
- Symptomatic epilepsies with generalised myoclonus:
  - cerebral anoxia
  - cerebral infections (particularly prion disease)
  - drugs, toxins, poisoning.
- Symptomatic epilepsies with focal myoclonus.
- Occipital lobe epilepsy and frontocentral epilepsy.
- Progressive myoclonic epilepsies:
  - Unverricht–Lundborg disease
  - ceroid lipofuscinosis
  - dentate-rubro-pallido-luysian atrophy (DRPLA)
  - lafora body disease
  - mitochondrial disease (MERRF)
  - sialidosis.

- Most myoclonic seizures are generalised, although focal myoclonus does occur in occipital lobe and frontocentral epilepsies.
- The drugs usually used to treat myoclonus are valproate, clonazepam, clobazam, phenobarbital, topiramate and lamotrigine. Levetiracetam has a good effect, although currently is not licensed for this indication. Piracetam is a related drug with excellent effects in some patients with severe myoclonus, particularly in the progressive myoclonic epilepsies (at high doses, occasionally up to 32 g/day).
- Some antiepileptic drugs can exacerbate myoclonus, notably vigabatrin, gabapentin, tiagabine, carbamazepine and oxcarbazepine.
- The prognosis and response to treatment of these epilepsies depend on the syndrome type and underlying aetiology.

Treatment of epilepsy in women

Fertility

Fertility is reduced by about 30% in women with treated epilepsy. The reasons include:

- social effects (low rates of marriage, marry late, social isolation and stigmatisation)
- personal choice (avoidance of pregnancy because of the risk of epilepsy or drug treatment to the offspring)
- impaired personality and cognitive development
- genetic factors and adverse antiepileptic drug effects also lead to reduced fecundity
- possible association between the polycystic ovarian syndrome and valproate, although evidence is contradictory.

Contraception

Care is needed in choosing the appropriate method, in view of potential interactions with antiepileptic drugs.

- Combined oral contraceptive pill:
  - Antiepileptic drugs that induce hepatic enzyme activity (barbiturates, phenytoin, primidone, oxcarbazepine, carbamazepine) increase the metabolism of the oestrogen and progesterone components of the pill (sometimes by 50%), thereby reducing its efficacy.
  - Topiramate lowers the level of oestrogen by 30% by a different mechanism.
  - Patients comedicated with these drugs therefore need higher doses of the pill to achieve contraceptive effect – a pill with at least 50 μg oestradiol should be given initially, or two 30 μg oestradiol pills.

- Alternatively, 'tricycling' a 50 µg oestrogen preparation can be employed (daily intake of 50 µg pill for 3 months without a break, followed by 4 days off).
- Lamotrigine has also been shown to reduce contraceptive efficacy by a different mechanism.
- Breakthrough bleeding (midcycle bleeding) is a useful sign of inadequate oestrogenic effect, but contraceptive failure can occur without midcycle bleeding.
- Women should be advised that, even with higher dose preparations, there is still a higher risk of contraceptive failure (3 failures per 1000 women-years compared to 0.3 per 1000 in the general population).
- There is no risk with non-enzyme-inducing drugs (clobazam, gabapentin, levetiracetam, pregabalin, valproate, vigabatrin) – a 30 µg oestradiol compound can be taken safely.
- The combined contraceptive pill tends to lower lamotrigine levels by about 50%.
- Progesterone only pills (the 'mini-pill') are affected in a similar manner to the combined oral contraceptive pill and patients should take at least double the usual dose, or use other forms of contraception.
- Injectable contraceptives (medroxyprogesterone acetate (Depo-Provera)) – has no interaction with antiepileptic drugs and can be used. The progestogen implant (Implanon) should be avoided.
- Postcoital contraception (the morning-after pill) – the first dose should be doubled and a second single dose given 12 hours later.
- Intrauterine contraception (coils) – unaffected by enzyme inducing drugs.

Menstruation and catamenial epilepsy

- In many women, the pattern of seizures is related to the menstrual cycle.
- Occasionally, intermittent therapy around the high-risk days can reduce seizure frequency (e.g. with clobazam 10 mg/day oral), although this approach is usually disappointing.

Teratogenicity of antiepileptic drugs

Studies have been largely confined to the older drugs. There is very little information about the risks of the newer drugs but general advice from the manufacturers is that their use in pregnancy should be avoided.

- Risk of major malformations:
  - The most common malformations associated with traditional antiepileptic drugs (phenytoin, phenobarbital, primidone, benzodiazepine, valproate, carbamazepine) are cleft palate and cleft

lip, cardiac malformations, neural tube defects, hypospadias and skeletal abnormalities.
- Because most studies have been of women on multiple drug therapy, the risks of many of the individual drugs are not known.
- The background population risk of spina bifida is approximately 0.2–0.5% with geographic variation. Valproate is associated with a 1–2% risk of spina bifida aperta, and carbamazepine about 0.5–1%.
- The risk of malformations was thought to be particularly high with phenytoin, although recent studies of phenytoin monotherapy have shown a very low risk of major defects. Phenytoin is clearly associated with neuroblastoma in the infant, although the absolute risk is very small.
- It is not clear to what extent benzodiazepines have any teratogenic effects.
- About 95% of significant neural tube defects can be detected prenatally by ultrasound scan, as can cleft palate and other midline defects, and major cardiac and renal defects.
- Other developmental abnormalities
  - Less severe dysmorphic changes ('fetal syndromes') may exist, although there is little agreement about their frequency: hypertelorism and distal digital hypoplasia, craniofacial abnormalities, minor skeletal changes and growth retardation.
  - Recent interest has focused on a 'valproate syndrome', which in one study was said to occur in up to 50% of infants born to mothers on valproate, resulting in developmental delay and learning disability. However, the evidence is inconclusive, but caution is advisable with valproate in pregnancy.

Pregnancy

Epilepsy increases by up to three-fold the risks of various common complications of pregnancy, and the perinatal mortality is about twice that of the general population.
- Pregnancy has an unpredictable effect on seizure frequency. In about one-third of women seizures become less frequent, but in another third seizure frequency increases.
- There is inconclusive evidence that a fetus is affected by the hypoxia or metabolic changes during a seizure. However, in the later stages of pregnancy a convulsion carries the risk of trauma to the placenta or fetus, especially if the woman falls. Partial seizures without secondary generalisation are unlikely to have any deleterious effects on the fetus.

- Many of the enzyme-inducing antiepileptic drugs reduce serum folate level. Folate supplementation to lessen the risk of neural tube defects is therefore recommended (folic acid 5 mg/day oral).
- There is a risk of infantile deficiency of vitamin K dependent clotting factors (II, VII, IX and X) and protein C and S where the mother is taking enzyme-inducing antiepileptic drugs. This predisposes to infantile haemorrhage, including cerebral haemorrhage:
  - the neonate should therefore receive 1 mg of vitamin K im at birth, and again at 28 days
  - it is also sometimes recommended that the mother take oral vitamin K (20 mg/day) in the last trimester, although the evidence is rather contradictory
  - if any two of the clotting factors fall below 50% of their normal values, im vitamin K and fresh frozen plasma should be given to the baby
  - if neonatal bleeding occurs, or if concentrations of factors II, VII, IX or X fall below 25% of normal, an emergency infusion of fresh frozen plasma is required.
- The development of epilepsy by chance during pregnancy is not uncommon. Specific causes include meningiomas and arteriovenous malformations, which are said to grow during pregnancy, ischaemic stroke, subarachnoid haemorrhage, intracranial venous thrombosis and various infections including *Listeria*, *Toxoplasma*, human immunodeficiency virus (HIV) and other viruses.
- Occasionally, epileptic seizures occur only during pregnancy (gestational epilepsy), but this is rare.
- The treatment of new-onset epilepsy follows the same principles in the pregnant as in the non-pregnant patient.

Eclampsia and pre-eclampsia

- Most new-onset seizures in the late stages of pregnancy (after 20 weeks) are caused by eclampsia.
- Magnesium sulphate (iv infusion of 4 g, followed by 10 g im, and then 5 g im every 4 hours as required) is more effective than phenytoin and/or diazepam.

Labour

- About 1–2% of women with epilepsy have tonic–clonic seizures during delivery and this can clearly complicate labour.
- The fetal heart rate can be dramatically slowed by a seizure, and fetal monitoring is recommended during vaginal delivery.

SOCIAL EFFECTS OF EPILEPSY

Epilepsy has potential social consequences which can cause greater disability than the immediate effects of individual seizures. 'Being epileptic' can be far worse than simply having seizures. Patients with epilepsy have higher rates of anxiety and depression, social isolation, unmarried status and are more likely to be unemployed or registered as permanently sick.

- A holistic approach to therapy is essential, of which drug treatment is often only a small part.
- A good patient–doctor relationship, counselling, psychological therapy and lifestyle advice are all important.
- The overall aim is to encourage as normal a lifestyle as possible, and to balance the risks incurred by normal activities against the risks imposed by the epilepsy.
- Lifestyle and treatment decisions should be made ultimately by patients and carers, and the role of the treating physician is to assist decision-making by providing information and advice.

GENETIC COUNSELLING

About 1% of epilepsies are due to a monogenic cause where counselling depends on the penetrance and mode of inheritance. Most other epilepsies have complex inheritance patterns and genetic advice depends on the frequency of epilepsy in the family.

- Idiopathic generalised epilepsy:
  - the risk of developing epilepsy in a first-degree relative is 5–15%, while the risk in a second-degree or more distant relative is close to that of the general population
  - monozygotic twins have a concordance rate of about 70–80%, increasing to 90% when EEG changes are included with clinical features
  - risk for siblings is 6%, increasing to 8% if photosensitivity is found in the proband or if a parent has epilepsy, 12% when a parent also shows generalised EEG abnormalities, and 15% when the sibling shows a generalised EEG trait
  - the risk to the offspring of an affected individual is about 5% (9% in female and 2% in male offspring)
  - occasional large families have many affected members and these families have higher risks.
- Benign epilepsy with centrotemporal spikes:
  - the genetics are complex and ill-understood

- concordance in monozygotic twins varies from 0% to 100% in different studies
- for most sporadic cases the risk of developing epilepsy in first-degree relatives is about 15%, rising to 30% if centrotemporal EEG abnormalities are found.

■ Febrile seizures:
- inheritance seems polygenic, although there are a few large families with dominant inheritance; from the counselling point of view it is therefore important to gain a detailed family history before estimating risk
- there is 35–70% clinical concordance in monozygotic twins
- there is increased risk for first-degree relatives, ranging from 8% in whites to 20% in Japanese.

Serum-level monitoring

Some pharmacokinetic properties of individual antiepileptic drugs are shown in Table 2.6.

Factors affecting serum drug levels are shown in Box 2.4, and the value of monitoring individual drugs in Table 2.8. Blood level monitoring of some antiepileptic drugs is indicated to:

■ assess blood levels where there is a poor therapeutic response in spite of adequate dosage
■ identify the cause of adverse effects where these might be drug induced
■ monitor phenytoin dose changes in view of the non-linear kinetics and lack of predictability of the phenytoin dose–blood level relationship
■ measure pharmacokinetic changes in the presence of physiological or pathological conditions known to alter drug disposition (e.g. pregnancy, liver disease, renal failure, gastrointestinal disease, hypoalbulinaemic states)
■ identify and minimise the consequence of adverse drug interactions in patients receiving multiple drug therapy
■ identify which drugs require dosage changes to optimise therapy in patients on antiepileptic drug polytherapy
■ assess changes in bioavailability when a drug formulation has been changed
■ identify poor compliance.

Although the levels of any drugs can be measured, the relationship between effect (efficacy or adverse effects) and blood level varies between drugs, and blood level monitoring is generally useful only for certain drugs (see Table 2.7).

Table 2.6   Pharmacokinetic properties of antiepileptic drugs

Drug	Oral bio-availability*	Metabolism	Half-life[†] (hours)	Protein binding	Active metabolite
Carbamazepine (CBZ)	Moderate	Hepatic	5–26[e]	75%	CBZ epoxide
Clobazam	Moderate	Hepatic	10–77 (50[a])	83%	N-DMC
Clonazepam	Moderate	Hepatic	20–80	86%	None
Ethosuximide	High	Hepatic	30–60[d]	10%	None
Gabapentin	Moderate[e]	None	5–7	None	None
Lamotrigine	High	Hepatic	12–60[d]	55%	None
Levetiracetam	High	Non-hepatic	6–8	None	None
Oxcarbazepine	High	Hepatic	8–10[a, d]	38%[a]	MHD
Phenobarbital	Moderate	Hepatic	75–120[d]	45–60%	None
Phenytoin	Moderate	Hepatic	7–42[b, d]	85–95%	None
Pregabalin	Moderate	None	6	None	None
Primidone	High	Hepatic	5–18[d] (75–120[a])	25%	Pheno-barbital
Tiagabine	High	Hepatic	5–9[c, d]	96%	None
Topiramate	High	Hepatic	19–25[d]	15%	None
Valproate	High	Hepatic	12–17[d]	85–95%	None
Zonisamide	High	Hepatic	49–69[d]	30–60%	None

*High = 95% or more, moderate = 75–95%.
[†]Half-life in healthy adult.
[a]Value for active metabolite.
[b]Phenytoin has non-linear kinetics, and so half-life can increase at higher doses.
[c]Absorption of tiagabine is markedly slowed by food, and the drug should be taken at the end of meals.
[d]Half-life varies with comedication.
[e]Absorption of gabapentin is by a saturable active transport system, and the rate will depend on the capacity of the system.
N-DMC, N-desmethylclobazam; MHD, monohydroxy derivative.

Box 2.4 Factors affecting blood levels of antiepileptic drugs

- Drug factors:
  - formulation
  - comedication.
- Patient factors:
  - genetic/constitutional factors (absorption, metabolism, excretion)
  - disease states (renal, hepatic, changes in plasma proteins, gastrointestinal disturbance)
  - others (pregnancy, nutritional status, body weight changes).

Table 2.7 Value of measuring antiepileptic drug levels in determining dose

Drug	'Target level' (µmol/l)	Value of blood level measurements in routine practice
Carbamazepine	20–50	***
Ethosuximide	300–700	***
Lamotrigine	10–60	**
Oxcarbazepine	50–140[a]	*
Phenobarbital	50–130	**
Phenytoin	40–80	***
Primidone	25–50[b]	**
Topiramate	10–60	*
Valproate	300–700	**
Zonisamide	30–140	*
Benzodiazepine	–	0
Gabapentin	–	0
Levetiracetam	–	0
Pregabalin	–	0
Tiagabine	–	0

***, Very useful, drug level closely related to drug effects (efficacy and adverse effects), measurements should be frequently made.

**, Useful, measurements often required, drug levels loosely related to drug effects.

*, Limited usefulness, measurements occasionally required, levels loosely related to drug effects.

0, No general utility, measurement only required in exceptional circumstances (or to check compliance), drug levels generally not clearly related to drug effect.

[a]Monohydroxy derivative (MHD).

[b]Measurement of derived phenobarbital levels is more useful.

Drug level monitoring is frequently misused, and measurements made unnecessarily or interpreted incorrectly. There is marked individual variability and the 'therapeutic ranges' are average figures only. The importance of 'treating the patient, not the serum level' cannot be overstated. It is a mistake (commonly made) to:

- increase the dose in patients fully controlled simply because the serum level is below the therapeutic range
- lower the dose in patients who are experiencing no adverse effects because the serum level is above the therapeutic range
- ignore adverse effects because the levels are within the therapeutic range.

Pharmacokinetic drug interactions

The most important antiepileptic drug interactions (Table 2.8) are those mediated by the P450 and the UGT hepatic enzyme systems. These enzymes can be induced or inhibited by antiepileptic drugs. Autoinduction (induction of the drug's own metabolism) can occur.

Table 2.8 Pharmacokinetic drug interactions	
Level of interaction	**Drug**
Commonly require dose changes due to interactions with other drugs	Carbamazepine Ethosuximide Lamotrigine Oxcarbazepine Phenobarbital Primidone Phenytoin Tiagabine Topiramate Valproate Zonisamide
Generally minor interactions. Dose	Clobazam
changes only occasionally required	Clonazepam
Rarely (if ever) interact with other drugs	Gabapentin Levetiracetam Pregabalin

- Carbamazepine, phenytoin and phenobarbital are amongst the most potent enzyme-inducers in the pharmacopoeia.
- Pharmacokinetic interactions between antiepileptics (and other drugs) are therefore very common and can have a major impact on clinical therapeutics.
- Interactions with other non-antiepileptic drugs include:
  - antipsychotic drugs
  - antidepressants
  - antibiotics
  - theophyllin
  - warfarin
  - antifungal drugs
  - antihypertensive drugs
  - cardiovascular drugs.
- The list of known interactions is very long, and before any comedication is considered, the potential for drug interaction should be checked.

Less important pharmacokinetic interactions are in relation to:
- protein binding
- drug absorption
- excretion or drug transport.

FIRST AID

Short-lived tonic–clonic seizures do not require emergency drug treatment, but:
- the patient should be made as comfortable as possible, preferably lying down (or eased to the floor if seated), the head should be protected and tight clothing or neckwear released
- injury should be avoided (e.g. from hot radiators, top of stairs, hot water, road traffic)
- no attempt should be made to force anything between the teeth
- *after* the convulsive movements have subsided, roll the patient into the recovery position, check the airway is not obstructed and that there are no injuries
- ensure there is no apnoea and that the pulse is maintained
- when fully recovered, the patient should be comforted and reassured.

Non-convulsive seizures are less dramatic but can still be disturbing and embarrassing. If consciousness is impaired, injury should be avoided (e.g. from wandering about). However, attempts at restraint often increase confusion and cause agitation or occasionally violence.

EMERGENCY DRUG TREATMENT OF SEIZURES
Prolonged convulsions or serial seizures

If a tonic–clonic seizure continues for 5–10 minutes it is usual to give benzo-diazepines intravenously (or rectally):

- undiluted iv diazepam is given at a rate not exceeding 2–5 mg/min, using the Diazemuls formulation
- the adult bolus iv or rectal dose is 10–30 mg
- in children the equivalent bolus dose is 0.2–0.3 mg/kg
- iv lorazepam is an alternative with some advantages over iv diazepam (longer duration of action, less risk of cardiovascular collapse): 4 mg in adults, 0.1 mg/kg in children.

Seizures occurring in clusters

Acute therapy after the first seizure can be given in an attempt to prevent subsequent attacks. Oral clobazam 10–20 mg is a common choice and will take effect within 1–2 hours and last for 12–24 hours.

TONIC–CLONIC STATUS EPILEPTICUS

Status epilepticus is defined as a prolonged continuous seizure, or rapidly repeating seizures without recovery in between. Tonic–clonic status epilepticus carries a high risk of morbidity and mortality. It is a medical emergency and the seizures should be controlled with the utmost urgency. If tonic–clonic status epilepticus is allowed to persist for more than about 2 hours there is a substantial risk of seizure-induced cerebral damage. The risk rises the longer the seizures continue. For this reason, the drug treatment of tonic–clonic status epilepticus is best divided into three stages:

- the first stage (early status) is defined as the first 30 minutes of seizure activity
- the second stage (established status) is reached if early-stage treatment fails
- the third stage (refractory status) is reached if seizures continue for more than 1–2 hours after initiating therapy, despite early/established stage therapy.

A systematic protocol-driven approach is important in this emergency situation. The choice of drug regimen is somewhat arbitrary. A protocol favoured by the author is shown in Box 2.5, and details of the drugs used are given in Table 2.9. It is important not to forget to initiate, or continue, oral antiepileptic drugs.

There are other published protocols with equal claims to effectiveness.

Box 2.5   The treatment of tonic–clonic status epilepticus in adults

Stage of early status (0–30 minutes)

Lorazepam 4 mg iv bolus (can be repeated once).

↓ *If seizures continue after 30 minutes*

Stage of established status (30–60/90 minutes)

Phenobarbital iv infusion 10 mg/kg at 100 mg/min.

or

Phenytoin iv infusion 15 mg/kg at 50 mg/min.

or

Fosphenytoin iv infusion 15 mg phenytoin equivalents (PE)/kg at 100 mg PE/min.

or

Valproate iv infusion 25 mg/kg at 3–6 mg/kg/min.

↓ *If seizures continue after 30–90 minutes*

Stage of refractory status (> 60/90 minutes: general anaesthesia)

Propofol: iv bolus 2 mg/kg, repeated if necessary, and then followed by a continuous infusion of 5–10 mg/kg/hour initially, reducing to a dose sufficient to maintain a burst suppression pattern on the EEG (usually 1–3 mg/kg/hour).

or

Thiopental: iv bolus 100–250 mg given over 20 seconds with further 50 mg boluses every 2–3 minutes until seizures are controlled, followed by a continuous iv infusion at a dose sufficient to maintain a burst suppression pattern on the EEG (usually 3–5 mg/kg/hour).

or

Midazolam: iv bolus 0.1–0.3 mg/kg at a rate not exceeding 4 mg/minute initially, followed by a continuous iv infusion at a dose sufficient to maintain a burst suppression pattern on the EEG (usually 0.05–0.4 mg/kg/hour).

When seizures have been controlled for 12 hours, the anaesthetic drug should be withdrawn slowly (over up to 12 hours). If seizures recur, the general anaesthetic agent should be given again for another 12 hours, and then withdrawal attempted again. This cycle may need to be repeated until seizure control is achieved.

Table 2.9   Drugs used in the stages of early and established tonic–clonic status epilepticus

Drug	Route of administration	Adult dose	Paediatric dose
Diazepam	iv bolus (not exceeding 2–5 mg/min)	10–20 mg	0.25–0.5 mg/kg
	Rectal administration	10–30 mg	0.5–0.75 mg/kg*
Midazolam	im or rectally	5–10 mg*	0.15–0.3 mg/kg*
	iv bolus	0.1–0.3 mg/kg at 4 mg/min*	
	iv infusion	0.05–0.4 mg/kg/h	
Clonazepam	iv bolus (not exceeding 2 mg/min)	1–2 mg at 2 mg/min*	250–500 µg
Fosphenytoin	iv bolus (not exceeding 100 mg phenytoin equivalents(PE)/min)	15–20 mg PE/kg	–
Lorazepam	iv bolus	0.07 mg/kg (usually 4 mg)*	0.1 mg/kg
Phenytoin	iv bolus/infusion (not exceeding 50 mg/min)	15–20 mg/kg	20 mg/kg at 25 mg/min
Phenobarbital	iv bolus (not exceeding 100 mg/min)	10–20 mg/kg	15–20 mg/kg
Valproate	iv bolus	15–30 mg/kg	20–40 mg/kg

*May be repeated.

Acknowledgements

Many details in this text are taken, with permission, from Shorvon SD. *Handbook of Epilepsy Treatment: Forms, Causes and Therapy in Children and Adults*. Blackwell, Oxford, 2005.

Further reading

Arzimanoglou A, Guerrini R, Aicardi J. Aicardi's epilepsy in children, 3rd edn. Lippincott, Williams and Wilkins, Philadelphia, 2003.

Shorvon SD. Handbook of epilepsy treatment: forms, causes and therapy in children and adults. Blackwell, Oxford, 2005.

Shorvon SD, Perucca E, Fish D, Dodson E (eds). The treatment of epilepsy, 2nd edn. Blackwell, Oxford 2004.

Wallace SJ, Farrell K (eds). Epilepsy in children. Arnold, London, 2004.

3 SLEEP DISORDERS

Paul Reading and Adam Zeman

Despite their generally low profile in neurology education programmes, patients with sleep problems often present to neurologists. This can occur directly, most commonly for the assessment of excessive daytime sleepiness or the evaluation of nocturnal motor and behavioural disturbance, or indirectly because sleep disorders may exacerbate many common neurological disorders such as epilepsy, migraine and Parkinson's disease.

The International Classification of Sleep Disorders has recently been substantially revised (ISD-2). It recognises the following categories:

- *Sleep-related breathing disorders* – this group largely comprises obstructive and the less common central sleep apnoeas.
- *Hypersomnias not due to a sleep-related breathing disorder* – narcolepsy with and without cataplexy is the most important example here.
- *Insomnias* – acute and chronic forms are recognised. The latter include idiopathic, psychophysiological and paradoxical (i.e. misperceived) insomnias. Neurologists will often see 'insomnia secondary to a chronic condition', such as Parkinson's disease.
- *Circadian rhythm disorders* – primary and more common secondary forms are described, all reflecting a misalignment between the subject's sleep pattern and the societal norm, such that sleep and/or wakefulness is difficult when desired, needed or expected.
- *Parasomnias* – disorders of behaviour or experience occurring predominantly during sleep. Most are disorders of arousal from sleep and are classified according to the stage of sleep from which they arise, including sleep onset.

■ *Sleep-related movement disorders* – restless legs syndrome and periodic limb movement disorder are the commonest examples that will present to neurologists.

EXCESSIVE DAYTIME SLEEPINESS

About 5% of the population complain of persistent and troublesome sleepiness in situations in which they would expect to be alert. The overwhelming majority with significant excessive daytime sleepiness (EDS) have an identifiable cause for their symptoms. A confident diagnosis may sometimes be made on the history alone, but appropriate investigation is often required. Although there is increasing public awareness of EDS and the associated potential dangers, it can present in a variety of ways:

■ lethargy
■ irritability
■ poor concentration
■ memory impairment
■ clumsiness
■ low mood
■ personality change
■ worsened headaches
■ marital disharmony
■ impotence.

The most common cause of mild EDS is chronic sleep deprivation due to insufficient sleep, diagnosed by a thorough history and a sleep diary. In a sleep clinic population, in decreasing order of likelihood, EDS is due to:

■ fragmented or poor quality sleep (e.g. obstructive sleep apnoea, periodic limb movements during sleep, restless legs syndrome)
■ a primary sleep disorder (e.g. narcolepsy)
■ circadian rhythm misalignment (e.g. shift work sleep disorder).

Certain drugs can exacerbate nocturnal sleep fragmentation and should be avoided if possible:

■ alcohol and its sudden withdrawal
■ beta-blockers can disrupt sleep and cause nightmares
■ tricyclic antidepressants are generally sedative but may increase nocturnal motor disorders, such as periodic leg movements, and cause insomnia
■ selective serotonin reuptake inhibitors may worsen sleep quality
■ venlafaxine may decrease total sleep time in some patients
■ lithium can worsen the restless legs syndrome and periodic leg movements

- levodopa can produce nocturnal dyskinesia and a fragmented sleep pattern.

OBSTRUCTIVE SLEEP APNOEA

Obstructive sleep apnoea is by far the commonest cause of EDS resulting from fragmented sleep. There are usually clear clues to suggest the diagnosis:
- older age
- male sex
- central obesity with recent weight gain
- collar size over 43 cm (17 inches)
- deviated nasal septum
- enlarged tonsils
- receding chin
- unrefreshing sleep
- choking during sleep
- severe snoring with pauses in breathing
- morning 'hangover' with dry mouth.

Children, patients who live alone, or who are not obese can present a diagnostic challenge.

Management
- Continuous positive airway pressure (CPAP) is an established and effective treatment for symptomatic patients.
- Advice on lifestyle and weight reduction should be given, but is rarely effective.
- Selected patients may benefit from mandibular advancement devices.
- Palatal surgery is rarely advisable.
- For the small minority intolerant of CPAP or those with significant EDS despite optimal treatment, some physicians recommend wake-promoting agents such as modafinil in the dose used for narcolepsy (see below).

NARCOLEPSY SYNDROME (PRIMARY NARCOLEPSY)

Narcolepsy is best considered a disorder of sleep regulation. The prevalence in white populations is about 1 in 2000 and a significant proportion of sufferers are undiagnosed. Most patients develop symptoms in their late teenage years with little remission subsequently. The primary complaint usually reflects an inability to stay awake for more than 3 or 4 hours. The need to sleep can be irresistible and, in the instance of sudden 'sleep attacks', poorly recalled subsequently. Most patients report sleep episodes at unusual times such as during activities, including meals. Nocturnal sleep is characteristically disrupted and a variety of parasomnias may be associated with the condition:

- sleep fragmentation
- REM sleep paralysis
- disturbing nightmares
- hallucinatory experiences at sleep onset or on waking
- periodic limb movements during sleep
- REM sleep behaviour disorder
- non-REM parasomnia, such as sleep walking and more complex behaviours including eating.

Management of the excessive sleepiness

- The daytime naps of most narcoleptic patients last less than an hour and are usually restorative. If the patient's lifestyle permits, planned short naps, particularly in the afternoon, are recommended.
- Some evidence suggests that large carbohydrate meals can exacerbate sleepiness. Small, regular meals and the avoidance of refined foods rich in carbohydrates can improve sleepiness, anecdotally.
- Most patients benefit from medication to improve daytime wakefulness and alertness (Table 3.1).
  - Modafinil is first-line therapy in newly diagnosed narcolepsy; 100 mg oral, morning and lunchtime is the usual starting dose, increasing as required to 200 mg twice daily (some patients take higher doses with apparent benefit).
  - Although there are no good direct comparisons between modafinil and amphetamine-like drugs, the latter are now considered second-line therapy for when modafinil causes unacceptable adverse effects, or is ineffective.
  - Dexamphetamine taken in three divided doses through the day is most commonly used; starting daily dose of 15–30 mg oral, and increasing if necessary over several months to 45–60 mg/day.
  - Some authorities recommend methylphenidate in a dose range 30–120 mg/day, taken in 2 or 3 divided doses, as an alternative.
  - Many patients with severe sleepiness may benefit from both modafinil and dexamphetamine simultaneously.
  - If amphetamine is inappropriate or not tolerated, less potent stimulant medication such as selegiline (10–20 mg/day oral, morning and

Table 3.1 Drug treatment of excessive daytime sleepiness

	Modafinil	Amphetamine-like drugs
Mechanism of action	Unknown, possible direct stimulation of posterior hypothalamus	Mostly via indirect release of catecholamines, particularly dopamine resulting in non-specific cortical activation
Duration of action	Around 5 hours	Around 2 hours
Rebound hypersomnia on discontinuation	Rare	Common
Main adverse effects	Headache, usually transient; gastric upset	Agitation; cardiovascular problems such as hypertension; euphoria; weight loss and reduced appetite
Precautions	Increased dose of oestrogen-containing oral contraceptives required	Can be used recreationally; a controlled drug
Effects on cataplexy	Minimal	Moderate suppression
Expense	Around €300 per month	Around €70 per month for an average dose of dexamphetamine
Cognitive effects	May improve executive function, particularly in tasks requiring planning	Speed of responding increased; increased impulsivity
Typical dose	100–200 mg twice daily	10–20 mg three times daily dexamphetamine

lunchtime) can be used (but not SSRIs, to avoid the risk of the serotonin syndrome).
- Patients often self-medicate with caffeine or stimulant drinks, which should be encouraged unless excessive or contraindicated.
- Most narcoleptics remain somewhat prone to excessive sleepiness despite optimal therapy. Involvement in self-help groups can be helpful in selected cases. The provision of educational material, possibly via the Internet, should also be encouraged.

– Gamma-hydroxybutyrate is a naturally occurring metabolite which appears to increase total sleep time, particularly the deep slow wave stages. It has been available in the USA since 2002 and is likely to receive a licence for cataplexy in most European countries in early 2006. It may be useful in resistant cases, especially when disturbed nocturnal sleep is a major symptom. It appears to improve cataplexy and daytime somnolence, with maximum effects occurring only after several weeks of treatment. It is taken before bed as a liquid preparation with a second dose around 4 hours after initial sleep onset. A total dose of 4.5–9 g per night is usual. Its main drawbacks are its short duration of action and potential for abuse. Nausea, weight loss and nocturnal confusion can be limiting adverse effects.

Cataplexy

Approximately 70% of narcoleptic patients complain of cataplexy – transient partial or total paralysis occurring suddenly and in clear consciousness, most often triggered by a positive emotion such as laughter or its anticipation. Most antidepressants (see Chapter 13) are effective against cataplexy:

- fluoxetine 20–60 mg once daily, but dry mouth, nausea, sexual dysfunction
- clomipramine 10–100 mg/day in 1 or 2 divided doses, but dry mouth, weight gain, constipation, drowsiness
- venlafaxine, 37.5–300 mg/day in 1 or 2 divided doses, but anorexia, insomnia, hypertension
- gamma-hydroxybutyrate is also used for resistant cases (see above).

Sleep-associated hallucinations

Around 10% of narcoleptic patients have frequent and disturbing hallucinatory experiences occurring around sleep or sometimes during full wakefulness. Medications for cataplexy usually suppress these hallucinations.

Sleep paralysis

Infrequent episodes of sleep paralysis at sleep onset or at the point of awakening are reported by at least 50% of narcoleptics. This requires reassurance and not specific medication.

Poor sleep

Disturbed or fragmented nocturnal sleep can be a prominent feature of some narcoleptics, reflecting the dysregulation of normal sleep mechanisms.

A benzodiazepine such as low-dose clonazepam (0.5–1 mg oral, before bed) can be helpful with occasional improvement in daytime wakefulness.

Parasomnias

Some patients have additional parasomnias, including REM sleep behaviour disorder or severe periodic limb movements, requiring specific therapy (see below).

Significant obstructive sleep apnoea is probably more common in the narcoleptic population and should not be overlooked.

SECONDARY NARCOLEPSY

Structural abnormalities in the region of the hypothalamus or third ventricle may present in a similar way to idiopathic narcolepsy, but often with atypical features or resistance to therapy. Examples include tumours, such as those arising from the pituitary, and hydrocephalus due to a variety of causes. Treatment should clearly be directed at the underlying pathology where possible.

IDIOPATHIC HYPERSOMNOLENCE

Idiopathic hypersomnolence is a rare and poorly characterised condition that may affect up to 10% of severely somnolent patients initially referred with a possible diagnosis of narcolepsy. It is a diagnosis of exclusion, although it does have characteristic features. The treatment options are limited to:

- symptomatic control
- wake-promoting agents (modafinil and amphetamine) can be partly effective
- any associated mood disorder may require specific treatment.

OTHER NEUROLOGICAL CAUSES OF EXCESSIVE DAYTIME SLEEPINESS

Unwanted EDS, as opposed to fatigue or simple lethargy, may be a prominent symptom in patients with a variety of neurological conditions:

- parkinsonian syndromes
- dementias
- multiple sclerosis
- myotonic dystrophy

- head injuries
- encephalitis.

Treatable causes such as significant obstructive sleep apnoea or nocturnal dystonia in the case of Parkinson's disease should always be considered. Some patients with evidence of prominent sleep fragmentation as a cause of EDS may benefit from a low-dose benzodiazepine such as clonazepam 0.25–1 mg at night. The risks of long-term dependence must be weighed against the underlying condition and any success of treatment.

Modafinil appears to be a safe drug when used long term and has a licence in the UK for all causes of excessive sleepiness due to an underlying chronic pathological condition. Some evidence suggests that it can be useful for EDS in the neurological conditions outlined above, in the dose range used for narcolepsy.

CIRCADIAN RHYTHM SLEEP DISORDERS
Extrinsic causes

Difficulties with sleep or alertness due to shift work or jet lag are normal responses to abnormal situations. However, because the resulting symptoms may be so troubling in certain individuals, treatment may be necessary, especially if the consequences of fatigue are dangerous. Although some individuals tolerate shift work better than others, advancing age invariably undermines this ability to adapt.

- Short spells of night shift with time for recovery should be encouraged.
- Light therapy during the night can help in specific circumstances.
- Wake-promoting agents such as caffeine or even modafinil (see above) may be justified in selected cases.
- Melatonin mimics the effects of darkness on the circadian system. Although there is no good evidence, many authorities recommend it to aid daytime sleep. A typical adult dose is 3–5 mg taken around 2 hours before sleep is required.
- If the spell of shift work is brief, intermittent use of short-acting hypnotic agents such as temazepam can be helpful to aid sleep onset.

Intrinsic causes

The four types of intrinsic circadian rhythm disorder thought to reflect dysfunction of the endogenous circadian pacemaker are:
- Delayed sleep phase syndrome:
  - commoner in young adults

- 5% of all cases who are referred with insomnia
- subjects cannot sleep before 1 am or later
- overnight sleep normal or long
- extreme difficulty with morning waking
- possible genetic basis.
- Advanced sleep phase syndrome:
  - rare
  - typical bedtime 6–9 pm
  - cannot sleep after 4 am
  - genetic abnormality established in some.
- Non-24-hour sleep phase syndrome:
  - sleep–wake cycle wholly reliant on intrinsic biological rhythm with periodicity of around 25 hours
  - no response to external time cues
  - total desynchrony alternates with complete conformity in 3–4 week cycles
  - rare in subjects who are not totally blind.
- Irregular sleep–wake pattern:
  - seen mostly in severely brain damaged subjects
  - sleep and wake times totally disorganised
  - 3 or 4 naps over 24 hours typical
  - total daily sleep time normal.

The delayed sleep phase syndrome is the most common type of intrinsic circadian rhythm disorder seen in neurological practice:
- it is important to recognise as it can cause significant difficulties in the workplace or in an educational setting
- treatment is difficult and specialist input should be sought if available
- a combination of behavioural training with melatonin (3–5 mg oral) given mid-evening may be helpful
- some authorities recommend phototherapy given early in the morning.

PARASOMNIAS

Sleep–wake transition disorders

- Unpleasant symptoms at the point of sleep onset may be severe or frequent enough to produce a referral to neurological services, usually to exclude an epileptic phenomenon.
- Most people report occasional jerks or a sensation of falling just at the point of sleep onset. Rarely, this type of symptom can occur several times a week or have a more dramatic quality, sufficient to cause concern.

Complaints such as loud bangs, visual flashes, or 'explosions' in the head (exploding head syndrome) require reassurance of their benign nature. Intermittent courses of short-acting hypnotics or tricyclic medication can be used in severe cases.

Non-REM parasomnias

Around 1% of young adults report abnormal behaviours that arise from sleep and occur on a regular basis. The vast majority are due to a non-REM parasomnia and are thought to reflect an intrinsic abnormality of the arousal mechanisms from deep sleep:

- childhood history of prominent sleep-talking, sleep-walking or night terrors
- positive family history of the above
- disturbances occur within 90 minutes of sleep onset and rarely recur
- no recollection of events
- subjects often retire back to bed spontaneously
- behaviours can be complex and sometimes dangerous, ranging from simple arousals to complex acts that appear to involve planning, such as cooking meals
- eyes usually open and limited verbal communication possible
- worse if stressed or sleep deprived, and after alcohol.

Management

- After recognition of the diagnosis, reassurance and simple measures to improve safety are often all that is needed.
- Subjects should be advised about general sleep hygiene and to avoid excessive alcohol before bedtime.
- Short courses of benzodiazepines such as clonazepam (0.25–1 mg at night) may be used for severe symptomatic spells, or if there are concerns when sleeping away from home.

REM sleep parasomnias

Sleep paralysis

Some individuals appear predisposed to episodes of isolated REM sleep paralysis, usually occurring at wake onset. If severe or frequent, medication used to treat cataplexy and suppress REM sleep phenomena can be used intermittently.

REM sleep behaviour disorder

Prominent jerks or brief violent behaviours arising from deep sleep in an elderly male patient may suggest this disorder. It can occur in an idiopathic form or as part of a neurodegenerative syndrome, most commonly Parkinson's disease or multiple system atrophy. The characteristic features are:

- strong preponderance of elderly male subjects (male/female ratio10:1)
- behaviours brief and usually aggressive, often with vocalisation
- injuries to subject or bed partner may be severe
- on arousal, immediate dream recall common
- strong association with parkinsonian syndromes if long follow-up
- consequent daytime somnolence not usually severe.

■ Certain drugs, including most antidepressants, may exacerbate this condition and should be used with caution.

■ Sudden withdrawal of benzodiazepines or alcohol can also precipitate symptoms.

■ Treatment with clonazepam (0.25–3 mg at night) is usually successful and required long term.

■ If clonazepam or an alternative benzodiazepine is unsuccessful or not tolerated, anecdotal success with levodopa, melatonin, carbamazepine and gabapentin has been reported.

Other parasomnias and related disorders

Sleep-related panic attacks cause recurrent awakening with panic or fear, often associated with a feeling of impending death or choking, usually from non-REM stage 2 or 3 sleep. There is often, but not always, a history of daytime anxiety and panic. The patient becomes fully alert on waking.

Sleep medicine is not immune to 'functional' presentations: patients with nocturnal dissociative disorder present with abnormal behaviour from sleep, which turns out, on investigation, to have a psychogenic basis.

Further reading

Kryger MH, Roth T, Dement WC. Principles and practice of sleep medicine, 4th edn. Saunders, Philadelphia, 2005.

Parkes JD. Sleep and its disorders. WB Saunders, London, 1985.

Silber MH, Krahn LE, Morgenthaler TI. Sleep medicine in clinical practice. Taylor & Francis, London, 2004.

4   STROKE

Helen M. Dewey, Brian R. Chambers and Geoffrey A. Donnan

DEFINITION OF STROKE AND TRANSIENT ISCHAEMIC ATTACK

- The World Health Organisation (WHO) definition of stroke is the sudden onset of a focal neurological deficit lasting more than 24 hours in which causes other than vascular have been excluded. A transient ischaemic attack (TIA) has the same definition but lasts less than 24 hours, often just for a few minutes.
- Subarachnoid haemorrhage (SAH) is the exception to this definition and usually presents without focal neurological deficits.
- Some definitions of stroke and TIA incorporate brain imaging (changes thought to be due to infarction or haemorrhage, seen on computed tomography (CT) or magnetic resonance imaging (MRI)).

EPIDEMIOLOGY

- Stroke is the third most common cause of death worldwide (after coronary heart disease and all cancers combined) and the major cause of disability.

Table 4.1   Causes of intracerebral haemorrhage

Cause	Usual features
Rupture of small, deep perforating arteries	Deep location (basal ganglia, thalamus, cerebellum, brainstem) Frequently associated with hypertension Age ≥ 45 years
Cerebral amyloid angiopathy	Lobar (or multiple) Less likely to be hypertensive Age ≥ 70 years
Arteriovenous malformation or cavernoma	Variable location Typical 'target' MRI appearance of cavernomas Most common cause in those < 45 years
Saccular aneurysm	Suggestive pattern and position of lobar haemorrhage Associated subarachnoid haemorrhage
Coagulopathy	Anticoagulants Antiplatelet drugs Thrombolytic treatment Thrombocytopenia Clotting factor deficiency
Tumour	Most common: melanoma, lung carcinoma, renal carcinoma, choriocarcinoma, testicular carcinoma, glioblastoma
Trauma	Bilateral frontal ± temporal lobar haemorrhage Subarachnoid or subdural haemorrhage Widespread brain contusions History of trauma but not always severe
Intracranial venous thrombosis	Younger age; frequently female Associated seizures, headache Multiple haemorrhages
Infective endocarditis with mycotic aneurysm	Systemic features of bacterial endocarditis
Drugs	Alcohol Amphetamines Cocaine
Acute hypertension	Clinical setting including acute renal failure, eclampsia

- Stroke is a heterogeneous condition with many causes; in whites, approximately 85% are ischaemic, 10% due to intracerebral haemorrhage, and 5% due to SAH (intracerebral haemorrhage is more common in Japanese and Chinese).
- The incidence of stroke varies somewhat from region to region, but has been accurately measured in only a few populations. The best data are from western countries where age-standardised incidence for people aged 55 years or more ranges from about 4.2 to 6.5 per 1000 population per annum.
- 20% of stroke patients die within 1 month and about 30% within 1 year. About one-third remain disabled; the remaining third either recover fully or regain independence of daily living.
- Intracerebral haemorrhage (Table 4.1) and SAH have a higher 30-day case fatality (around 50%) and greater long-term disability among survivors.
- While stroke mortality and incidence are declining in many western countries, they may be increasing in Eastern Europe and Asia.

DIAGNOSIS OF STROKE/TIA

- The diagnosis of stroke/TIA requires a compatible history and neurological examination backed up by brain imaging to exclude mimics (Box 4.1).
- Brain MRI with diffusion weighted imaging (DWI) identifies most acute ischaemic strokes within the first few hours but is not widely available. However, DWI is not infallible and imaging may be normal in patients with small strokes, particularly in the posterior fossa.

Box 4.1   Some conditions mimicking stroke/TIA

- Epileptic seizure.
- Sepsis (including meningoencephalitis).
- Toxic/metabolic disorder (e.g. hypoglycaemia, hyperglycaemia, hyponatraemia).
- Space-occupying lesion (e.g. tumour, abscess).
- Syncope/presyncope.
- Peripheral vestibulopathy.
- Migraine.
- Subdural haematoma.
- Multiple sclerosis.
- Peripheral nerve lesion.
- Bell's palsy.

- Urgent assessment of stroke is required so that appropriate treatment can be started at once.
- Urgent assessment of TIA is also required to determine the most likely underlying mechanism, because the risk of stroke in the first hours to days is very high, and there is a unique opportunity to instigate appropriate secondary prevention strategies. Crescendo events without cortical symptoms (capsular warning syndrome) have a high risk (40%) of lacunar stroke within 1 month.

History

- The key features are an *abrupt* onset of a clearly *focal* neurological deficit in a patient who is generally well. A clear time of onset makes stroke/TIA more likely and is *critical* information when considering eligibility for acute stroke treatment.
- SAH is the exception to the requirement for a focal neurological deficit. Sudden onset of severe headache ('like an explosion') is the key symptom, often accompanied by photophobia, neck stiffness and nausea.

Examination

- A neurological deficit that can be readily localised to a specific vascular territory predicts stroke (other than SAH).
- A number of features make a stroke mimic more likely:
  - confusion frequently indicates systemic illness or metabolic derangement
  - dysarthria is common in sick, edentulous patients, and in alcoholics
  - vertigo alone more commonly indicates peripheral vestibulopathy than stroke.
- Previous stroke and pre-existing cognitive deficits complicate assessment.
- Worsening of existing stroke neurological deficits frequently occurs with systemic illness (e.g. sepsis) or as a result of epilepsy.
- Neck stiffness is the key finding in SAH but takes some hours to develop, and in some patients may not develop at all.

Initial investigations to exclude stroke mimics

- Blood sugar should be checked in all patients with suspected stroke/TIA. Hypoglycaemia and, less often, hyperglycaemia may present with focal neurological deficits.
- Other metabolic derangements should be excluded with (at a minimum) assessment of renal function, electrolytes and full blood examination.
- If sepsis is suspected, a systematic search for the underlying cause should be made.

PATHOLOGICAL TYPE AND TOPOGRAPHY OF STROKE/TIA

There are no clinical features that reliably distinguish between ischaemic and haemorrhagic stroke, so brain imaging is mandatory in all cases. Even for TIA it is not possible to exclude a small intracerebral haemorrhage or TIA mimic as a cause for rapidly resolving symptoms just on clinical grounds – brain imaging is always required (unless ocular attacks only).

Confirmation of intracerebral haemorrhage

- CT and MRI (particularly gradient echo sequences) have high sensitivity for acute intracerebral haemorrhage. However, small intracerebral haemorrhages resolve quickly and may not be visible on CT for more than a few days after onset. Blood products remain visible long term on MRI, so this is the best test to distinguish haemorrhage from ischaemia in patients presenting after a delay.
- Angiography is required when saccular aneurysm or arteriovenous malformation (AVM) is suspected.
- The causes of intracerebral haemorrhage are listed in Table 4.1.

Confirmation of subarachnoid haemorrhage

- SAH is most commonly (85%) due to rupture of an intracranial saccular aneurysm.
- CT is highly sensitive (95%) to SAH within the first 24–48 hours, but becomes negative in a matter of a few days.
- If CT scan is normal, lumbar puncture is essential. The diagnostic finding is xanthochromic CSF which may take up to 12 hours to develop *in vivo*. Xanthochromia persists for up to 2 weeks after SAH but may disappear sooner.
- When a patient presents late with a history very suggestive of SAH, catheter or CT angiography should be performed (note that any aneurysm detected might not in fact have ruptured but be incidental).

Confirmation of ischaemic stroke

- MRI is the imaging investigation of choice in acute ischaemic stroke. DWI demonstrates diagnostic high signal within the first few hours after onset and angiography sequences provide information about the status of intracranial (± cervical) vessels. Unfortunately, MRI has limited availability, is slow (compared to standard CT) and it is difficult to scan unstable and critically ill patients.

- CT imaging is frequently normal very early after ischaemic stroke but may show subtle changes that tend to be more obvious with larger areas of infarction.
- If initially normal, and there is any doubt of the clinical diagnosis, CT can be repeated after 3–7 days or MRI performed.

Clinical classification of ischaemic stroke

The Oxfordshire Community Stroke Project clinical classification is useful for bedside application (Table 4.2). It provides a simple prognostic tool and helps guide further investigations.

Table 4.2   Simplified version of the Oxfordshire Community Stroke Project classification of ischaemic stroke

Subtype	Defining features	Usual cause and prognosis
TACI (total anterior circulation infarct)	Ipsilateral motor and/or sensory deficit *and* higher cortical dysfunction (e.g. dysphasia), neglect *and* homonymous hemianopia	Large middle cerebral artery infarct due to embolism from the heart or proximal arterial source, high likelihood of death and long-term dependency
PACI (partial anterior circulation infarct)	Two of three deficits necessary for TACI *or* higher cortical dysfunction alone *or* restricted motor/ sensory deficit (e.g. confined to one limb or face and hand)	Smaller infarct but same causes as TACI, better prognosis for recovery but high risk of early recurrence
LACI (lacunar infarct)	Pure motor hemiparesis Pure sensory stroke Sensorimotor stroke Ataxic hemiparesis	Small deep infarct due to small-vessel disease, relatively good prognosis
POCI (posterior circulation infarct)	Brainstem signs *or* cerebellar dysfunction without ipsilateral long-tract signs (i.e. not ataxic hemiparesis), *or* isolated homonymous hemianopia, *or* combinations	Infarct in the posterior cerebral hemisphere, brainstem or cerebellum, due to large- or small-vessel disease or cardiac embolism, variable prognosis

Infarct topography defined by imaging

Another classification of ischaemic stroke is based on infarct topography seen on brain CT or MRI. This allows further insight into the underlying mechanism and prognosis. The distribution of these infarct patterns is largely based on the arterial vascular territory (Fig. 4.1).

- Infarction within the territory of a cerebral artery or major cerebral branch artery, and striatocapsular infarction, are most commonly due to artery-to-artery embolism or embolism from the heart.
- Lacunar infarction is mainly due to *in situ* thrombosis within a single small penetrating artery.
- Infarction within the territory of the anterior choroidal artery, and white matter medullary infarction, have various mechanisms.

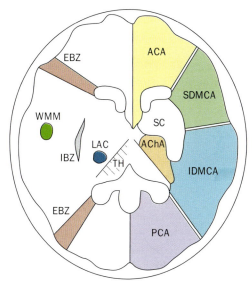

EBZ	External border zone	SC	Striatocapsular
IBZ	Internal border zone	IDMCA	Inferior division middle
WMM	White matter medullary		cerebral artery
LAC	Lacune	AChA	Anterior choroidal artery
TH	Thalamic	PCA	Posterior cerebral artery
ACA	Anterior cerebral artery		
SDMCA	Superior division middle		
	cerebral artery		

Fig. 4.1   Infarct topography defined by brain imaging.

- Thalamic infarction may be lacunar or due to artery-to-artery or cardiac embolism.
- Although border-zone infarcts often suggest a haemodynamic mechanism (acute fall in blood pressure), they can be caused by extracranial artery occlusion, embolic intracranial artery occlusion or small vessel disease.

DEFINING THE CAUSE OF STROKE

Theclassification developed for the Trial of ORG 10172 in Acute Stroke Treatment (TOAST) has become the most commonly used mechanistic ischaemic stroke classification and is based on five subtypes:

- large artery atherothromboembolism   35%
- embolism from the heart   24%
- small vessel disease   18%
- uncertain cause   18%
- rare causes   5%

- Common causes of embolism from the heart are atrial fibrillation, mural thrombus post-myocardial infarction or complicating cardiomyopathy, endocarditis, and patent foramen ovale with atrial septal aneurysm.
- Aortic arch atheroma is also an important source of embolism.
- In western societies, extracranial carotid bifurcation atherosclerosis is an important cause of stroke. Plaque inflammation and rupture causing secondary thrombosis leads to artery-to-artery embolism. Obstruction to flow may also give rise to haemodynamic cerebral infarction, typically involving external and/or internal border-zone territories.
- Small-vessel disease generally results in lacunar syndromes, the most common being pure motor hemiparesis.
- The clinical features and brain imaging should be used to guide further investigations to determine the most likely underlying stroke/TIA mechanism (Fig. 4.2 and Table 4.3).

ACUTE TREATMENT OF TIAs

- Antiplatelet therapy with aspirin as first line (see below).
- Some clinicians administer iv heparin aiming for an activated partial thromboplastin time (APTT) of 1.5–2.5 times normal values for 24–72 hours, as a short-term measure in cases of symptomatic severe carotid or vertebrobasilar stenosis, or crescendo events (e.g. capsular warning syndrome), although there is no good evidence to support this.

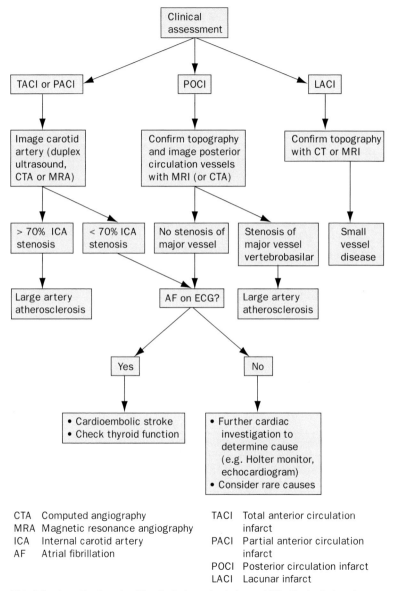

CTA   Computed angiography
MRA   Magnetic resonance angiography
ICA   Internal carotid artery
AF   Atrial fibrillation

TACI   Total anterior circulation infarct
PACI   Partial anterior circulation infarct
POCI   Posterior circulation infarct
LACI   Lacunar infarct

Fig. 4.2   Investigation algorithm for ischaemic stroke and TIA after brain imaging has excluded haemorrhage.

■ Early carotid endarterectomy for symptomatic severe carotid stenosis (see below).

ACUTE TREATMENT OF STROKE

■ Stroke is a medical emergency now there is effective, time-critical therapy that improves outcome.
■ There are three proven acute interventions:
  – Stroke unit care for all stroke types: 20 treated to prevent one death or dependency.
  – Aspirin within 48 hours of stroke onset for ischaemic stroke: 77 treated to prevent one death or dependency.

Table 4.3 Rarer causes of ischaemic stroke	
Cause	Identifying tests
Arterial dissection	Imaging (catheter angiography, MRI and MRA, CT angiography, duplex ultrasound)
Arteritis (including Takayasu's arteritis, giant cell arteritis, polyarteritis nodosa, allergic angiitis, granulomatis arteritis, systemic lupus erythematosus, rheumatoid arthritis)	Imaging (catheter angiography, sometimes MRA), vasculitic markers in the blood, temporal artery biopsy
Intracranial venous thrombosis	Imaging (CT delta sign, MRV)
CADASIL	Skin biopsy, genetic test
Infective endocarditis	Blood cultures, echocardiogram
Antiphospholipid syndrome	Antiphospholipid antibody, lupus anticoagulant, anticardiolipin antibody
Other prothrombotic states	Full blood count, ESR, prothrombin time, antithrombin III, protein C, protein S, factor V-Leiden, antinuclear antibodies, haemoglobin electrophoresis, fibrinogen, platelet aggregation

CADASIL, cerebral autosomal dominant arteriopathy with subcortical ischaemic stroke and leukoencephalopathy; ESR, erythrocyte sedimentation rate; MRA, magnetic resonance angiography; MRV, magnetic resonance venography.

- Alteplase (tissue plasminogen activator) within 3 hours of stroke onset for ischaemic stroke: 10 treated to prevent one death or dependency.

■ Since the introduction of proven interventions, it is now much more important to streamline the assessment and management of acute stroke patients:
  - more rapid assessment means more eligible patients will benefit from thrombolysis; door to needle time of 60 minutes is achievable and should be the benchmark
  - efficient delivery of alteplase (Box 4.2) to eligible patients requires locally appropriate, rapid-response protocols; a dedicated acute stroke team; excellent team work with emergency services, emergency department and radiology department personnel; and much enthusiasm.

Stroke unit care

■ Outcomes for stroke patients are improved by stroke unit care, regardless of patient age, stroke type or stroke severity.

■ The features of stroke unit care responsible for the improved outcomes are probably:
  - expert evidence-based multidisciplinary care (nursing, medical and allied health practitioners)
  - patients located in a geographically defined unit
  - regular, multidisciplinary team meetings for management decisions and effective discharge planning

---

Box 4.2   Alteplase checklist

- Stroke onset definitely < 3 hours previously.
- Significant neurological deficit.
- CT scan excludes intracranial haemorrhage, cerebral neoplasm, other stroke mimics.
- BP below 185/110 and stable (may require antihypertensive agents, see below).
- Hypo- and hyperglycaemia, thrombocytopenia and coagulopathy excluded.
- No recent head trauma, stroke or myocardial infarction.
- No surgery or haemorrhage within the past month that might lead to unmanageable haemorrhage.
- No recent arterial puncture at non-compressible site.
- Menstruation is probably not a contraindication.

– functional and goal directed rehabilitation
– continuing education and support for staff
– family and carer involvement in care and discharge planning.

Aspirin for ischaemic stroke

Aspirin (150–300 mg oral, rectal or iv) is modestly beneficial when given within 48 hours of ischaemic stroke onset. Given its low cost and good safety profile (there is a small increased risk of intracranial and extracranial haemorrhage), it is appropriate in most cases.

Thrombolysis with alteplase for ischaemic stroke

- The extremely short time window (≤ 3 hours) for success underlines the urgency of stroke assessment.
- Benefits decline over time, with every 5 minutes wasted leading to a 5% reduction in the likelihood of a good outcome.
- The dose is 0.9 mg/kg iv with 10% given as a bolus and the remainder over an hour.
- The use of alteplase is associated with a 6–7% symptomatic intracerebral haemorrhage rate (three-fold increase above natural history). The predictors may include early ischaemic change on CT and poor blood pressure control.

Surgery for ischaemic stroke

- Cerebellar infarction may be complicated by oedema that develops 48–72 hours after onset, causing brainstem compression and acute hydrocephalus. Depression of conscious state is the cardinal clinical feature. Urgent posterior fossa surgical decompression and a ventricular shunt can prevent further deterioration and death.
- Total middle cerebral artery infarction may be complicated by massive oedema, leading to raised intracranial pressure, brainstem compression and death, particularly in young patients. Hemicraniectomy may be life-saving and result in an acceptable outcome for some patients.

TREATMENT OF INTRACEREBRAL HAEMORRHAGE

- In general, patients with haemorrhagic stroke should be managed in a stroke unit as for ischaemic stroke.
- Palliation may be the most appropriate management (see below) for elderly patients with impaired consciousness and large volume haemorrhage, as the outlook for good recovery is very poor.

- There is evidence that high initial blood pressure (mean arterial pressure > 120 mmHg) is associated with haematoma expansion and worse outcomes. Thus there is a reasonable rationale to control blood pressure more rigorously than for ischaemic stroke (see below): < 160/90 at all times.
- Recombinant factor VIIa attenuates haematoma growth but is associated with thromboembolic complications. It is not a routine treatment.
- Compression stockings should be used for deep venous thrombosis prophylaxis, and antithrombotic drugs avoided.
- Routine surgical evacuation of intracerebral haematoma should not be performed.
- Surgical evacuation of intracerebral haematoma may be life-saving in the setting of definite or suspected aneurysmal haemorrhage, and for cerebellar haemorrhage with brainstem compression and obstructive hydrocephalus.
- Although there is little evidence for benefit, surgical evacuation may be considered in selected patients if a cerebral haemorrhage is superficial, and recent clinical deterioration has occurred.
- There is no evidence from randomised controlled trials to guide management of patients presenting with intracerebral haemorrhage due to an arteriovenous malformation; clinical practice varies widely across the world. Reported annual re-bleed rates range from 6% to 18% and are highest in the first 6–12 months after the first bleed. Current interventional approaches are endovascular embolisation, surgical removal, stereotactic radiation therapy or some combination of two of these, or even all three.
- Nor is there any evidence how to treat cavernomas – surgical removal is the only option other than do nothing.

TREATMENT OF SUBARACHNOID HAEMORRHAGE

- Close monitoring for the early detection and management of complications.
- Reduced consciousness at presentation, older age and higher volumes of subarachnoid blood are associated with poorer outcome.
- The amount of subarachnoid blood correlates with vasospasm associated with delayed cerebral ischaemic deficits, hydrocephalus, and other complications.
- Early re-bleeding is an important cause of a poor outcome.

Aneurysm management

- Occlusion of the ruptured aneurysm may be achieved via an open surgical approach or an endovascular technique (usually detachable coils).

- Open surgical management remains standard in many places for most ruptured aneurysms. Operation within the first 3 days is generally advocated with the aim of reducing the risk of early re-bleeding and to allow intensive management of vasospasm (see below) should this develop.
- Endovascular occlusion of aneurysms is less invasive than open surgery, leads to better short-term outcomes and less epilepsy, but the long-term risk of re-bleeding remains uncertain.
- Early surgical evacuation of any associated large intraparenchymal haematoma and/or treatment of acute hydrocephalus (see below), may be life-saving.

General care
Prior to aneurysm occlusion

- Patients should be nursed strictly in bed in quiet, darkened surroundings and provided with sufficient analgesia to avoid pain-related blood pressure surges. Aspirin should be avoided. Constipation and straining should be prevented.
- Intravenous hydration with normal saline (about 3 l/day) is recommended to counteract cerebral salt wasting and to avoid hypovolaemia that may predispose to delayed cerebral ischaemia.
- Antihypertensive medication is generally avoided unless the systolic blood pressure is so high that re-bleeding is considered likely (e.g. > 160–180 mmHg). Rapid or excessive blood pressure lowering may contribute to delayed cerebral ischaemia.
- Graduated compression stockings should be used for prevention of deep venous thrombosis.

After aneurysm occlusion

- To reduce the risk of vasospasm, it is commonly recommended that systolic blood pressure is prophylactically elevated to 140–160 mmHg or to 20% above baseline levels.

Diagnosis and management of complications
Delayed cerebral ischaemia

- Effective measures for reducing the risk of cerebral ischaemia assumed to be due to vasospasm, include adequate salt and water intake, avoidance of antihypertensive treatment, and routine calcium antagonists (e.g. nimodipine 60 mg oral every 4 hours for 3 weeks).

- Presentation is with new focal neurological deficits, reduction in level of consciousness, or both. Alternative causes of deterioration (e.g. hydrocephalus and re-bleeding) must be excluded with CT.
- Transcranial Doppler ultrasound is diagnostic of vasospasm if velocities are in the clearly abnormal range.
- Treatment includes induced hypertension (increase systolic blood pressure by at least 20%; a systolic blood pressure of 180–200 mmHg may be appropriate in some individuals), hypervolaemia (central venous pressure 10–12 cm) and normal to low haematocrit (Hb 80–100; Hct low 30s) – so-called 'triple H therapy'.
- Transluminal angioplasty and intra-arterial papaverine have been reported to be of benefit in some centres.

Acute hydrocephalus

- This occurs in about 20% of patients.
- Presentation is with decreasing consciousness.
- The usual approach is repeated lumbar puncture, and external ventricular drainage via a catheter, inserted through a burr hole if necessary.

Systemic complications

- These include hyponatraemia (usually due to salt depletion rather than inappropriate secretion of antidiuretic hormone), cardiac arrhythmias and neurogenic pulmonary oedema.

Asymptomatic intracranial aneurysms

- 1 in 20 people aged > 30 years has an unruptured cerebral aneurysm.
- A family history of aneurysmal SAH in at least two first-degree relatives, or polycystic kidney disease with a family history of SAH, substantially increase the risk of having an aneurysm, and screening for asymptomatic aneurysms is appropriate in these individuals if treatment would be seriously contemplated.
- There is a negligible risk of rupture of aneurysms < 7 mm diameter within the anterior circulation and, in those with no prior history of SAH, they do not require treatment.
- CT angiography and magnetic resonance angiography (MRA) both reliably demonstrate aneurysms > 5 mm and can be used for screening. The choice will depend on local availability and expertise.
- People aged < 50 years with unruptured aneurysms > 7 mm are offered treatment with clipping or coiling, as the reduction in risk of SAH

outweighs the risks of intervention. A more conservative approach is used in older people because the risk of intervention is higher.

■ In people aged > 50 years with no history of SAH, only aneurysms > 12 mm should generally be treated with clipping or coiling, as the risk of poor outcome after intervention is higher at older ages.

MANAGEMENT OF RARE STROKE SYNDROMES

Arterial dissection

■ There is no evidence from randomised controlled trials to guide management of carotid and vertebral dissection. Therefore practice varies widely.

■ Some clinicians routinely administer iv heparin (in full anticoagulation doses) or low-molecular-weight heparin for up to 2 weeks and continue with 3–6 months of warfarin anticoagulation, perhaps followed by aspirin as an antithrombotic drug for some months longer. However, there is no evidence that this is more effective than alternative approaches.

■ Other clinicians use an antiplatelet agent alone (usually aspirin), perhaps for a few months.

■ Others use no antithrombotic therapy unless the patient is worsening.

Intracranial venous thrombosis

■ Intracranial venous thrombosis should be considered as the cause of stroke in women on the oral contraceptive pill, during pregnancy and the puerperium, in association with intracranial, ear or sinus infections and in patients with cancer and haematological disorders.

■ Epileptic seizures and headache are common features.

■ MRI with magnetic resonance venography (MRV) is the investigation of choice to confirm the diagnosis. However, magnetic resonance venograms can be difficult to interpret and there is considerable interobserver variation. CT venography or catheter angiography may be required.

■ Treatment comprises management of any predisposing underlying condition (e.g. infection), anticoagulation and lowering any intracranial hypertension. Full-dose anticoagulation with iv heparin aiming for an APPT of 1.5–2.5 normal for no more than 7 days or low-molecular-weight heparin (e.g. nadroparin 0.6 ml, sc every 12 hours for 1–3 weeks) is used acutely. This should be followed by warfarin, aiming for an International Normalised Ratio (INR) of 2–3 for 6 months.

PALLIATION

- For patients with a devastating stroke and no potential for a good neurological recovery, the approach is to ensure patient comfort and avoid unnecessary investigations and interventions.
- Depending on local circumstances, a palliative care team may assist with patient management. Expert nursing care with attention to hygiene, skin, mouth and eye care, and changes of position are each important, together with adequate analgesia (e.g. sc morphine 2.5–5 mg or more as required) provided regularly (3–4 hourly).
- In the dying stroke patient, abnormal respiration patterns, noisy breathing and retained secretions may be of great concern to relatives and friends. It is important to provide adequate explanation and reassurance.

GENERAL MANAGEMENT OF ACUTE STROKE

- Observation of neurological status and vital signs allow early detection of deterioration and prompt investigation for treatable causes of worsening:
  - conscious level using the Glasgow Coma Score
  - neurological status (e.g. National Institutes of Health Stroke Scale)
  - physiological parameters (blood pressure, pulse, oxygenation, respiratory pattern, temperature, fluid status, blood sugar).
- Monitoring should be frequent early after stroke (hourly) and subsequently dictated by each individual patient's status.
- Neurological worsening is common and reported in up to 40% of cases, and may be due to stroke-related factors or systemic complications (Table 4.4).

Management of physiological parameters

Blood sugar

Hyperglycaemia is associated with a poor outcome following stroke but it is uncertain whether aggressive control of blood sugar levels improves outcome. Pragmatically, blood sugar should be monitored, any frank diabetes treated, and glucose-containing intravenous fluids avoided early after stroke.

Supplemental oxygen

Hypoxic patients should receive oxygen supplementation, but this is not otherwise routinely required.

Table 4.4 Causes of neurological worsening after stroke	
Stroke-related causes of worsening	**Systemic causes of worsening**
Progressing ischaemia	Infection: pneumonia, urinary, venous/arterial access site
Expanding haematoma	
Recurrent stroke event	Hypoxia: consider pneumonia, pulmonary embolism
Ischaemic cerebral oedema (usually 24–72 hours)	
Hydrocephalus	Metabolic derangement (e.g. hyponatraemia)
Epilepsy	Acute coronary syndromes
Haemorrhagic transformation of infarct	
Vasospasm	

Intravenous fluids

Maintenance of normovolaemia is probably beneficial. Intravenous fluids should be started early after stroke in dehydrated patients and in those likely to have inadequate oral intake.

Nutrition

Enteral feeding via a nasogastric tube should be considered for dysphagic patients during the first week after stroke, rather than later. Feeding via a percutaneous gastronomy tube should be reserved for those with contra-indications to nasogastric feeding, and may be considered in those with persisting dysphagia.

Dysphagia

- Dysphagia occurs acutely in > 50% of hospitalised stroke patients and increases the risk of aspiration, respiratory infection and poor outcome.
- It is more common after large hemispheric, brainstem or bilateral stroke, in patients with impaired consciousness and in the elderly.
- A moist or bubbly voice, weak or absent cough, abnormal tongue or palatal movement, reduced palatal sensation and poor sitting balance make dysphagia more likely.
- A simple bedside test of swallow is to observe the patient attempting to swallow small volumes of water. Coughing, gagging and the development of a wet voice suggest aspiration.
- Most patients spontaneously recover safe swallowing ability.

Management of fever

Pyrexia is associated with a poor outcome after stroke. Fever should be treated with antipyretics and the underlying cause (aspiration pneumonia, urinary tract infection, venous access site infection, deep venous thrombosis, etc.) sought and treated.

Blood pressure control

- There is little evidence to guide blood pressure management after acute stroke.
- Early blood pressure lowering should generally be avoided because this may worsen ischaemia in at-risk peri-infarct brain tissue (the penumbra).
- In patients already receiving medication, oral antihypertensive agents may be continued.
- In patients with severe persistent hypertension ($\geq$ 230/120 mmHg) or hypertension associated with acute end organ damage (e.g. left ventricular failure, aortic dissection), blood pressure lowering may be appropriate:
  - cautious reduction (perhaps by 10–20% at first) should be the aim and the patient closely monitored for neurological deterioration
  - parenteral agents are appropriate as they can be carefully titrated (but do require close haemodynamic monitoring of the patient in a high dependency unit)
  - in the absence of definitive evidence, labetolol, sodium nitroprusside and glyceryl trinitrate (GTN) are all reasonable choices (transdermal GTN patches can be easily titrated)
  - sublingual agents (e.g. calcium antagonists and angiotensin converting enzyme inhibitors) should be avoided because of their tendency to cause precipitous and unpredictable hypotension.

General nursing care

Skilled and attentive general nursing care remains a fundamental aspect of good stroke care.

Skin care

Maintenance of clean and dry skin and frequent repositioning are important to prevent pressure areas. The need for hands-on care is not obviated by the use of pressure-relieving mattresses or other devices.

Bladder care

- Bladder dysfunction occurs frequently after stroke and may be due to detrusor areflexia (resulting in acute urinary retention with overflow incontinence) or hyperreflexia (resulting in urgency and frequency ± incontinence).
- Acute urinary retention is common early after stroke and is managed initially with an indwelling catheter. Intermittent catheterisation is impractical. Factors that increase the risk of retention include benign prostatic hypertrophy, pre-existing bladder dysfunction, diabetes, bed rest, constipation and decreased consciousness.
- Stroke patients with decreased consciousness are appropriately managed with an indwelling catheter in the acute stage, with subsequent management dictated by the patient's neurological status.
- Fluid input and output should be monitored in all acute stroke patients for at least 24 hours and symptoms of bladder dysfunction (e.g. inability to void, frequency, urgency, incontinence) actively sought.
- When bladder dysfunction is suspected, ultrasound should be used to assess bladder volume non-invasively: above 500 ml should be avoided and the patient catheterised if necessary. Detrusor muscle overstretch injury may lead to long-term, disabling bladder dysfunction.
- Bladder training and anticholinergic medications (e.g. oxybutynin) may be useful for detrusor hyperreflexia once urinary retention has been excluded (see Chapter 17).

Bowel care

- Constipation is common following stroke: predisposing factors include pre-existing constipation, inactivity, poor oral intake and medications.
- Adequate hydration should be ensured.
- Osmotic agents (e.g. sorbitol) are the most appropriate laxatives.
- Severe constipation should be treated vigorously along the usual lines (see Chapter 17).

Mouth and eye care

Regular mouth and dental care is important for patient comfort. In the unconscious patient and in patients with lower motor neuron facial weakness, the eyes must be protected from injury.

COMPLICATIONS OF ACUTE STROKE

Medical complications occur in more than 50% of hospitalised stroke patients and are associated with poor outcome and increased length of hospital stay. The most frequent complications are falls, chest and urinary tract infections, and pressure sores (see General management of acute stroke, p. 103).

Pneumonia

- Chest infections occur in up to one-third of patients and are associated with a two-fold increased risk of hospital death and poorer long-term outcome.
- Risk factors include mechanical ventilation, stroke involving the vertebrobasilar territory or multiple vascular territories, dysphagia and abnormal admission chest X-ray.
- Prohibition of oral intake in dysphagic patients and enteral feeding (via nasogastric or percutaneous gastrostomy tube) reduces, but does not abolish, the risk of aspiration.
- Early mobilisation and maintenance of a semi-upright or upright posture may reduce the risk of pneumonia, but there are no data to prove the effectiveness of these strategies.
- Antibiotic treatment for stroke-related pneumonia is selected on the assumption that aspiration has occurred and should include an agent active against anaerobic infection (e.g. benzyl penicillin + metronidazole). Broader antibiotic cover is necessary for patients with pneumonia receiving mechanical ventilation, or otherwise managed on an intensive care unit.

Deep venous thrombosis and pulmonary embolism

- Deep venous thrombosis (DVT) occurs in 4–75% of stroke patients not receiving prophylactic treatment, depending on the population studied but more on how the diagnosis is made.
- Pulmonary embolism (PE) occurs much less commonly, with reported frequencies ranging from 1% to 6%.
- Low-dose aspirin (75–150 mg/day), full-length graduated compression stockings and anticoagulation are all effective prevention strategies in non-stroke populations.
- Anticoagulation with unfractionated or low-molecular-weight heparin is effective in preventing DVT and PE in stroke patients, but this is at the expense of an increased risk of cerebral haemorrhage.
- It is best to use graduated compression stockings in all bed-bound and paretic patients and to reserve anticoagulation (typically unfractionated heparin 5000 units sc bd) for patients considered to be at particularly high risk (e.g. those with a personal or family history of venous thrombosis, those with dense lower limb paresis).

Falls

- Physical and cognitive deficits after stroke increase the risk of falls; checklists may be helpful in identifying those most at risk.
- Environmental modifications reduce fall risk (e.g. non-slip floor surfaces) and the risk of serious fall-related injury (e.g. soft floor surfaces).
- A home hazard assessment and home modifications (e.g. adequate lighting, non-slip surfaces, hand rails) may improve safety.

Spasticity

- Spasticity is common after stroke.
- Muscle shortening promotes and exacerbates spasticity and so postures that encourage this should be avoided.
- Prolonged positioning of muscles in a lengthened position may assist to maintain a full range of motion (e.g. positioning the ankle in a dorsiflexed posture maintains calf muscle length).
- As post-stroke spasticity is a focal phenomenon, systemic medications such as benzodiazepines and baclofen have virtually no role (see Chapter 9).
- Botulinum toxin injections into spastic muscles in combination with physical therapy is the most effective treatment. Botulinum toxin reduces the development of contracture and so improves the ease of caring for people with stroke via improved hygiene, dressing and comfortable positioning of the limb.
- Other effective interventions include dynamic splinting, vibration, stretch and biofeedback. Intrathecal baclofen may also be very effective in selected patients with severe spasticity.

Seizures and post-stroke epilepsy

- Epileptic seizures occur in about 10% of stroke patients.
- Cortical and haemorrhagic stroke are associated with increased risk for seizures, as is severe stroke.
- Seizures are effectively managed with standard medications (see Chapter 2).

Mood disorder

- Post-stroke depression and anxiety (including agoraphobia) are very common.
- Depression is associated with a poor outcome and an increased risk of death.

- Antidepressants and behavioural therapy are effective treatments (see Chapter 13).
- It is often difficult to diagnose post-stroke depression, particularly in patients with dysphasia or cognitive impairment. Therefore, it is reasonable to give a trial of antidepressants when depression is suspected (e.g. change in appetite and social interaction, unexplained late neurological worsening or slowing of improvement).

Shoulder pain

- Shoulder pain is common in hemiplegic stroke patients. There are many contributing causes and each patient requires individual assessment.
- Rotator cuff injury is present in about 50% and may be due to injury around the time of stroke, or be pre-existing. Skilled manual handling is essential to avoid shoulder trauma.
- Subluxation of the shoulder is associated with shoulder pain. Strategies to prevent or stabilise subluxation (e.g. lap trays) are generally used, although there is little evidence for their effectiveness.
- Overhead pulley exercise should not be used as this has been shown to increase shoulder pain.

Deconditioning and fatigue

Deconditioning, poor fitness and fatigue are common problems for stroke survivors and contribute to long-term disability and handicap. Prolonged bed rest should be avoided and patients should be mobilised as soon as possible after stroke.

Carer burden

Care of disabled stroke survivors is a burdensome task and carers may develop anxiety and depression. Education and training in the care of the disabled stroke patient may reduce carer burden. Practical support (e.g. home care, community nursing, respite services) are of undoubted benefit.

REHABILITATION

- Stroke rehabilitation (provided as an organised inpatient, outpatient or home-based programme) improves outcome.
- The number-needed-to-treat with a period of inpatient rehabilitation started in the subacute period after stroke to ensure that one extra patient returns home is about 20.

- The appropriate rehabilitation programme for a given individual depends on numerous factors, including: local service availability, stroke severity and disability, patient and carer preference, availability of family support, transport and cultural issues.
- It remains uncertain which components of rehabilitation are the most important in producing good outcomes and how these should be best applied to individual patients.
- No particular philosophical approach to physical therapy has been shown to be more effective than any other, although there is evidence that a functional, goal-directed approach is effective (e.g. if independent walking is the goal, walking is the activity to practise).
- Patients experiencing difficulty with activities of daily living (ADL) benefit from interventions specifically targeting ADL.
- High-quality evidence for the efficacy of aphasia therapy remains limited.
- Disabled patients may require specialised assessment of their ability to drive.
- The usual approach to work is to return part-time with a gradual increase in hours and duties under the supervision of the treating physician.
- The cost of rehabilitation is about one-third the total lifetime costs of stroke.

SECONDARY PREVENTION
Risk factors for stroke

The risk factors for stroke are similar to those for other vascular diseases, with the exception of atrial fibrillation and carotid artery stenosis (Table 4.5). Identification of modifiable and causative risk factors is important for secondary prevention of stroke, and the prevention of stroke after TIA.

Secondary prevention interventions (Table 4.6)
Antiplatelet drugs (Fig. 4.3)

- The antiplatelet drugs effective in secondary prevention are aspirin alone, clopidogrel, and aspirin with modified-release dipyridamole, all of which achieve about a one-fifth odds reduction in the risk of stroke/myocardial infarction/vascular death in patients with prior stroke or TIA.
- Low-dose aspirin (75–150 mg/day) is as effective as high-dose aspirin, and has less gastrointestinal adverse effects, including bleeding. Up to 10% of patients do not tolerate aspirin because of gastrointestinal adverse effects (indigestion, nausea, constipation).

Table 4.5	Risk factors for stroke
Non-modifiable	**Modifiable**
Age	Hypertension
Gender	Smoking
Genetic factors	Atrial fibrillation
Ethnicity	Diabetes
	Heavy alcohol intake
	Carotid artery stenosis
	Obesity
	Heart disease
	Hypercholesterolaemia
	Lack of exercise

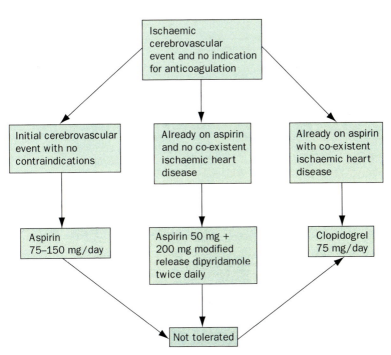

Fig. 4.3 Suggested algorithm for long-term antiplatelet treatment.

- Aspirin (50 mg bd) plus modified-release dipyridamole (200 mg bd) may be more effective than aspirin alone in preventing recurrent stroke, but not myocardial infarction. Up to 20% of patients do not tolerate this combination because of severe headache or gastrointestinal symptoms.
- Clopidogrel (75 mg/day) is as effective as, and may even be slightly more effective than aspirin when used for the secondary prevention of vascular events in high-risk patients. It is better tolerated than aspirin, with a lower risk of indigestion but higher risk of diarrhoea, and it is significantly more expensive.

Table 4.6	Effective prevention strategies for stroke patients	
Approach	Eligibility	Treatment options
Blood pressure lowering	'Hypertensive' and 'normotensive' patients	Perindopril ± indapamide
	Ischaemic and haemorrhagic stroke, TIA	Ramipril Low salt diet
Antiplatelet drugs	Ischaemic stroke, TIA	Aspirin, clopidogrel, aspirin + dipyridamole
Warfarin	Ischaemic stroke or TIA + atrial fibrillation or other high risk cardiac source of embolism	Warfarin (or aspirin if warfarin contraindicated)
Carotid revascularisation	Ischaemic stroke or TIA + moderate to high grade ipsilateral carotid stenosis	Carotid endarterectomy ? Carotid angioplasty
Cholesterol lowering	Stroke patients with prior ischaemic heart disease, and perhaps even those without	Statins Diet
Smoking	All smokers	Cease
Diabetes	All diabetics	Tight control with diet ± medication
Obesity	Overweight	Diet
Inactivity	All patients	Regular exercise

- There is currently no evidence supporting the combination of aspirin plus clopidogrel in the secondary prevention of stroke.
- Patients who have had gastrointestinal bleeding while taking aspirin can be as safely managed (after ulcer healing) with a combination of aspirin with a proton pump inhibitor as with changing to clopidogrel.

Anticoagulation

The risk of embolism in patients with non-valvular atrial fibrillation and the suggested management is shown in Table 4.7.

- All ischaemic stroke survivors and TIA patients in atrial fibrillation should ideally be anticoagulated with warfarin.
- However, there are often contraindications (falls, cognitive problems, etc.), in which case aspirin still provides some risk reduction.
- Patients with paroxysmal atrial fibrillation have a similar risk of recurrent stroke as those with chronic atrial fibrillation and should be anticoagulated.
- In most patients, warfarin should be continued indefinitely, irrespective of whether or not antiarrhythmic drugs are used in an attempt to maintain sinus rhythm.
- In patients with a stroke occurring in the setting of recent myocardial infarction and left ventricular mural thrombus, anticoagulation is usually maintained for 3–6 months before reverting to aspirin.

Table 4.7   Antithrombotic treatment for patients in atrial fibrillation

Stratification of risk based on level of accompanying risk factor	Stroke risk (% per year)	Recommended therapy
Any high-risk factor* or more than 1 moderate risk factor	6–12	Warfarin, INR 2.0–3.0
One moderate risk factor†	2–5	Warfarin, INR 2.0–3.0; or aspirin 75–325 mg/day
No risk factors	≤ 1	Aspirin 75–325 mg/day

*High-risk factors are previous stroke or TIA, hypertension on treatment, reduced left ventricular function, age > 75 years, mitral stenosis, prosthetic heart valve.
†Moderate risk factors are age 65–75 years, diabetes, coronary heart disease.
INR, International Normalised Ratio.

- Acute ischaemic stroke patients with a mechanical heart valve and atrial fibrillation should receive aspirin 100 mg/day plus warfarin (INR 3.0–4.5).
- There is some evidence that direct thrombin inhibitors may be an effective alternative to warfarin. Monitoring of INR is unnecessary. However, there are concerns about hepatotoxicity.

Blood pressure lowering

- Clinical trials have shown that treatment of patients with TIA or stroke using perindopril 4 mg plus indapamide 2.5 mg or ramipril 10 mg/day reduces the incidence of stroke, myocardial infarction and vascular death by about one-quarter, irrespective of the baseline blood pressure down to about 130/70 mmHg.
- Other antihypertensive regimens are probably as beneficial for the same reduction in blood pressure.
- Not all stroke patients tolerate these medication regimens because of symptomatic hypotension, in which case reduce the dosage until better tolerated or try alternative drug regimens.
- When to initiate blood pressure lowering is an important consideration. In 'normotensive' patients it is generally best to wait until there are signs of substantial recovery in perhaps a week or two. In 'hypertensive' cases, treatment can be started sooner. In both instances, gentle titration is recommended.

Carotid endarterectomy

- Patients with a carotid territory TIA or non-disabling stroke that are found to have ipsilateral carotid artery stenosis should be considered for carotid endarterectomy.
- There is a gradient of increasing benefit with increasing stenosis (except for post-stenotic collapse, critical stenosis and trickle flow, where there is little reduction in stroke risk although TIAs are reduced).
- Most patients with ≥ 70% stenosis are appropriately treated with surgery.
- Patients with 50–69% stenosis may also be considered if there is plaque ulceration and no satisfactory alternative cause for the stroke.
- Catheter angiography remains the gold standard for defining degree of stenosis but is associated with about 0.5% risk of stroke, myocardial infarction or death. Duplex sonography, CT angiography or MRA are acceptable alternatives provided there is good quality control.
- Surgery should only be performed in centres where surgeons have demonstrated expertise in performing the operation skilfully and with an acceptably low complication rate.

- The risk of stroke recurrence is maximal in the first few weeks after a stroke/TIA, and so the earlier surgery is done the better, except in neurologically unstable patients where the risk of surgery is excessive.
- Carotid angioplasty and stenting, incorporating distal neuroprotection, may prove to be a safe and effective alternative to carotid surgery, and trials are in progress.
- Carotid endarterectomy has a role in selected patients with asymptomatic carotid disease, particularly in younger age groups. The role of carotid angioplasty and stenting is uncertain at present.

Cholesterol lowering

- Several trials have shown that statins in patients with angina and myocardial infarction lower the risk of stroke.
- There is currently only indirect evidence that statins in patients with TIA or stroke reduce their risk of stroke.
- However, *coronary events* are reduced by statins in stroke survivors.

It is reasonable to prescribe a statin (e.g. simvastatin 40 mg/day oral) to all stroke/TIA survivors if only to prevent myocardial infarction. Myopathy and abnormal liver function are uncommon, but important, adverse effects.

Diabetic control

- Diabetes is a potent risk factor for ischaemic stroke.
- Although there is no direct evidence that good glycaemic control reduces the risk of subsequent stroke, microvascular and non-vascular complications are reduced.

FOLLOW-UP

- Stroke patients and carers find the early post-discharge period difficult and report dissatisfaction with post-discharge services and the information they have received about stroke.
- Early outpatient follow-up is helpful to provide additional information about stroke and to fine tune secondary prevention strategies.
- Ongoing regular review of disabled survivors allows assessment and management of any emerging problems (e.g. spasticity, mood disorder).
- Functional decline is common long-term after stroke. This may be prevented or improved with a period of 'top-up' rehabilitation.
- 10–20% of stroke survivors require long-term residential care. The decision to place a stroke survivor in residential care is often traumatic

for both the survivor and his or her family, and these individuals require emotional support.

■ Providing long-term care to a disabled stroke survivor is a burdensome task. Respite services (either provided in the community or as residential care) are commended by carers and vital in allowing families to continue to care for disabled stroke survivors long-term in the community.

Further reading

Donnan G, Norrving B, Bamford J, Bogousslavsky J. Subcortical stroke, 2nd edn. Oxford University Press, Oxford, 2002.

Hankey GJ. Stroke – your questions answered. Churchill Livingstone, Edinburgh, 2002.

Warlow CP, Dennis MS, van Gijn J, Hankey GJ, Sandercock PAG, Bamford JM, Wardlaw JM. Stroke. A practical guide to management, 2nd edn. Blackwell Science, Oxford, 2001.

5   DEMENTIA

David Neary

DEFINITION AND CLASSIFICATION

Dementia is a generic term referring to various specific neuropsychological syndromes which themselves are determined by the topographical distribution of the pathology in specific cerebral diseases (encephalopathies).

These encephalopathies can be classified as:
- Cortical encephalopathies:
  - Alzheimer's disease
  - frontotemporal dementia.
- Subcortical encephalopathies:
  - subcortical ischaemic vascular dementia
  - Huntington's disease
  - normal pressure hydrocephalus.
- Corticosubcortical dementias:
  - dementia with Lewy bodies
  - corticobasal degeneration.
- Multifocal encephalopathy:
  - Creutzfeld–Jakob disease (CJD).

NEUROPSYCHOLOGICAL SYNDROMES

Cortical dementia

In Alzheimer's disease involvement of the posterior neocortex and limbic

social gatherings, crowds, prolonged travel, unfamiliar holidays and hotels, and exposure to strangers
- avoid unnecessary admissions to hospital, general anaesthetics and unnecessary minor surgical procedures
- withdraw or limit drugs with sedative effects (e.g. opiates, hypnotics, antidepressants, antiepileptic drugs)
- advice on sleep hygiene with fixed nocturnal sleeping routines and afternoon naps; use of a bedside lamp to prevent nocturnal confusion.
- Drug treatment of confusion:
  - avoid routine neuroleptics, especially in dementia with Lewy bodies, to reduce the risk of neuroleptic malignant syndrome
  - use atypical antipsychotics (risperidone, quetiapine, olanzapine, clozapine)
  - anticholinesterase inhibitors (donepezil, rivastigmine, galantamine; see below) can be used in the confusional state of dementia with Lewy bodies.

Symptoms of language impairment

Aphasia leads to impairment of expression, word finding, comprehension, reading, writing and calculation. This is highly characteristic of Alzheimer's disease and can be the presenting symptom.
- Treatment:
  - referral to speech and language therapist for analysis of aphasia, therapy and psychological support.

Symptoms of visuospatial impairment

Visuospatial disorder causes inability to recognise and locate objects, to locate unfamiliar and familiar surroundings, and to dress and carry out complex activities such as cooking. These problems are also highly characteristic of Alzheimer's disease.
- Management:
  - exclude primary ocular problems such as cataract and glaucoma
  - advise that the patient's symptoms are due to failure of the complex 'camera work' of the brain and not to an abnormality of the lens of the eye and so spectacles cannot help
  - advise simplification of the layout of the home, preferably with 'open-plan'
  - ensure the patient is not endangered in the kitchen because of visual disturbance or loss of sense of smell (common in Alzheimer's disease and frontotemporal dementia).

Symptoms of disorders of praxis

Apraxia leads to loss of skilled movements of the arms and hands, and in walking. It is common in Alzheimer's disease and corticobasal degeneration.

■ Management:
- exclude orthopaedic disorders (e.g. osteoarthritis of the hips or knees)
- refer to occupational therapy for appropriate aids in the home to help manual performance and mobility, and diminish the danger of falls
- there are no drug treatments for apraxia.

Symptoms of memory disorder

Amnesia leads to forgetfulness, particularly of recent events, inability to name individuals and recognise familiar places, loss of belongings and the patient's whereabouts. Severe amnesia is characteristic of Alzheimer's disease.

■ Management:
- maintain strict and familiar daily routines
- advise the use of written memos on boards, calendars and a diary, or of sound cues on a mobile phone
- carry a mobile phone when out of doors alone
- advise carers not to respond angrily to the patient's often repetitive questions in order to avoid causing irritability and aggression, as well as loss of confidence and depression.

Symptoms of failure of executive functions

Dysexecutive syndrome leads to cognitive failures in judgement, planning, insight and the organisation of social and occupational life in addition to affective and behavioural disorders. These problems are characteristic of frontotemporal dementia and occur only in the late stages of Alzheimer's disease and subcortical ischaemic vascular dementia.

■ Management:
- advise carers to resolve any legal issues as soon as possible (e.g. power of attorney, testamentary capacity)
- the altered personality and behaviour of the patient must be explained to carers and their children in scientific and non-moralistic terms; this will reduce the considerable stressful load on carers which can lead to family breakdown and mental illness in the carers
- encourage carers to be frank about the diagnosis to other family members and friends, since the behavioural disorder with disinhibition and overactivity can lead to social embarrassment and criminal offences if not understood

- the apathy and lack of motivation in frontotemporal dementia and subcortical ischaemic vascular dementia can be misinterpreted as depression refractory to drug treatment
- on the other hand, depression in Alzheimer's disease may lead to apathy and the magnification of cognitive symptoms, but these can respond to antidepressants
- depression (see Chapter 13) should be treated with selective serotonin reuptake inhibitors (SSRIs); tricyclic antidepressants should be avoided since they can lead to confusion
- stereotypic behaviours with repetitive movements, gestures, hoarding, wandering and clock-watching characterise frontotemporal dementia; some patients respond to SSRIs
- overeating, food fads, gluttony and hyperoral behaviour require control of the food supply by carers and advice from dieticians
- the stereotypic wandering and pacing behaviour of frontotemporal dementia can be harnessed into therapeutic routines (e.g. housework, accompanied walks).

Wandering in Alzheimer's disease is secondary to the confusional state and usually requires drug therapy (see atypical antipsychotics, above). However, admission to hospital is necessary for permanent care.

MANAGEMENT OF SPECIFIC DISEASES CAUSING DEMENTIA

Alzheimer's disease

In Alzheimer's disease there is a deficiency of acetylcholine synthesis in the brain.

- Anticholinesterase inhibitors are recommended for moderate to mild disease – Mini-Mental State Examination (MMSE) 12–24/30:
  - donepezil (Aricept) 5 mg/day oral at bedtime, increasing to 10 mg
  - rivastigmine (Exelon) 1.5 mg oral bd, increasing gradually if necessary to 3 mg bd
  - galantamine (Reminyl) 4 mg oral bd increasing gradually to 12 mg/day in 2 divided doses if tolerated.
- Because of the cholinergic effects the patient must be screened for cardiac dysrhythmia with electrocardiography (ECG) before starting treatment. Cardiac disorder is a contraindication to treatment.
- The adverse effects are the predictable gastrointestinal consequences of excess cholinergic activity (e.g. nausea, colic, diarrhoea).

- Memantine (Ebixa), a glutamate antagonist, has been developed for moderately severe to severe Alzheimer's disease (MMSE 5–14/30). This drug has not yet been approved by the National Institute for Health and Clinical Excellence (NICE) in the UK.

In Alzheimer's disease there is also abnormal deposition of amyloid (Aβ) material in the brain and cerebral blood vessels. However, immunisation against Aβ failed because of the development of aseptic meningo-encephalitis, but oligonucleotide therapeutics are being developed to prevent amyloid deposition.

Frontotemporal dementia

This is a clinical syndrome arising from frontotemporal lobar degeneration. Some familial cases are due to a mutation of the tau gene on chromosome 17.
- There is no specific drug therapy for this disorder.
- The stereotypical behaviours characteristic of the condition can sometimes be modified by SSRIs.

Subcortical ischaemic vascular dementia

Disease of the small penetrating arteries supplying the subcortical white matter causes lacunar infarcts and diffuse ischaemic degeneration of the white matter, leading to a subcortical dementia that is insidious and progressive, and not necessarily related to obvious stroke-like events.
- Prevention, by reducing the levels of vascular risk factors (see Chapter 4):
  - hypertension
  - diabetes mellitus
  - atrial fibrillation
  - hypercholesterolaemia
  - smoking.
- Some trials of the following drugs have suggested improvement, but await confirmation: aspirin, galantamine, rivastigmine, donepezil, memantine and nimodipine.

Huntington's disease

This is an autosomal-dominant inherited disease due to a CAG repeat genetic mutation on chromosome 4. Chorea and dystonia occur along with subcortical dementia with a dysexecutive syndrome, robbing the patient of insight.
- Management: see Chapter 6.

Dementia with Lewy bodies

This leads to parkinsonism with akinesia, resting tremor and a fluctuating confusional state with visual hallucinations and secondary delusions.

■ Management:
 – treatment of the parkinsonism requires very low doses of levodopa to avoid mental confusion and may be of some help (see Chapter 6)
 – conventional neuroleptics should not be used in the treatment of the confusional state because of the high risk of the neuroleptic malignant syndrome, which can be fatal
 – anticholinesterase inhibitors are successful in treating the confusional state, but are not licensed in Europe as yet
 – atypical antipsychotic agents (e.g. quetiapine, olanzapine, risperidone, clozapine) can help the confusion
 – future treatments are aimed at altering the metabolism of synuclein, which constitutes the Lewy body and contributes to neuronal cell death.

Corticobasal degeneration

This leads to highly asymmetrical akinesia, rigidity and dyskinesia of one upper limb with profound apraxia of the arm together with the alien limb phenomenon. The disorder spreads eventually to the other limbs and to buccofacial apraxia.

■ Management:
 – antiparkinsonian medication is usually ineffective but it is worthwhile trying selegeline and amantidine, and later small doses of levodopa (see Chapter 6)
 – referral to speech and language therapy, physiotherapy and occupational therapy.

Creutzfeld–Jakob disease

CJD can be sporadic, familial, iatrogenic and, in the new variant, secondary to ingestion of prion material in infected meat. Neurological symptoms and signs and psychological failure develop rapidly and the disorder is usually fatal within 6 months to 2 years. No effective treatments for CJD have been confirmed, although claims have been made for various interventions such as oral quinacrine and intraventricular pentosan polysulphate.

MILD COGNITIVE IMPAIRMENT

Mild cognitive impairment in the elderly is an active research area in old-age psychiatry aimed at differentiating the impaired cognition, chiefly of memory, of 'normal ageing', from the earliest stages of Alzheimer's disease and subcortical ischaemic vascular dementia. The neurologist is not usually faced with this dilemma, since the very elderly are less likely to be referred to a neurological diagnostic clinic. However, it is best for the neurologist to suspect that the earliest forms of Alzheimer's disease and subcortical ischaemic vascular dementia must exist, and to be sceptical of the notion of normal ageing. Magnetic resonance imaging (MRI) evidence of cerebral and hippocampal atrophy, or widespread evidence of white matter disease in individuals with vascular risk factors, suggest the earliest stages of Alzheimer's disease or subcortical ischaemic vascular dementia, respectively.

The neurologist in the general outpatient clinic as well as the diagnostic dementia centre is more likely to be referred young individuals complaining of poor memory. These 'well but worried' individuals are a common and stressful problem, particularly for junior neurologists.

- Usually they are youthful without vascular risk factors.
- There may be an obscure and distant family history of dementia which has concerned them.
- They have often learned and developed fears about dementia from newspapers and the media.
- They arrive at the clinic punctually, smartly dressed and usually unaccompanied.
- They give a comprehensive and highly detailed account of their memory problems and often describe embarrassing slips of memory which have caused them, but not others, concern.
- Their memory problems are usually relatively unapparent to family members, colleagues and employers.
- Their occupational performance may not have declined and they may even have succeeded financially.
- The neurological examination is normal.
- On careful questioning a history is discovered of domestic, social and occupational stress, insomnia, anxiety and depression, recurrent headaches and other pain problems, and the ingestion of large quantities of analgesics and sedatives, and excessive quantities of alcohol to reduce anxiety, stress and insomnia.

Management

- Full and frank explanation of the way in which concentration is reduced by such a lifestyle leading to secondary and inevitable problems in memory, together with reassurance, can often successfully resolve the consultation.

- A fulsome description of the severe symptoms of Alzheimer's disease in which there is diminished insight, in contrast to the well worried's complaints and self-assurance, reinforces prognostic optimism.
- For the obsessional individual a normal computed tomography (CT) brain scan result, reported directly and shown to the patient, can be eminently therapeutic.
- The offer of an opportunity for review in a further year, should symptoms persist or worsen, expressed in a highly confident manner, is usually well-received, but not subsequently taken up.
- This offer is important because a minority of these individuals will have something to worry about and may subsequently present with an early form of dementia, usually Alzheimer's disease.

Further reading

Baldwin R, Murray M. Services for younger people with dementia. In: Dementia (O'Brien J, Ames D, Burns A, eds), 2nd edn. Arnold, London, 2000, pp. 253–259.

Brown M, Godber C, Wilkinson D. Services for dementia: a British view. In: Dementia (O'Brien J, Ames D, Burns A, eds), 2nd edn. Arnold, London, 2000, pp. 291–297.

deCarli C. Mild Cognitive Impairment: procedure, prognosis, aetiology and treatment. Lancet, Neurology 2003; 2: 15–21.

deLeeuw F-E, van Gijn J. Vascular dementia. Practical Neurol 2003; 3: 86–91.

McKeith I, Mintzer J, Harsland D, et al. Dementia with Lewy bodies. Lancet, Neurology 2004; 3: 19–28.

Neary D, Snowden JS. Sorting out the dementias. Practical Neurol 2002; 2: 328–339.

O'Brien JT, Erkinjunti T, Reisberg B, et al. Vascular cognitive impairment. Lancet, Neurology 2003; ii: 89–98.

Rockwood K. Size and treatment effect on cognition of cholinesterase inhibition in Alzheimer's disease. J Neurol Neurosurg Psychiatry 2004; 75: 677–685.

Roman GC, Erkinjunti T, Wallin A, et al. Subcortical ischaemic vascular dementia. Lancet, Neurology 2002; i: 426–436.

Silverberg GD, Mayo M, Saul T, et al. Alzheimer's disease, normal pressure hydrocephalus and senescent changes in CSF circulatory physiology: a hypothesis. Lancet, Neurology 2003; ii: 506–511.

Simpson SA. The management of Huntington's disease. Practical Neurol 2004; 1: 204–211.

6 PARKINSON'S DISEASE AND OTHER MOVEMENT DISORDERS

Victor S. C. Fung and John Morris

Chapter contents

To manage a patient with a movement disorder it is necessary to:

- Classify the clinical phenomena: is it mainly a hypokinetic (e.g. akinesia, rigidity) or hyperkinetic (e.g. tremor, chorea, dystonia, myoclonus) movement disorder? Note: several different abnormal movements may occur in the same patient.
- Formulate a syndromal diagnosis, taking into account other neurological (e.g. pyramidal, cerebellar, cognitive) and non-neurological (e.g. ocular abnormalities, organomegaly) features, age of onset, temporal course of the disease and family history (e.g. sporadic, late-onset, slowly progressive, akinetic/rigid syndrome with rest tremor = a parkinsonian syndrome).
- Generate an aetiological differential diagnosis based on the syndromal diagnosis.

Treatment involves not only appropriate drug therapy, but also counselling, allied health intervention and, commonly, management of cognitive and psychiatric comorbidity.

PARKINSONISM

- Parkinsonism is a syndrome characterised by the triad of tremor, rigidity and bradykinesia.

- In terms of management, patients can be divided into two groups: those with Parkinson's disease (who respond well to levodopa) and those with atypical parkinsonism (who do not).
- In Parkinson's disease, there is loss of dopaminergic substantia nigra neurons, but preservation of striatal neurons.
- In atypical parkinsonian syndromes, there is loss of striatal neurons in addition to nigral neurons.
- The relative involvement of each region in individual patients and diseases determines the degree of dopa responsiveness.

PARKINSON'S DISEASE
Epidemiology

- Parkinson's disease affects over 1% of all people > 50 years old.
- 5–10% of patients with Parkinson's disease present at age < 40 years.
- There is a similar incidence in males and females.
- All ethnic groups are equally affected.

Diagnosis

The diagnosis is clinical. Investigations are required only if there is doubt about the diagnosis. Magnetic resonance imaging (MRI) is more sensitive than computed tomography (CT), for example in detecting infarcts or focal gliosis or atrophy (as occurs, for example, in the putamen in multiple system atrophy). In patients < 50 years old, serum copper and caeruloplasmin levels (Wilson's disease) and HIV serology should be checked.

The way that patients are given their diagnosis can have a lasting influence on their attitude to their illness and subsequent quality of life. It is useful to point out that:

- Parkinson's disease progresses slowly over many years, in younger patients over decades.
- Although there is no cure, there is very effective and long-lasting treatment to control the symptoms.
- Because the disease advances slowly, there will be time to make any necessary adjustments to the illness.
- Progression is very variable, and many patients retain normal or near-normal function for many years.

Younger patients often have great difficulty in coming to terms with the diagnosis; there is little point in prescribing drugs until the patient has accepted the diagnosis and wants treatment.

Genetic causes

- Parkinson's disease is usually sporadic.
- There are rare families with autosomal-dominant or autosomal-recessive patterns of inheritance, but genetic testing is not widely available.
- More than half of juvenile-onset patients (< 20 years) have a recessively inherited defect in the Parkin gene. They can be remarkably responsive to small doses of levodopa. Dystonia may be prominent, leading to the misdiagnosis of dopa-responsive dystonia.

Medical management

- The aim of initial treatment is to reduce motor disability while minimising the risk of medium- to long-term complications of therapy.
- No treatment has been shown to slow disease progression.
- Conversely, no drug (including levodopa) has been shown to worsen disease progression. This is important to emphasise because many patients have concerns about potential drug toxicity based on theoretical and laboratory data obtained from the internet and other sources.

Management can be divided into three stages:
- early stage of good symptom control
- mid-stage, when the 'honeymoon' ends and problems such as motor fluctuations and dyskinesias appear
- late-stage, when problems resistant to levodopa such as falls and dementia emerge.

The available drugs, their doses, mechanisms of action and adverse effects are summarised in Table 6.1. Some important points include:
- As with any drug, a balance must be struck between achieving maximal improvement and minimal adverse effects.
- When first started, levodopa is best given with food to reduce nausea. It is absorbed from the small intestine but not the stomach. Later in the disease when reliable rapid absorption becomes more important, it is best taken on an empty stomach.
- Dietary amino acids from protein metabolism compete with levodopa for entry into the bloodstream and also into the brain, so avoiding heavy protein meals may improve the therapeutic effect.
- Slow titration (over weeks or months) upwards of all dopaminergic drugs minimises dose-limiting nausea and dizziness.
- Domperidone 10–20 mg oral tds is a peripherally acting dopamine antagonist that can reduce drug-induced nausea. It does not cross the blood–brain barrier, although in high doses it can cause central

Table 6.1   Drugs used in the management of Parkinson's disease

Class of drug	Generic name	Introductory dose	Common maintenance dose	Mechanism of action	When to use	Adverse effects: common or serious/ potentially life-threatening*
Levodopa	Levodopa/ benseraside	100/25 mg 0.5–1 tablet tds	Dopa 100–200 mg tds	Converted in brain to dopamine	To reverse motor symptoms in early or late disease	Nausea/vomiting; postural hypotension; insomnia; hallucinations; dyskinesias (together these are referred to as dopaminergic adverse effects)
	Levodopa/ carbidopa	100/25 mg 0.5–1 tablet tds	Dopa 100–200 mg tds			
Ergot-derived dopamine agonists	Bromocriptine	2.5 mg/day	5 mg tds	Ergot alkaloids, which stimulate dopamine receptors	When used in early Parkinson's disease to delay need for levodopa, may delay or reduce likelihood of developing dopa-induced	Dopaminergic adverse effects (more likely to provoke hallucinations, confusion and psychosis than levodopa); peripheral oedema. These are ergot alkaloids. Contraindicated in patients
	Cabergoline	0.5 mg/day	2–6 mg/day			
	Pergolide	0.125 mg/day or qds	0.5–1 mg tds			

dyskinesias.
Ameliorates
motor
fluctuations in
later disease

with unstable coronary
heart disease or
peripheral vascular
disease, pulmonary
fibrosis or evidence of
pulmonary asbestosis
because of vasospastic
and fibrotic properties.
**Up to 3% of patients
develop pulmonary
or, less commonly,
retroperitoneal
fibrosis. Around 33%
of patients on
pergolide develop
cardiac valvular
fibrosis.**
Check chest X-ray,
ESR, ECG and renal
function; regular
symptomatic review
and cardiac and
pulmonary auscultation
should be performed
in all patients

Continued

Table 6.1 *Continued*

Class of drug	Generic name	Introductory dose	Common maintenance dose	Mechanism of action	When to use	Adverse effects: common or serious/ potentially life-threatening*
Non-ergot-derived dopamine agonists	Pramipexole	0.125 mg tds	0.5–1.5 mg tds	Non-ergot alkaloids which stimulate dopamine receptors	When used in early Parkinson's disease to delay need for levodopa, may delay or reduce likelihood of developing dopa-induced dyskinesias. Ameliorates motor fluctuations in later disease	Dopaminergic adverse effects (more likely to provoke hallucinations, confusion and psychosis than levodopa); peripheral oedema. **Excessive drowsiness more common than with levodopa or ergot agonists; can cause sudden onset of sleep ('sleep attacks') without warning; patients should be warned about potential to occur when driving.** Not known to have fibrotic complications
	Ropinirole	0.25 mg tds	3–7 mg tds			

Apomorphine	2.0 mg sc	2–8 mg 1–10 times daily	Stimulates dopamine receptors	Ameliorates sudden motor fluctuations in later disease. Must be given subcutaneously, effect emerges within 5–10 minutes and lasts ~60 minutes	Patients must be pretreated for 3 days with domperidone and then continue in short to medium term to prevent severe vomiting and hypotension; injection-site pain, erythema and nodule formation
Catechol-O-methyltransferase (COMT) inhibitors	Entacapone	200 mg with each dose of levodopa	Maximum 2000 mg/day	Inhibits COMT, an enzyme involved in the breakdown of levodopa to inactive metabolites in gut and blood	Ameliorates motor fluctuations. Must be taken at same time as levodopa, has short half-life so effect lasts only for that dose	Enhanced dopaminergic adverse effects (can be managed by reducing levodopa intake); urine discoloration (harmless); diarrhoea

Continued

Table 6.1 *Continued*

Class of drug	Generic name	Introductory dose	Common maintenance dose	Mechanism of action	When to use	Adverse effects: common or serious/ potentially life-threatening*
COMT inhibitors *(continued)*	Tolcapone (restricted use, available only in some countries)	100 mg tds	100–200 mg tds	Inhibits COMT, an enzyme involved in the breakdown of levodopa to inactive metabolites in gut and blood	Ameliorates motor fluctuations. Has longer half-life than entacapone, therefore taken 2 or 3 times daily	As above; **very rare reports of severe or fatal hepatic failure (patients must have fortnightly measurement of liver function during first 4 months of treatment, monthly thereafter)**
NMDA antagonist	Amantadine	100 mg/day	100 mg morning or midday, or tds	Multiple actions, not well understood	To suppress dyskinesias, also has minor beneficial effect on reversing motor symptoms	Livedo reticularis (common, harmless); nightmares, hallucinations and confusion, anticholinergic adverse effects (see below)
Monoamine oxidase B inhibitors	Selegiline	5 mg/day	5 mg morning and midday	Selective inhibitor of MAO-B, an	Ameliorates motor fluctuations (modest	Nightmares, hallucinations and confusion, worsening

				enzyme involved in the break-down of levodopa and dopamine to inactive metabolites in brain	effect), also has minor beneficial effect on reversing motor symptoms	of dyskinesias, potential for cheese effect or serotonin syndrome when used in combination with other MAO (including MAO-A) inhibitors or serotonergic drugs (MAO also metabolises serotonin)
Anticholinergics	Benzhexol	1 mg/day	2 mg tds	Block-acetylcholine receptors	Adjuvant treatment for rest tremor in younger patients	Dry mouth; memory impairment; confusion; constipation; blurred vision and exacerbation of glaucoma; urinary retention (together these are referred to as *anticholinergic* adverse effects); may be difficult to wean after long-term use; avoid sudden cessation to prevent cholinergic crisis
	Benztropine	0.5 mg/day	2 mg tds			

*Serious/potentially life-threatening adverse effects are shown in bold type.
ECG, electrocardiogram; ESR, erythrocyte sedimentation rate.

dopamine blockade. It may prolong the QT interval and should not be used in combination with other drugs that have this property.

■ Metoclopramide and prochlorperazine are contraindicated because of their central dopamine antagonist actions.

■ Sudden withdrawal or reduction in dosage of levodopa or dopamine agonists can induce the parkinsonism–hyperpyrexia syndrome, a neurological emergency with clinical features similar to the neuroleptic malignant syndrome (see below).

■ There is no maximum dose of levodopa. The aim is to keep the dose as low as possible, compatible with reasonable benefit. However, in younger patients it is best to try to keep the daily dose below 600 mg/day and to add an agonist before going above this dose.

Early stage treatment

There are several considerations when deciding which drug to start first:

■ Levodopa is the most effective symptomatic treatment.

■ Early treatment with a dopamine agonist, with or without supplemental levodopa, is associated with ~30% less chance of dyskinesias after 3–5 years of therapy.

■ Younger-onset patients are more likely to have troublesome dyskinesia.

■ Dopamine agonists are rarely adequate as sole therapy for more than a year or two.

■ Dopamine agonists are more prone than levodopa to cause hallucinations, postural hypotension and confusion, and should therefore be used with particular caution in the elderly and those with cognitive impairment.

The options should be discussed with the patient. If a maximal therapeutic benefit is the priority (e.g. employment is threatened) then levodopa is the preferred drug. A dopamine agonist can then be added if the total daily levodopa dose of 600 mg/day has been reached and the response is inadequate. In younger patients with mild symptoms, where a maximal response to treatment is not necessarily required, treatment can be started with a dopamine agonist and then, when necessary, levodopa substituted or added.

Management points

■ In early disease, dopaminergic therapy reliably improves the most disabling problem (bradykinesia), so improving hand function and gait.

■ Rest tremor often breaks through at times of stress even on high doses of levodopa.

- In younger patients, an anticholinergic drug is sometimes added to control tremor if the response to levodopa is unsatisfactory. This class of drug is best avoided in the elderly because of its effects on memory and propensity to induce psychosis.
- The time to reach maximal benefit from a particular dose level of levodopa can be 4–8 weeks. The initial recommended maintenance dose is ½ a 100 mg levodopa (plus dopa decarboxylase inhibitor) tablet tds, building up to 1–2 tablets tds depending on the response.
- If there is a poor response to one dopamine agonist it may be worth trying another.
- Ergot-based dopamine agonists should be avoided in patients with a history of pulmonary fibrosis or asbestos exposure because of the risk of pleuropulmonary fibrosis. Retroperitoneal fibrosis can also occur. Monitor with regular chest auscultation and be alert for unexplained urinary tract symptoms or severe leg oedema (mild ankle swelling is a relatively common adverse effect of dopamine agonists).
- Cardiac valvular fibrosis has been reported in 30–45% of patients taking pergolide. The risk with other dopamine agonists is unknown. In patients on ergot agonists, monitor for symptoms of heart failure and listen to the heart at each visit. It may be wise to obtain an echocardiogram (ECG) at some point on these patients until we know more about the incidence of this complication.
- Excessive drowsiness and sudden onset of sleep can occur with any dopaminergic therapy, but especially with the newer, non-ergot agonists pramipexole and ropinirole. Patients should be warned about the risk of falling asleep while driving.

Mid-stage treatment

In the first few years of treatment, motor function remains stable throughout the day. Very responsive patients may have no signs of the disease at all. If they forget a dose, it does not matter; indeed, deterioration may not occur for several days should the patient stop taking the drug. But, sooner or later, this 'honeymoon' ends and a number of problems emerge.

Motor fluctuations

Motor fluctuations have two aspects:

- reappearance of parkinsonian symptoms and signs as the effect of each dose of levodopa wears off, or doses fail to work throughout the day
- appearance of abnormal involuntary movements in response to dopaminergic therapy (dyskinesias and dystonia).

Reappearance of parkinsonism

In most patients the first manifestation of motor fluctuations is 'wearing off' of the benefit of each dose of levodopa before the next tablet is due:

- On a three times daily dosage schedule, this happens after each dose so the patients find themselves waiting for the next dose to kick in – so-called 'end of dose failure'.
- 'Sleep benefit' is lost and patients complain of being markedly slow until their first dose of levodopa in the morning has started to work (early morning akinesia).
- During the night, patients may have difficulty turning in bed or getting to the toilet (nocturnal akinesia).
- A dose of levodopa may take an hour or two to have effect or fail altogether, particularly if the patient has taken it after a protein meal or has been emotionally upset ('delayed ons' and 'dose failures').
- Fluctuations may occur suddenly and without warning. Like a light switch, the patients may change from being 'on' (functioning well) to 'off' (slow, stiff and immobile).

These problems are thought to reflect loss of the 'long-duration effect' of levodopa whereby it continues to be released from dopamine stores for several days after levodopa administration has ceased. Patients now increasingly depend on reliable gut absorption and steady plasma levels of levodopa, something that is hard to achieve with a drug with a plasma half-life of only 1 hour.

There are several approaches to the management of this problem:

- Take levodopa more frequently. The advantage is that this is simple and, in the early stages, effective. The disadvantage is that it probably increases the risk of developing dyskinesias.
- Add a dopamine agonist that has a longer half-life than levodopa and buffers the rise and fall in plasma levodopa levels.
- Add an enzyme inhibitor to reduce the breakdown of levodopa or dopamine:
  - COMT (catechol-O-methyltransferase) inhibitors (entacapone and tolcapone) add about 90 minutes of 'on time' each day to patients with motor fluctuations. The duration of effect of each dose of levodopa may be increased by up to 0.5–1 hour.
  - Selegiline inhibits monoamine oxidase B (MAO-B), which breaks down dopamine centrally. In practice, this is not very effective.
- Slow-release preparations of levodopa can be used at bedtime to

improve nocturnal mobility. They are not particularly effective for most patients in managing daytime motor fluctuations.

For patients with sudden severe or unpredictable 'offs', rescue apomorphine is useful. Apomorphine is derived from the production of morphine but is a dopamine agonist, *not* an opiate, something which has to be explained to patients who are anxious about its name:

- Apomorphine is as potent as levodopa and has the same adverse effects.
- It is given by subcutaneous injection, takes effect in 5–10 minutes, and works for about an hour.
- The dose is determined by individual titration.
- It is a potent emetic, and when it is first introduced domperidone has to be given also.
- For patients with fluctuations that cannot be controlled by levodopa or other agonists, there is a place for continuous subcutaneous infusion of apomorphine delivered by a portable pump. Local inflammation at the site of the infusion is lessened by using a plastic cannula, but can be a limiting adverse effect.

Dyskinesias

Most patients treated with levodopa eventually develop involuntary movements (dyskinesias) in response to therapy. Dyskinesias can be choreiform, ballistic, dystonic or varying combinations of all three.

- Except for early disease, especially in younger patients in whom exercise-induced dystonia can be a presenting symptom, dyskinesias do not occur unless the patient is taking dopaminergic therapy.
- Dopamine agonists, other than apomorphine, usually cause no or only mild dyskinesias when used alone. They may worsen dopa-induced dyskinesia when first added to the regimen, necessitating a lower dose of levodopa.
- Peak-dose dyskinesias:
  - occur 1–2 hours after a dose at a time when motor benefit is maximal
  - they are usually choreiform and occasionally, if severe, ballistic
  - they are often mild and asymptomatic, indeed the patient may sometimes not be aware of them
  - they often do not require treatment or dose modification
  - if they are severe enough to warrant treatment, try reducing the amount of each dose of levodopa; to prevent worsening of parkinsonism, a dopamine agonist can be added or the dosing interval of levodopa shortened.

- Dyskinesias can also occur as the motor benefit begins to take effect or as it wears off (intermediate-dose dyskinesias, also known as diphasic dyskinesias as they commonly occur at both dose onset and offset). Diphasic dyskinesias are commonly a mixture of chorea and dystonia.
- End-of-dose dystonia occurs later in the dose cycle and coincides with a wearing off of benefit. The same phenomenon is seen before the first dose of levodopa in the morning. It is relieved by taking another dose of dopa. The pain associated with end-of-dose dystonia may target a region of the body which is painful for other reasons (e.g. prolapsed disc, previous surgery). Differentiating end-of-dose dystonia from peak-dose dyskinesias is very important because the appropriate treatment strategy for the former is to *increase* rather than decrease dopaminergic treatment.
- Amantadine up to a maximum dose of 100 mg tds can partially suppress dyskinesias in around two-thirds of patients. Unfortunately, the benefit is often short-lived, lasting about 6 months.
- Many patients are unable to distinguish their dyskinesias from their 'tremor'. Ask the patient to tell you when the problems occur in relation to each dose and to mimic his or her movements. Observation through a dose cycle by an experienced nurse can help to sort out this problem.
- Dyskinesias without any motor benefit suggest the possibility of multiple system atrophy.

Surgery for Parkinson's disease

- The dopaminergic deficit leads to neuronal overactivity in the subthalamic nucleus and globus pallidus pars interna.
- Functional surgery interrupts output from these nuclei, either with a lesion or with an implanted deep brain stimulation device that delivers high-frequency impulses.
- The main benefit is a reduction in both the severity and duration of motor fluctuations.
- Best 'on period' function is not improved by surgery except through reduction in dyskinesias, which is usually marked following both bilateral pallidal and subthalamic surgery (the latter through postoperative reduction in levodopa requirements).
- Therefore, the two main indications for surgery are severe motor fluctuations, and/or severe dyskinesias unresponsive to medical therapy.
- Patients who do not respond to levodopa will not benefit from surgery.
- Dementia, uncontrolled psychosis or depression, advanced age and a parkinsonian syndrome, other than idiopathic Parkinson's disease, are contraindications to surgery.

Late-stage Parkinson's disease

Patients with long-standing disease eventually develop problems that are partly or completely levodopa-resistant. These include:

- freezing of gait, when the feet involuntarily stick to the ground
- loss of postural reflexes and falls
- speech and swallowing disturbance.

NON-MOTOR SYMPTOMS IN PARKINSON'S DISEASE

Non-motor symptoms are common and a major cause of morbidity.

Depression

- Depression can occur at any stage, even before motor dysfunction, and has a major impact on quality of life.
- It commonly appears after a year or two and ultimately affects around 50% of patients.
- The risk of depression is independent of motor disability.
- Both depression and Parkinson's disease itself cause patients to complain of lack of energy. Sleep disturbance and loss of appetite are more useful markers of depression.
- If a patient appears to respond to levodopa but continues to complain of debilitating symptoms, consider the possibility of depression.
- Treatment (see Chapter 13):
  - levodopa does not usually improve depression
  - depression can be effectively treated with selective serotonin reuptake inhibitors (SSRIs)
  - tricyclic antidepressants can also be useful, especially if there is sleep disturbance or nocturia, but they cannot be combined with SSRIs because of the risk of provoking the serotonin syndrome (see section below)
  - the antidepressant doses required can be lower than those used in psychiatric practice.

Hallucinations/delusions

About 30% of patients with advanced disease experience visual hallucinations or delusions.

- The hallucinations are vivid and well formed (e.g. people, insects) and mainly occur at night. Patients soon realise their nature and are not frightened by them. They often herald the early stages of parkinsonian dementia but can occur in the presence of normal cognition.

- More troublesome are delusions where, for example, the patient becomes convinced that their spouse is having an affair or intruders are trying to enter their house.
- Hallucinations and delusions may escalate into frank psychosis, leading to aggression or self-injury. Psychosis usually occurs in patients with coexistent cognitive impairment.
- Hallucinations that do not affect the patient's behaviour and do not trouble them do not require treatment. If necessary:
  - nocturnal hallucinations can be reduced by keeping a low light on in the bedroom
  - in the past, the only treatment option for troublesome hallucinations or delusions leading to aggressive or aversive behaviour was gradual withdrawal of all antiparkinsonian medication other than levodopa; this approach can (but curiously, does not always) result in worsening motor disability
  - quetiapine 25–100 mg/day oral in 2 divided doses or low-dose olanzapine 2.5–7.5 mg/day oral can effectively control hallucinations and delusions without adversely affecting motor function very much
  - clozapine 6.25–50 mg/day oral in 2 divided doses has least effect on motor problems, but is hampered by the need for fortnightly blood tests to monitor the low risk of serious leukopenia.

Psychosis

- Severe, acute psychosis is a medical and psychiatric emergency.
- Ideally, the patient should be admitted to a unit specialising in managing this type of problem.
- Patients should be managed in a single room with the mattress on the floor and a nurse present at all times.
- Exclude a metabolic or infective trigger for the disorder (most commonly, urinary or chest infection).
- Atypical neuroleptics are usually inadequate in achieving rapid control of the acutely psychotic parkinsonian patient.
- It may be necessary to use low-dose parenteral haloperidol im or iv, at doses much lower than in the usual psychiatric setting (2.5–5.0 mg, repeated as required).
- An oral atypical neuroleptic should be started and haloperidol withdrawn as soon as improvement begins.
- There is a risk of provoking the neuroleptic malignant syndrome and, if this occurs, the appropriate treatment is electroconvulsive therapy, which will also help the psychosis.

■ Benzodiazepines such as diazepam are useful as adjuvant therapy in the setting of an acute psychosis.

Dementia

Almost all patients eventually develop cognitive impairment: varying degrees of memory disturbance, hallucinations, fluctuations in attention and cognitive ability, confusion and behavioural change. Acetylcholinesterase inhibitors provide modest improvement in some patients (see Chapter 5).

Autonomic symptoms

■ Symptomatic postural hypotension is common in advanced disease and made worse by most of the antiparkinsonian drugs, particularly levodopa and the dopamine agonists. If symptomatic:
  – withdraw antihypertensives
  – minimise or withdraw dopamine agonists
  – add dietary salt and elevate the head of the bed as much as is tolerable
  – add fludrocortisone, oral, gradually in 0.1 mg increments up to a maximum dose of 1 mg/day, taken in the morning (need to monitor electrolytes for hypernatraemia and hypokalaemia)
  – add midodrine 5–10 mg oral 4 hourly during waking hours
  – monitor closely for the unwanted and potentially dangerous adverse effect of supine hypertension.
■ Bladder disturbance and erectile dysfunction are also common. Their management is dealt with in Chapter 17.

DRUG-INDUCED PARKINSONISM

In the past, many patients on long-term traditional neuroleptic therapy had signs of mild parkinsonism with reduced arm swing, stooped posture, slight rigidity and bradykinesia. With the move towards using atypical neuroleptics in schizophrenia, this is now less of a problem. Still an issue is the development of parkinsonism or tardive dyskinesia, particularly in the older patient, as a result of the inappropriate use of neuroleptic agents such as prochlorperazine and metoclopramide as a treatment for dizziness and nausea.

Management

■ Withdrawal of the offending drug, allowing its effect to wear off without taking other measures (this may take a year or two).

- In psychosis, where continued therapy is necessary, traditional neuroleptics can be replaced with the atypical neuroleptics such as quetiapine or clozapine.
- Antiparkinsonian drugs such as levodopa are not usually effective in the presence of dopamine blockade and may worsen psychosis.
- Anticholinergic drugs have been used for generations but have never been proven to be effective in double-blind studies.
- In practice, unless the parkinsonism is severe, no specific drug treatment is needed other than lowering the dose of the offending drug.

ATYPICAL PARKINSONIAN SYNDROMES

The atypical parkinsonian syndromes are all characterised by degeneration in not just the substantia nigra, but also in the corpus striatum and globus pallidus. This explains the poor response to levodopa therapy.

Multiple system atrophy (MSA)

MSA presents as three clinical phenotypes:
- parkinsonian (MSA_p)
- cerebellar (MSA_c)
- autonomic (MSA_a).

In the late stages, the three forms may merge.
- Patients with MSA_p may be indistinguishable from those with Parkinson's disease in the first few years.
  - Early falls (within the first 1–2 years), rapid progression, myoclonus of the fingers, and autonomic features (impotence, postural hypotension and incontinence of urine) are distinguishing features.
  - The motor response to levodopa is variable. Some show no benefit at all, yet may get dopa-induced dyskinesia (characteristically affecting the face). Others respond well for a year or two and then lose the benefit. Rare patients have an excellent response, although this also wanes with time.
  - Therefore, all patients should have a trial of levodopa, titrating cautiously to the highest tolerated dose as it may exacerbate postural hypotension.
- The autonomic features (MSA_a) should be treated (see postural hypotension, above, and Chapter 17).
- There is no specific drug treatment for MSA_c, but rehabilitation and allied health support is useful.

It is important not to abandon these patients but to see them and their families on a regular basis to provide support and encouragement.

Progressive supranuclear palsy

This produces an akinetic rigid syndrome with early falls, often in the first year, rigidity which is greater in the neck than the arms, and frontal dementia. The hallmark, which may not appear for some years, is slowing of saccadic eye velocity and, later, loss of downward gaze.

- While it is always worth giving the patient a trial of levodopa, particularly in the early stages when the diagnosis is still uncertain, the response to antiparkinsonian medication is poor.
- It is important not to abandon these patients to their fate. A regular visit to the clinic helps them and their family understand and cope with the disease.
- Patients often have heavy falls, refusing or forgetting to use a frame or wheelchair which they clearly need.

DRUG-INDUCED MOVEMENT DISORDERS PRESENTING WITH HYPERTONIA

Neuroleptic malignant syndrome

- A clinical triad of rigidity, dysautonomia and alteration in mental status that develops within days to weeks of starting or increasing the dose of neuroleptic medications.
- Commonly misdiagnosed as meningitis or sepsis, which must always be considered in the differential diagnosis, because of the high fever and tachycardia.
- Treatment:
  - withdraw the neuroleptic drug in mild to moderate cases
  - in moderate to severe cases add a dopaminergic agent (e.g. bromocriptine 2.5 mg stat as a test dose, titrated over 48 hours to 5–10 mg oral tds or via nasogastric tube)
  - ± the muscle relaxant dantrolene 25 mg oral tds, or iv (initial dose 1 mg/kg)
  - if oral administration of a dopaminergic drug is not possible, subcutaneous apomorphine is effective, with pretreatment with rectal domperidone.
- Supportive care to maintain hydration and prevent complications such as renal failure secondary to rhabdomyolysis, deep venous thrombosis and pneumonia.
- In severe cases intensive care admission for endotracheal intubation, muscle paralysis and ventilatory support may be necessary.
- An identical syndrome can occur in patients with Parkinson's disease after sudden withdrawal or reduction in dose of dopaminergic therapy.

Serotonin syndrome

- Similar presentation to neuroleptic malignant syndrome, except that clonus, myoclonus and seizures are much more common.
- Usually occurs within hours to days (as opposed to days to weeks with neuroleptic malignant syndrome) of drug exposure. Commonly precipitated by coadministration of serotonergic drugs (e.g. tramadol prescribed for a patient already taking a serotonin reuptake inhibitor).
- In mild to moderate cases, withdrawal of the offending drug(s) usually results in rapid resolution of symptoms within 24 hours.
- In patients with a severe or prolonged syndrome, specific therapy with the serotonin antagonist cyproheptadine should be instituted: initial dose 4–8 mg oral, with a repeat dose in 2 hours. If no improvement occurs, it is discontinued, but if a response occurs it should be maintained up to a dose of 32 mg/day in 4 divided doses until resolution of the symptoms.
- Benzodiazepines should be used to reduce anxiety.
- Supportive care and, for severe cases, muscle paralysis and mechanical ventilation may be required.

TREMOR

Tremor refers to involuntary movements that are rhythmic and oscillatory. The diagnosis of tremor relies on when it occurs, and the body part affected (Table 6.2).

Essential tremor

- This is seen in the outstretched hands and is usually symmetrical.
- The tremor worsens slowly over many years.
- Disability may be mainly one of social embarrassment.
- Many patients require no treatment other than reassurance that they do not have Parkinson's disease.
- Useful drugs are listed in Table 6.3, but rarely if ever abolish the tremor.
- Propranolol is the drug of first choice, but cannot be given if there is a history of asthma.
- Primidone is also effective if introduced slowly, but may be poorly tolerated by the elderly.
- For patients with severe, disabling tremor, contralateral thalamotomy can be performed, but bilateral thalamotomy is contraindicated because of the high risk of speech and cognitive disturbance.
- For bilateral cases, deep brain stimulation can be performed.
- For both unilateral thalamotomy and bilateral thalamic deep brain

stimulation there is about an 80% chance of significant improvement and 30% chance of adverse events, in particular dysarthria or ataxia, with a 1–2% risk of haemorrhage or death.

Dystonic tremor

- Dystonic tremor is a more irregular asymmetrical tremor than essential tremor and is associated with dystonia in the affected body part.
- There is an increased frequency of postural upper limb tremor in patients with any dystonia, referred to as 'tremor associated with dystonia'.
- Many patients presenting with isolated head/neck tremor or isolated postural tremor of the upper limbs have subtle, asymptomatic abnormal posturing. This may represent a *forme fruste* of dystonic tremor.
- Other clues that a tremor is dystonic are task specificity (e.g. writing), positional dependence and improvement with a sensory trick.
- The treatment of choice for dystonic head/neck tremor is botulinum toxin injections, which cause weakness by inducing reversible chemical denervation of the injected and overactive muscle(s).
- The results of treatment for distal upper limb tremor are disappointing because the doses required to alleviate the tremor cause weakness.
- Botulinum toxin is also effective for tremulous laryngeal dystonia: transient worsening of speech and/or swallowing disturbance occurs in a small minority of subjects.
- Drug therapy is disappointing in most patients. Anticholinergics can occasionally be useful, as can primidone or gabapentin.

Primary orthostatic tremor

- Patients present with unsteadiness or tremor in the legs that increases with prolonged standing. The symptoms are relieved by sitting or walking. Misdiagnosis as an anxiety disorder is common.
- The diagnosis is easily confirmed with surface electromyography from leg muscles while standing, which demonstrates high frequency 13–18 Hz muscle bursting, not seen in any other condition.
- Clonazepam, primidone and gabapentin can each be effective in reducing symptoms but are generally disappointing.
- The occasional patient responds to levodopa.

Palatal tremor

- Essential and occasionally symptomatic forms (with brainstem pathology) are recognised.

Table 6.2   Tremors and their causes and treatments

Tremor type	Body part affected	Tremor diagnosis	Comment	Treatment
Rest	Arms, legs, chin/tongue	Parkinsonian tremor	Little else causes true rest tremor	See section on Parkinson's disease
Postural	Upper limbs	Enhanced physiological	Should be moderate to high frequency. Look for underlying cause such as hyperthyroidism, anxiety, drugs	Of the underlying disorder
		Essential tremor	Should be reasonably symmetrical	See section on essential tremor and Table 6.3
		Dystonic tremor syndrome	Suspect if very asymmetrical, tremor shows positional dependence. Look for evidence of dystonic posturing in upper limbs, and elsewhere, e.g. neck	Anticholinergics, primidone, gabapentin (anecdotal; little evidence on which to base recommendations)
		Parkinsonian tremor	Common in Parkinson's disease in combination with other parkinsonian signs, but can be isolated or the presenting feature. Suspect diagnosis if very asymmetrical	See section on Parkinson's disease
	Head/neck	Dystonic tremor (cervical dystonia)	Look for subtle dystonic posturing in neck. If absent, positional dependence and presence of a sensory trick are clues	Botulinum toxin injections is treatment of choice. Drugs rarely effective

Intention	Upper limbs			
	—	Essential tremor	Can be more prominent than postural component, but latter should also be present. Is often the most disabling aspect of essential tremor	See section on essential tremor and Table 6.3
		Cerebellar tremor	Other cerebellar signs usually present. Often reduces if patient performs movement with eyes closed	None effective
Mid-action (kinetic)		Essential tremor	—	See section on essential tremor
		Dystonic tremor syndrome	Suspect if very asymmetrical, tremor shows task specificity or positional dependence. Look for evidence of dystonic posturing in upper limbs but also elsewhere, e.g. neck	See section on dystonic tremor
		Cerebellar tremor	Other cerebellar signs usually present	None effective
		Primary orthostatic tremor	Leg and truncal tremor that appears on standing and disappears with walking. Has unique high frequency (13–18 Hz) which makes it difficult to see	Clonazepam, gabapentin, primidone, levodopa help some patients (anecdotal; little evidence on which to base recommendations)

Table 6.3	Drugs for essential tremor		
Drug	**Dose range**	**Adverse effects**	**Comment**
Propranolol	Initial dose 10 mg bd. Titrate up to 40–240 mg/day in 2–3 divided doses	Fatigue and exercise intolerance; hypotension; bradycardia; impotence; nightmares; bronchospasm. Contraindicated in asthmatics	–
Primidone	Initial dose 62.5 mg nocte. Titrate up to 250–750 mg/day in 2–3 divided doses	Drowsiness; fatigue; dizziness; unsteadiness; reduces effectiveness of oral contraceptive pill	20–25% of patients experience a profound idiosyncratic reaction characterised by nausea, vomiting, drowsiness and even obtundation. Patients should be warned about this possibility and advised not to take their first dose while alone
Alprazolam	0.5–1.5 mg/day in 2–3 divided doses	Drowsiness; unsteadiness and falls; benzodiazepine can be associated with tolerance and addiction	Intermittent prn dosing can be effective
Gabapentin	600–1800 mg/day in 2–3 divided doses	Unsteadiness; abdominal bloating and weight gain; memory disturbance	–
Topiramate	50–400 mg/day in 2 divided doses	Paraesthesia; weight loss; drowsiness; memory disturbance; confusion; unsteadiness	–

- Essential palatal tremor is a monosymptomatic illness which presents with self-audible ear clicks.
- Symptomatic, but not essential, palatal tremor is usually associated with a cerebellar syndrome which can be progressive. Self-audible ear clicks are usually absent.
- If the clicks are distressing to the patient, botulinum toxin injections into the soft palate may provide relief; these may cause transient swallowing disturbance in a small minority of subjects.

DYSTONIA

- Dystonia is a disorder of motor control causing abnormal posturing and involuntary movements, most obvious during voluntary activity but often also at rest.
- Dystonic movements include athetosis (writhing movements of the fingers and face), twitching and writhing movements (choreoathetosis), myoclonus, tics and tremor.
- Dystonia can be task specific, focal (confined to one body part), segmental (confined to several adjoining body parts) or generalised.
- It can develop at any age. The age of onset, pattern of spread, and associated neurological and systemic features all give clues to its cause (Table 6.4).

Treatment

- Treatment of dystonia can be divided into treating the underlying disease, and symptomatic treatment of the dystonia.

Dopa-responsive dystonia

There are two forms:

- A classical, autosomal dominantly inherited form (Segawa's disease) presents with varying combinations of dystonia and parkinsonism, the former in childhood and the latter mainly in adulthood. Other than hyperreflexia, there are no other neurological signs.
  - The diagnosis should be considered in every patient with childhood or early adult onset dystonia in whom a firm cause cannot be found. Presentation in later life (age > 50 years) is usually with parkinsonism without dystonia.
  - Patients may be misdiagnosed early in life as hereditary spastic paraplegia, cerebral palsy or an idiopathic dystonia.
  - Treatment with low doses of levodopa is very effective.

Table 6.4   Features of the dystonias

Feature	Comment
Age	
Infantile (< 2 years)	Wide differential diagnosis
Juvenile (3–20 years)	Wide differential diagnosis
Adult (> 21 years)	Usually focal and idiopathic, rarely generalises or is secondary, Wilson's disease should be excluded in every patient presenting with dystonia under the age of 50 years
Pattern	
Focal	When fixed dystonia occurs early, suspect secondary or psychogenic aetiology
Segmental	In adult-onset idiopathic dystonia, relatively common in craniocervical dystonia but uncommon following presentation with limb dystonia
Generalised	More likely with childhood onset, rarely occurs with adult onset and suggests secondary cause
Hemidystonia	Suggests contralateral structural lesion
Paroxysmal	Usually idiopathic with key triggers (e.g. sudden movement), but exclude metabolic causes such as hypocalcaemia, hypoparathyroidism, hypoglycaemia and (if unilateral) structural pathology (especially multiple sclerosis or vascular malformation)
Aetiology	
Primary	May be sporadic or familial, non-degenerative
Dystonia-plus syndrome	Non-degenerative but with associated neurological features (e.g. dopa-responsive dystonia with Parkinsonism, myoclonus–dystonia syndrome)
Secondary	May have pure dystonia (e.g. Hallervordern–Spatz disease, glutaric aciduria), but associated neurological or systemic features usually present
Key associated neurological features	
Nil	Should always be the case in primary dystonia
Supranuclear ophthalmoplegia	Exclude Wilson's disease, Huntington's disease, Niemann–Pick type C, chorea–acanthocytosis,

Table 6.4	*Continued*
	spinocerebellar ataxia (especially SCA 2 and 3); ataxia–telangiectasia
Retinopathy	Exclude inborn error of metabolism, Hallervordern–Spatz disease, mitochondrial cytopathy
Parkinsonism	Common in young-onset idiopathic Parkinson's disease and may be presenting feature; exclude Wilson's disease, Huntington's disease, Niemann–Pick type C, chorea–acanthocytosis, spinocerebellar ataxia (especially SCA 2, 3 and 6)
Encephalopathy	Wide differential diagnosis
Dementia	Should never be present in primary dystonia
Spasticity	Dopa-responsive dystonia can be misdiagnosed as hereditary spastic paraparesis
Cerebellar ataxia	Wide differential diagnosis
Peripheral neuropathy	Wide differential diagnosis
Myopathy	Consider mitochondrial disease, neuroacanthocytosis syndrome (asymptomatic elevated serum creatine kinase)
Key associated systemic features	
Nil	Should be the case in adult-onset idiopathic forms
Kaiser-Fleischer rings	Present in 95% (not 100%) of patients with neurological Wilson's disease
Organomegaly	Suspect storage disease

- A second, much rarer form of dopa-responsive dystonia is caused by a number of recessively inherited metabolic defects in various points of the biopterin or dopamine synthesis pathways.
  - Presentation of these recessive forms is usually in infancy and with a more non-specific neurological syndrome, including developmental delay, seizures, involuntary movements and hypotonia. A history of oculogyric crises is an important clue.
  - Dystonia may be absent in infancy but usually develops later in the course of the disease.

Symptomatic treatment

- Chorea is often mild or asymptomatic and so treatment is required only if there is disability, which may be predominantly motor or social.
- Chorea often responds to dopamine antagonists (e.g. haloperidol) at low doses. The role of the newer, atypical antipsychotics is currently uncertain.
- Tetrabenazine can be equally effective and should be considered alongside dopamine antagonists as first-line therapy. To maximise tolerability, it should be titrated slowly with dose increments of 6.25 mg (¼ tablet) every 4–7 days up to a maximum dose of 200 mg/day in 3 divided doses. Drowsiness and reversible parkinsonism occur in about a third and depression in about 15% of patients.
- If these agents fail or are not tolerated, carbamazepine and valproate should always be tried, and are regarded as first-line therapy in Sydenham's chorea.
- For patients in whom severe chorea–ballismus has developed acutely, a short-term benzodiazepine to relieve anxiety is helpful.
- Tetrabenazine is the treatment of choice for severe ballismus once a specific metabolic cause has been excluded.

HUNTINGTON'S DISEASE

- Diagnosis is by genetic testing, best in the setting of a specialised clinic where the neurologist works with clinical geneticists, psychiatrists, counsellors, occupational therapists and social workers.
- Presymptomatic diagnosis has profound implications for individuals, whether the test result is positive or negative, and should only be undertaken after formal counselling when individuals have reached adult age and have given their own informed consent.
- In Huntington's disease, there is often a mixed movement disorder, especially in children and younger adults. Upper limb disability can be due to coexistent bradykinesia and/or apraxia. Dystonia can also be prominent. Rigidity may be the major feature, particularly in younger patients. It is important to establish which of these movement disorders is the predominant cause of disability before embarking on therapy.
- Patients are often not aware of or troubled by their chorea, which therefore does not necessarily require treatment unless it is contributing to incoordination of movement:
  - tetrabenazine can be extremely effective, but adverse events, in particular parkinsonism and depression, need to be monitored for closely (for doses, see above)

- sulpiride 200–400 mg/day oral in 2 divided doses is another possibility, and extrapyramidal adverse effects are usually minimal
  - for troublesome chorea, olanzapine may be tried.
- For agitation, a benzodiazepine may be used; irritability and aggression respond to haloperidol in low dosage (0.5 mg bd).
- Often there is limited insight into the disease, and therefore patient self-reporting of ability for tasks such as driving should not be taken at face value.
- In the early stages after diagnosis, when intellect and insight are relatively preserved, as well as later, the possibility of depression and suicidal tendency needs to be considered and monitored for closely. Depression may require both medical therapy and counselling.
- With advancing disease, motor disability increases, especially problems with fine motor skills, gait, balance and swallowing:
  - difficulties in speech, swallowing and mobility require speech therapy, dietary advice (rarely gastrostomy) and physiotherapy
  - when frequent falls lead to injuries a wheelchair is necessary.
- Conventional neuroleptics should be avoided because they lead to sedation and an increase in dystonia.
- Transplantation of embryonic tissue into the corpus striatum is under investigation.

The effect on family and social circumstances can be devastating. Because of these issues, Huntington's disease is best managed in the setting of a multidisciplinary clinic.

MYOCLONUS

Myoclonus is defined as sudden, unpredictable, shock-like movements or jerks. It can be cortical, subcortical or spinal in origin, and focal, multifocal or generalised in distribution.

Myoclonus most commonly occurs as part of a metabolic encephalopathy such as renal or hepatic failure. Other common causes are drugs (e.g. SSRIs), or neurodegenerative diseases such as Alzheimer's disease and dementia with Lewy bodies.

Cortical myoclonus

- Often responds to piracetam up to 24 g/day oral in 3 divided doses, either as monotherapy or in combination with antiepileptic drugs such as valproate (doses up to 2000 mg/day in 2–3 divided doses) or primidone (up to 750 mg/day oral in 3 divided doses) and clonazepam.

- The role of newer antiepileptic drugs such as lamotrigine and levetiracetam is uncertain.
- Some antiepileptic drugs such as gabapentin, carbamazepine and phenytoin can *cause* myoclonic jerks or asterixis (sudden brief inhibition of muscle contraction, also known as 'negative' myoclonus).

Subcortical myoclonus

Responds best to clonazepam.

HICCUPS

- Hiccups are due to spontaneous sudden contractions of the diaphragm, and are usually a normal phenomenon.
- When persistent, investigations should be directed at intra-abdominal or, less commonly, thoracic, cervical spine or brainstem pathology.
- Severe persistent hiccups are hard to treat:
  - temporary relief may come from swallowing a glass of water with the head turned to the left
  - chlorpromazine, methylphenidate, baclofen and most recently gabapentin have all been used with varying degrees of success.

TICS

- Tics are jerks, grimaces and other rather sudden movements which mainly involve the face (but can affect any part of the body) and which are preceded by a feeling of compulsion on the part of the patient.
- They appear in childhood and often disappear by adulthood.
- When multiple tics are seen, particularly causing vocalisations, the condition is referred to as Tourette's syndrome.
- Tics usually cause social rather than physical disability and require no specific treatment.
- Rarely, violent motor tics can cause injury to cervical nerve roots or the cervical cord.
- Management is best directed at the behavioural aspects of the problem, such as obsessive–compulsive disorder, attention deficit hyperactivity disorder, and towards treating anxiety or depression.
- Treatment with the dopamine antagonists pimozide and haloperidol, the atypical antipsychotic risperidone, tetrabenazine, low-dose pergolide and botulinum toxin injections reduce tic severity in the short to medium term.

RESTLESS LEG SYNDROME

The restless leg syndrome is common, affecting up to 5–10% of the population. It is idiopathic in the vast majority of patients and associated with a positive family history in over half. However, it can be caused or unmasked by iron deficiency, renal disease, peripheral neuropathy, pregnancy or Parkinson's disease and mimicked by thyroid disease, and these conditions should always be excluded and managed appropriately if present.

- The treatment of choice for idiopathic restless leg syndrome is dopaminergic therapy.
- In mild cases, levodopa is usually effective but in many (but not all) patients eventually tolerance or rebound symptoms occur in the morning (a phenomenon known as augmentation).
- Dopamine agonists, which have a longer half-life, are extremely effective and regarded by some as first-line therapy because of the problem of levodopa augmentation. Usually only relatively low doses are required, as opposed to the doses required in the treatment of parkinsonism: cabergoline, pergolide, pramipexole, ropinirole and rotigotine are all effective (see Table 6.1).
- For patients intolerant of dopaminergic therapy, a long list of potential therapies may possibly be effective (valproate, carbamazepine, clonazepam, gabapentin, etc.).

Further reading

Jankovic J, Tolosa E (eds). Parkinson's disease and movement disorders, 4th edn. Lippincott, Williams & Wilkins, Philadelphia, 2002.
Lyon G, Adams RD, Kolodny EH (eds). Neurology of hereditary metabolic diseases of children, 2nd edn. McGraw-Hill, New York 1996.

7 CRANIAL NERVES, NEURO-OTOLOGY AND THE CEREBELLUM

Geraint Fuller

Many of the chapters in this book are about one disease, a group of diseases, or types of symptom. This chapter is different in that it covers the range of problems that involve part, or rather a series of parts, of the nervous system, including most of those dealt with by the subspecialties of neuro-ophthalmology and neuro-otology.

The emphasis here is on treatment, and on those conditions with a specific treatment. However, in many of the conditions falling within the remit of this chapter where there are no specific treatments, the importance of an exact diagnosis, to provide an understanding of the condition and the prognosis, cannot be underestimated, because for many incurable conditions this provides the framework within which patients are able to live their lives.

The cranial nerves

The individual cranial nerves are emphasised in teaching the neurological examination. However, this is a convenience that is rarely respected by disease processes, and in practical terms it makes more sense to link some together in this section (e.g. III, IV and VI as causing eye-movement problems).

OLFACTORY NERVE

There are many conditions that can alter the sense of smell and the more common are listed in Table 7.1.

Table 7.1   Causes of loss or alteration of smell

Condition	Comment
Common	
Nasal or paranasal sinus disease following upper respiratory infection	Managed by ear, nose and throat specialists
Head injury	Some recover spontaneously within 12 months
Neurodegenerative conditions such as Parkinson's disease	Common but rarely a significant symptom
Uncommon	
Drug related (mainly altered taste)	Many immunosuppressants, antimicrobials (especially metronidazole), some hypoglycaemic and hypotensive drugs
Toxin exposure	Especially nasal inhalation of glue and petrol, and drugs of abuse such as cocaine; cigarette smoking
Dental	Treated by dentist
Rare	
Olfactory groove meningioma	Surgical management

Treatment depends on identifying any cause that can be treated – which is unlikely to be neurological:

- Sinus and nasal disease is usually managed by ear, nose and throat specialists.
- Recognition and removal of drugs that can alter smell sensation.
- Most patients who have lost their sense of smell notice this as a loss of sense of taste, even though their taste sensation is in fact preserved. Advice about the modalities of taste that are still preserved (bitter, sweet, sour, salty) and the use of food with interesting textures may go some way to ameliorate the loss of pleasure in eating as a consequence of lack of smell sensation.

OPTIC NERVE AND EYE

For all patients with problems with vision, non-specific measures such as appropriate correction of any refractive error, assistance with low vision aids and registration of any disability should be attended to, usually by an optometrist or ophthalmology service.

Acute demyelinating optic neuritis

This is a common cause of acute monocular visual loss, either alone or as part of multiple sclerosis (see Chapter 9). Corticosteroids are indicated if there is:

■ Severe pain.
■ Severe visual loss in the affected eye.
■ Poor vision in the other eye.

Ischaemic optic neuropathy

■ Non-arteritic optic neuropathy typically presents as painless loss of vision, commonly noticed on waking, and the optic disc is usually swollen, often with haemorrhages. Treatment hinges on prevention of further ischaemic events in the eye and elsewhere (see Chapter 4).
■ Arteritic optic neuropathy is the most important, although an uncommon, manifestation of giant cell arteritis. The diagnosis needs to be considered in any patient > 55 years old with visual symptoms, however unlikely it might seem, as corticosteroids will allow recovery and potentially prevent devastating visual loss (see Chapter 9).

Nutritional/toxic optic neuropathy

Nutritional and toxic optic neuropathies are rare and usually occur in the setting of poor diet, alcohol abuse and smoking, leading to some of the names commonly given to the condition (e.g. tobacco–alcohol amblyopia). In other situations a specific drug or toxin can be identified:

■ Some drugs causing toxic optic neuropathy:
  – ethambutol
  – chloramphenicol
  – isoniazid
  – choloroqine
  – vigabatrin
  – amiodarone
  – ciclosporine.
■ Some toxins causing toxic optic neuropathy:
  – methanol
  – heavy metals
  – toluene (glue sniffing).

Treatment is to remove any toxins, and treat with parenteral hydroxy-cobalamin (1 mg im weekly), oral vitamin B and folate.

Optic nerve compression

- Treatment is to decompress the optic nerve – if this is possible, which depends on the cause of the compression – either surgically or, where the compression is by aneurysm, by endovascular techniques. Stereotactic radiotherapy is also used.
- However, this is not as simple as it sounds. Frequently there must be a compromise between the risks of any intervention against the likely progression of the disease. For example, stereotactic radiotherapy may slow progression of a meningioma but, on the other hand, it can cause radiation-induced optic neuropathy and visual loss.

Rarer causes of optic neuropathy

There are a number of infections and inflammatory conditions that can cause optic neuropathy, although usually as part of a systemic illness. Treatment is for the underlying condition.

- Infections:
  - Lyme disease (see Chapter 14)
  - cat-scratch disease
  - syphilis (see Chapter 14).
- In human immunodeficiency virus (HIV) infection and other immunodeficiency states (see Chapter 14):
  - cytomegalovirus (CMV)
  - varicella zoster
  - toxoplasma.
- Sarcoid (see Chapter 9).

Idiopathic intracranial hypertension

This uncommon condition almost always occurs in obese young women (see Chapter 8). It is important to exclude other causes of raised pressure such as: vitamin A intoxication; drugs, particularly roaccutane and tetracyclines; and intracranial venous thrombosis (see Chapter 8).

Glaucoma

There are two forms of glaucoma, both of which may present to neurologists:

- Chronic, or open-angle, glaucoma is a common treatable cause of chronic visual loss, which rarely presents to neurologists, but is easily missed when it does present with the characteristic pattern of

peripheral field loss, optic nerve cupping and raised intraocular pressure. Early disease may present with centrocecal field loss.
- Acute, or closed-angle, glaucoma is rarer and presents as unilateral headache/eye pain with halos around light sources, or monocular visual loss.

Both are treatable and are managed by ophthalmologists; the second is an ophthalmological emergency.

Pupillary syndromes

Horner's syndrome is of particular importance for the diagnosis of associated conditions. In contrast with with Holmes–Adie pupil recognition it is important to confirm that there is no significant associated pathology.

There are no specific treatments for the pupillary changes themselves.
- Some patients with Horner's syndrome are helped cosmetically by surgery to lift the upper eyelid.
- Patients with a Holmes–Adie pupil can be helped by information so they understand the nature of their problem and use sunglasses and other strategies to avoid symptoms such as glare in bright light.

Ptosis

Ptosis has many causes but only a modest number of solutions – mechanical aids (e.g. ptosis bars on glasses) or surgical correction.

Ptosis occurs unilaterally with:
- Horner's syndrome – usually mild, treatment is cosmetic with surgery to lift the eyelid.
- III nerve lesion – usually more marked ptosis, or complete eye closure, although with diplopia, which may limit the effectiveness of treating the ptosis itself.
- Aponeurotic dehiscence (also called age-related ptosis), which usually responds well to surgery if needed.

Ptosis occurs bilaterally with:
- Myopathies such as myotonic dystrophy (usually mild, although surgery may help), Kearns–Sayre (where surgery is disappointing and mechanical aids are usually advised) and oculopharyngeal dystrophy (where surgical correction is effective).
- Myasthenia gravis (treat the myasthenia; see Chapter 12).

EYE MOVEMENTS

Isolated III, IV or VI cranial nerve disorders

There are many causes for isolated involvement of the III, IV and VI nerves, including compression, ischaemia, inflammation, infiltration, trauma as well as the involvement of IV and VI as false localising signs with raised intracranial pressure. For all these the primary treatment is of the underlying pathology. It is worth emphasising the particular importance of urgent assessment of III nerve palsies, especially those with papillary involvement, to look for compression by a posterior communicating artery aneurysm.

There are useful symptomatic treatments for the diplopia itself:
■ Patching one eye or covering one lens of the patient's glasses with opaque tape.
■ Frenzel prisms can be applied to glasses to realign the visual axes – although this will not help any torsional element. As the patient recovers the strength of the prisms will need review.
■ For patients with stable diplopia these methods can be supplemented by:
  – botulinum toxin injection of the antagonist of the weak muscles
  – strabismus surgery.

Cavernous sinus and superior orbital fissure syndromes

The combination of III, IV and VI nerve and V lesions results from pathology in the cavernous sinus or superior orbital fissure:
■ Fungal infection (e.g. mucormycosis, treated with local debridement and amphotericin).
■ Carotid aneurysm, treated either neurosurgically or with endovascular techniques.
■ Tumours, direct spread of primary – from pituitary, nasopharynx – or metastatic spread, treated for the underlying tumour.
■ Tolosa–Hunt syndrome:
  – rare and always a diagnosis of exclusion
  – combination of orbital pain, ophthalmoplegia (III, IV or VI), perhaps with ophthalmic branch of V, and normal vision
  – imaging may demonstrate inflammatory mass, and biopsy chronic inflammation
  – responds dramatically to prednisolone 60–100 mg/day oral, and then tapered.

Thyroid eye disease

■ Normally managed by ophthalmologists rather than neurologists.

- Results from hypertrophy of the extraocular muscles and increase in orbital fat.
- Primary treatment is of the underlying thyroid disease.
- Additional treatments may include:
  - lubricants and artificial tears
  - systemic and local corticosteroids, given early in the course when patients present with rapidly progressive and painful proptosis
  - radiotherapy if steroids fail
  - decompressive surgery can be considered if non-surgical methods fail or if there is significant optic nerve compression
  - persistent double vision can be treated by surgically weakening the relevant extraocular muscle.

Opsoclonus

- This chaotic eye movement disorder occurs in adults, either as part of a paraneoplastic syndrome, usually along with myoclonus, or as a postinfectious condition.
- Those with paraneoplastic associated immune-mediated opsoclonus may respond to immunosuppression or plasma exchange (see Chapter 15).
- Some patients with idiopathic opsoclonus have been reported to respond to intramuscular ACTH.
- Clonazepam 0.5–2 mg/day oral in 2–3 divided doses may provide some symptomatic benefit.

Superior oblique myokymia

This rare syndrome presents with intermittent oscillopsia because the myokymia produces small-amplitude monocular torsional movements. Carbamazepine helps most patients. The dose should be titrated up from 100 mg/day oral (see Chapter 2).

TRIGEMINAL NERVE

Trigeminal neuralgia

This severe pain syndrome (prevalence 4–5 per 100,000) seems to be caused by compression of the intracranial part of the trigeminal nerve by an aberrant artery or vein, at least in some patients. About 2% of cases are due to multiple sclerosis. It rarely arises from compression of the nerve from other causes, such as meningioma. The latter is treated neurosurgically.

- There are three types of treatment:
  - drugs to control the pain

- destructive procedures that to varying degrees impair trigeminal nerve function (balloon compression or radiofrequency ablation of the trigeminal ganglion, glycerol injection into the trigeminal cistern, neurectomy and stereotactic gamma knife radiosurgery)
- posterior fossa microvascular decompression to remove the cause of the syndrome.

There are, however, very few randomised trials to guide the therapeutic choice.

■ The standard drug is carbamazepine, usually initiated at low dose, 100 mg bd oral (see Chapter 2), and titrated up over days or weeks against the pain and any adverse effects. If the pain is relieved without adverse effects, the drug should be continued for a month or two and then gradually reduced and withdrawn if the patient has gone into remission. If the drug is limited by adverse effects it is worth trying at least one second-line drug.

■ Second-line drugs include gabapentin, sodium valproate, phenytoin, topiramate, oxcarbazepine, baclofen and clonazepam (for doses and adverse effects, see Chapters 2 and 9). The same dosing strategy is used as for carbamazepine.

■ If drugs fail, then the destructive procedures should be considered, but they can all cause numbness and paraesthesia of the side of the face. The duration of benefit is very variable and a small number of patients develop severe painful sensory loss (anaesthesia dolorosa).

■ For younger and fit patients microvascular decompression may be preferable to the destructive procedures. It can render over two-thirds of patients free of pain at 10 years with only 1% with facial sensory loss. There are, however, risks and, as the procedure is operator dependent, not all centres achieve this level of success.

Trigeminal sensory neuropathy

There are no specific treatments for this condition. Positive sensory symptoms that are distressing can be helped by pain-modulating drugs such as amitriptyline, carbamazepine and gabapentin (see Chapter 18).

FACIAL NERVE

Bell's palsy

■ There is rather poor evidence that it is reasonable to give prednisolone acutely, usually an oral dose of 30–40 mg/day for a week, hoping to speed and enhance recovery. There is disagreement about just how long after onset it can still usefully be given – most consider within 48 hours. However, in a patient with severe facial weakness, little would be lost even after a greater delay.

- There is even less certainty about whether patients should be given antivirals, in particular aciclovir, which may possibly have an effect.
- With severe facial nerve weakness some suggest acute decompression of the nerve surgically. The balance between risks and benefits for this procedure is unclear.
- Prevention of corneal damage during the period of facial nerve recovery is perhaps the most important treatment:
  - liberal use of simple artificial tears, lacrilube overnight and patching will be sufficient in patients with mild weakness
  - glasses with side protection that prevent wind or dust reaching the cornea can be helpful
  - in patients unable to close their eye, lid weights or, in extreme cases, tarsorrophy may be needed.
- Pushing up the corner of the mouth on the weak side with a finger can make the voice much clearer, particularly on the telephone.
- Aberrant reinnervation may follow severe facial nerve weakness; blinking occurs when smiling, or eye closure when eating. Local injection of botulinum toxin into the responsible muscles can help these symptoms.
- If there is severe residual facial weakness, plastic surgeons can straighten the face to some extent with cosmetic procedures.

Hemifacial spasm

There are three treatment strategies:
- Just reassurance if the patient is untroubled by the movements.
- Botulinum toxin injection into the facial muscles, typically 20 units of Dysport at 3 or 4 sites, produces some symptomatic relief for 2–4 months. The dosing schedule and sites vary considerably according to response. It may produce temporary facial weakness.
- Posterior fossa microvascular decompression of the facial nerve is said to have a high chance of success, but the risk of the neurosurgical procedure must be balanced against a potential cure.

Facial myokymia

Local injection of botulinum toxin, 10–20 units of Dysport.

Gustatory sweating

This can occur after surgical procedures on the parotid gland. Aberrant reinnervation of surgically damaged parasympathetic nerves that should supply the parotid gland come to supply cutaneous sweat glands. Subcutaneous botulinum toxin at multiple sites over the area that sweats is effective in abolishing the sweating for 3–6 months.

Ramsay–Hunt syndrome

- Ramsay–Hunt syndrome, or herpes zoster oticus, is the combination, to varying degrees, of VII and VIII nerve palsies with herpetic vesicles in the external ear canal.
- Treatment is of the underlying infection (acyclovir 800 mg oral 5 times daily for 7 days) and of the secondary inflammatory cranial neuritis (prednisolone 40–60 mg/day oral for 7 days).
- Symptomatic treatment with vestibular sedatives may be needed for vertigo (see below).
- The cornea should be protected as in Bell's palsy.

VIII NERVE, BALANCE AND HEARING

Patients who present primarily with hearing difficulties, both hearing loss and tinnitus, fall within the remit of the ear, nose and throat specialist rather than the neurologist, and will not be considered here. From the neurological perspective the most important part of the VIII nerve is the vestibular nerve.

Acute peripheral vestibulopathy

Acute peripheral vestibular lesions are common and rarely is a specific cause found. They are often labelled as 'labyrinthitis', 'vestibular neuronitis' or 'vestibular labyrinthitis' providing an apparent, although spurious, diagnostic certainty as to the cause of the vestibular failure. Fortunately, most lesions are unilateral and recovery, largely through central compensation rather than peripheral vestibular recovery, is the rule.

- Diagnosis:
  - conditions with specific treatments must be excluded, in particular central vestibular syndromes where there are almost always other brainstem symptoms or signs
  - small cerebellar infarcts can be a particular diagnostic difficulty.
- Acute treatment:
  - Poor evidence that corticosteroids, either iv methylprednisolone or oral prednisolone (1 mg/kg daily reducing over 10 days), speed the resolution of symptomatic vertigo, which also clears in untreated patients.

  – At first, patients are very unwell, with severe nausea and vomiting, and often need antiemetics intramuscularly or by suppository (prochlorperazine or metoclopramide). Once the vomiting has settled, these should be switched to oral vestibular sedatives such as cinnarazine, betahistine or scopolamine, which have fewer adverse effects (Table 7.2). All vestibular sedatives should be phased out as

Table 7.2	Drugs used in the oral treatment of acute vertigo			
Drug	**Action**	**Dose**	**Primary symptom**	**Adverse effects and comments**
Prochlorperazine Metoclopamide	Dopamine antagonist	5 mg tds 10 mg tds	Nausea	Acute dystonic reactions in young and parkinsonism in older patients. Drowsiness. Available as oral, rectal or intramuscular preparations
Domperidone	Dopamine antagonist	10 mg tds	Nausea	Does not cross blood–brain barrier
Cinnarizine Cyclizine Meclozine	Antihistamine	30 mg tds 50 mg tds 12.5 mg/day	Dizziness	Drowsiness
Betahistine	Antihistamine	16 mg tds	Dizziness	Promoted as specific therapy for Menière's disease
Hyoscine	Anticholinergic	1 mg in 72 hours (as patch)	Dizziness	Dry mouth, blurred vision. Available as a patch
Diazepam	Benzodiazapine	2–5 mg up to tds	Anxiety	Drowsiness

soon as the symptoms resolve because they interfere with central compensation and may cause parkinsonism.

- Fortunately, after a unilateral vestibular lesion, even if severe, there is usually good functional recovery without the need for specific intervention.
- Patients should be encouraged to gradually increase their activities, and are usually helped if the process of compensation is explained to them.
- Some patients are also helped by physiotherapists advising them about vestibular rehabilitation (exercises described by Cawthorne and Cooksey are the most popular and consist of vestibular stimuli of gradually increasing complexity).

Uncompensated peripheral vestibulopathy

After an acute peripheral vestibular lesion some patients do not compensate as well as others – and frequently remain on long-term vestibular sedatives, particularly prochlorperazine, which may impede their recovery and cause parkinsonism. These patients often have additional symptoms of anxiety and may have significantly limited their day-to-day activities because of their dizziness. Sometimes there is a clear history of a vestibular upset, in others it is less clear and these patients may be labelled as having phobic postural vertigo. If alternative diagnoses are appropriately excluded the treatment includes:

- careful explanation of the nature of central compensation and the need for gradually increasing vestibular stimulation
- avoidance of vestibular sedatives
- vestibular rehabilitation by appropriately trained physiotherapists
- treatment of any associated anxiety or depression (see Chapter 13).

Benign positional vertigo

The most common form of benign positional vertigo is caused by otoconia (debris in the endolymph in the posterior semicircular canal). The otoconia lie at the bottom of the canal, so when the patient moves, the endolymph moves, carrying with it the otoconia. The otoconia then sink back into the lowest point in the canal, again provoking movement in the endolymph, which in turn stimulates the hair cells in the ampulla, provoking a sensation of vertigo. There are two approaches to treatment:

- Epley's manoeuvre (Fig. 7.1), a specific repositioning manoeuvre which clears the otoconia from the canal into the utricle. Patients can be taught to do this at home.

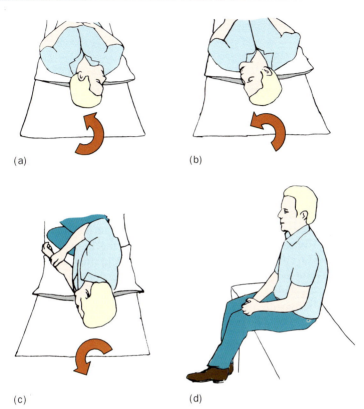

(a)   (b)

(c)   (d)

Fig. 7.1   Modified Epley's manoeuvre. Epley's manoeuvre is relatively acrobatic for older patients and this slight modification keeping the patient on the bed and extending the neck over a pillow (rather than having the head hanging off the end of the couch) makes it easier to do with older patients. The figure shows treatment for right ear benign positional vertigo. Start with the right ear down, neck slightly hyperextended (a). Then, without lifting the head, it is turned to the left (b). The patient then bends their knees and rolls onto their left side so they end up looking down into the couch (c). The patient then sits up (d).

■ Brandt–Daroff exercises (Fig. 7.2), a series of non-specific exercises that may work by clearing the otoconia, or by habituation. They are useful if the history is very suggestive, but Hallpike's manoeuvre is not diagnostic as to the affected side.

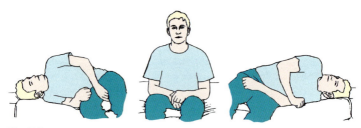

Fig. 7.2 Brandt–Daroff exercises. The patient is advised to swing from one side to the other as indicated, repeating this twice a day for 2 weeks.

Menière's disease

The diagnostic criteria for Menière's disease have been applied more rigorously in recent years making this apparently a much more uncommon disorder. Advice on treatment is hampered by the limited number of randomised trials and the high rate of remission in untreated patients. The main options are treatment of symptomatic dizziness with vestibular sedatives (see above), along with prevention using a low-salt diet, perhaps with bendrofluazide. Destructive procedures, either medical using intratympanic gentamicin or surgery, can be considered but, as the condition is often bilateral, only with the greatest of caution.

Bilateral vestibular failure

Gentamicin toxicity is the most common cause of bilateral vestibular failure, causing profound imbalance and oscillopsia on movement, usually without vertigo. In a patient recovering from severe sepsis this can be misleading, with the poor mobility being initially attributed to the debilitated state rather than bilateral vestibular failure. There is no specific treatment, although patients may compensate well with appropriate vestibular rehabilitation.

Nystagmus and oscillopsia

Oscillopsia is the symptom of movement of the visual world that may result from nystagmus. There are a few situations where there are some therapeutic opportunities:

■ If symptomatic, congenital nystagmus can be improved by ophthalmological and orthoptic manoeuvres, including correction of acuity, prisms and surgery on external ocular muscles.

■ Acquired nystagmus is generally not responsive to treatment unless directed at the underlying condition. There are a few exceptions:

- 3,4-Diaminopyridine 20–100 mg/day or 4-aminopyridine 10 mg/day can improve downbeat nystagmus. Other agents reported to have occasional benefit are gabapentin, clonazepam and baclofen.
- 4-Aminopyridine is also helpful in upbeat nystagmus.
- Acquired pendular nystagmus due to multiple sclerosis has been reported to respond to memantine, a glutamate agonist licensed for Alzheimer's disease (see Chapter 5). Clonazepam and sodium valproate (see Chapter 2) are also reported to help on occasion.
- Periodic alternating nystagmus, in which (as the name suggests) nystagmus switches direction every 2–3 minutes, is caused by a range of brainstem pathologies. Symptomatically it can be suppressed with baclofen (see Chapter 9).

IX, X AND XII NERVES, INCLUDING DYSARTHRIA, DYSPHONIA AND DYSPHAGIA

Isolated IX, X or XII lesions can result from trauma, local involvement with tumours, infection or inflammation. For all causes the treatment is of the primary pathology. In many patients dysarthria and dysphagia are important symptoms, and close liaison with a speech and language therapist is essential, to assess safety of swallowing and provide practical advice to assist communication. Longstanding unilateral vocal cord weakness can be improved by mechanical stiffening of the weakened cord.

Glossopharyngeal neuralgia

This rare neuralgia is treated with the same drugs used for trigeminal neuralgia (see above).

Spasmodic dysphonia

Spasmodic dysphonia is rare. There are two forms, with:
- adduction of the vocal cords when the voice becomes strangled, hoarse and strained
- hyperabduction, when the voice becomes breathy and soft.

Both forms can be helped by botulinum toxin injections given endoscopically into the affected muscles.

Progressive bulbar palsy and pseudobulbar palsy

Patients with progressive dysarthria and dysphagia from whatever cause should be referred to a speech and language therapist who can advise on strategies to:

- aid communication, from voice production to light-writers and more complicated communication aids
- aid swallowing, from advice on how to swallow, diet alterations and use of thickeners, leading up to percutaneous gastrostomy if necessary.

Cerebellar syndromes

There are many causes of cerebellar problems that are part of a more widespread neurological condition, while in others the cerebellar syndrome may appear in isolation. From a therapeutic perspective they can be classified into those syndromes where there is a specific treatment of the underlying cause (Table 7.3), and those where there is no specific treatment. Non-specific interventions include:

- For mild cerebellar syndromes:
  - physiotherapy to assess and assist gait
  - use of stick
  - occupational therapy review at home or work for safety, including appropriate rails, bathing assistance.
- For more severe cerebellar syndromes:
  - physiotherapy to review gait
  - use of wheeled rollator or wheelchair
  - safety of transfers, aids to assist transfers
  - occupational therapy review
  - speech therapy review to advise on improving communication and swallow assessment.

The locked-in syndrome

- The locked-in syndrome is defined by quadriplegia and anarthria with preservation of consciousness, it usually results from lesions in the ventral pons.
- It is caused by basilar artery occlusion, brainstem haemorrhage, multiple sclerosis, osmotic insult or head trauma.
- Initial therapy should be:
  - resuscitation (supporting airway, breathing, oxygenation)
  - treating the cause if possible (e.g. corticosteroids for multiple sclerosis relapse).
- Appropriate nursing support to avoid complications of immobility.
- The most important aspect is to develop a method of communication. Vertical eye movements are usually preserved and can be used as the basis for simple yes/no responses or for letter finding as well as the basis

Table 7.3   Some conditions that involve the cerebellum and for which there are specific treatments

Type of cerebellar syndrome	Potential therapy
Thiamine deficiency	Thiamine (see Chapter 16)
Vitamin E deficiency	Vitamin E (see Chapter 16)
Wilson's disease	Penicillamine, zinc (see Chapter 16)
Refsum's disease	Diet, plasma exchange (see Chapter 16)
Drug toxicity (e.g. phenytoin, carbamazepine, lithium)	Stop drug
Alcohol abuse	Stop alcohol, triamine
Periodic ataxias	Carbamazepine; acetazolamide
Dopa responsive dystonia	Levodopa (see Chapter 6)
Multiple sclerosis	Corticosteroids (see Chapter 9)
Postinfective cerebellitis	Corticosteroids
Lyme disease	Antibiotics (see Chapter 11)
Abscess	Neurosurgery; antibiotics (see Chapter 14)
Paraneoplastic	Treat tumour; immunosuppression (see Chapter 15)
Cerebellar infarct/haemorrhage	Many need posterior fossa decompression to avoid coning (see Chapter 4)
Tumour	Neurosurgery (see Chapter 15)

of more sophisticated patient–computer interfaces using infrared eye-movement sensors. This requires specialist speech therapy and environmental control advice.

Further reading

Baloh RW, Halmagyi GM. Disorders of the vestibular system. Oxford University Press, Oxford, 1996.

Glaser JL. Neuro-ophthalmology, 3rd edn. Lippincott Williams and Wilkins, Baltimore, 1999.

Halmagyi GM. Diagnosis and management of vertigo. Clin Med 2005:159–165.

Neurology in practice. Neuro-ophthalmology and neuro-otology. J Neurol Neurosurg Psychiat 2004; 75(Suppl IV): 1–53.

Smith E, Delargy M. Locked-in syndrome. Br Med J 2005; 330: 406–409.

Straube A. Pharmacology of vertigo/nystagmus/oscillopsia. Curr Opin Neurol 2005; 18: 11–14.

8 COMA, RAISED INTRACRANIAL PRESSURE AND HYDROCEPHALUS

Alejandro A. Rabinstein and Eelco F. M. Wijdicks

Coma

Coma is a state of profound unresponsiveness in which the patient lies motionless, with eyes closed, and cannot be aroused even by painful stimulation.

EMERGENCY MANAGEMENT BEFORE THE CAUSE OF COMA IS ESTABLISHED

Assess airway safety, adequacy of ventilation and circulatory status

- Endotracheal intubation is indicated when:
  - Airway patency is compromised (absent gag and cough reflexes, pooling of respiratory secretions, gurgling).
  - Gas exchange is poor. Pulse oximeter may quickly indicate poor oxygenation, $SaO_2 < 90\%$ (but arterial blood gases must be measured immediately to identify hypoxia, hypercapnia and type of acid–base imbalance).
  - Inefficient breathing pattern is present (irregular, gasping; note that Cheyne–Stokes pattern and central neurogenic hyperventilation are not incompatible with normal gas exchange).

- Fluid resuscitation and, in refractory cases, infusion of vasopressors is indicated when:
  - systolic blood pressure < 90 mmHg (12 kPa)
  - cerebral perfusion pressure (CPP) < 60–70 mmHg (8–9.3 kPa) in patients with traumatic coma (CPP = mean arterial pressure – intracranial pressure).
- All comatose patients must have their cardiac rhythm monitored continuously for potentially life-threatening arrhythmias.

Stabilise cervical spine if trauma suspected or documented

- Cervical collar.
- Obtain cervical spine X-ray or computed tomography (CT) scan.
- Neurosurgery consultation.

Consider treatable life-threatening diseases and, if present, initiate emergency therapy

- All patients in acute coma of uncertain cause must receive:
  - Thiamine 100 mg iv.
  - Dextrose 50% solution, 50 ml iv (after thiamine to prevent potential precipitation of Wernicke's encephalopathy in malnourished patients).
  - Naloxone 0.4–2 mg iv (may repeat in 2–3 minutes if incomplete response). Rapid reversal of opioid effects may result in arousal with delirium as a result of withdrawal.
- When other life-threatening diseases are recognised or suspected, specific emergency treatment must be initiated without delay (see treatment section below).

CAUSES OF COMA

The causes of coma are divided into two main categories: structural intracranial disease and diffuse cerebral dysfunction.

Structural causes of coma

Diseases in this category most often produce focal or lateralising signs on neurological examination and are associated with abnormal brain imaging. But, absence of focal deficits on examination does not necessarily exclude structural damage, as proven by cases of acute hydrocephalus, some cases of meningitis and encephalitis, and postresuscitation anoxic-ischaemic encephalopathy.

Anatomical classification of structural abnormalities that can produce coma

- Hemispheric mass lesion with brain herniation.
- Diffuse bihemispheric damage.
- Bilateral diencephalic lesions.
- Cerebellar mass lesion resulting in brainstem displacement.
- Brainstem lesion involving the ascending reticular activating system.

Pathophysiological classification of structural abnormalities that can produce coma

- Cerebrovascular disease:
  - large hemispheric infarction or haemorrhage with brain herniation
  - acute basilar artery occlusion (with extensive brainstem and/or bilateral thalamic infarction)
  - extensive brainstem haemorrhage
  - large cerebellar infarction or haematoma with brainstem compression
  - aneurysmal subarachnoid haemorrhage
  - intracranial venous thrombosis
  - hypertensive encephalopathy
  - global hypoxia/ischaemia.
- Trauma:
  - diffuse axonal injury
  - brain contusions
  - epidural, subdural, subarachnoid haemorrhage.
- Infections:
  - bacterial meningitis
  - viral encephalitis
  - brain abscess
  - epidural or subdural empyema.
- Immune disorders:
  - acute demyelinating encephalomyelitis
  - autoimmune cerebritis (e.g. lupus cerebritis)
  - cerebral vasculitis.
- Tumours (including pituitary apoplexy).
- Acute hydrocephalus.
- Osmotic myelinolysis (after rapid correction of hyponatraemia).
- Disseminated intravascular coagulation.
- Thrombotic thrombocytopenic purpura.

Coma due to diffuse cerebral dysfunction

This category includes toxic, metabolic, endocrine and other systemic disorders. The patients characteristically do not have focal neurological signs or radiological abnormalities. However, this general rule is not followed in cases of seizures with post-ictal deficits, some instances of severe hypoglycaemia, and certain intoxications.

- Toxic causes:
  - carbon monoxide
  - cyanide
  - ethanol
  - atypical alcohols
  - anticholinergic drug poisoning
  - cholinergic agents (organophosphates, nerve gases)
  - sedative–hypnotic drugs (benzodiazepines, barbiturates, chloral hydrate)
  - opioids (including heroin)
  - sympathomimetics (amphetamines, cocaine, theophylline)
  - psychedelics (lysergic acid diethylamide (LSD), mescaline, phencyclidine (PCP))
  - antidepressants (tricyclics, monoamine oxidase (MAO) inhibitors)
  - neuroleptics (butyrophenones, phenothiazines)
  - lithium.
- Metabolic and endocrine causes:
  - hypoglycaemia
  - diabetic ketoacidosis
  - non-ketotic hyperosmolar coma
  - acute adrenal failure (Addisonian crisis)
  - myxoedema
  - uraemia
  - liver failure with portosystemic shunt
  - sepsis
  - thiamine deficiency (Wernicke's encephalopathy)
  - hyponatraemia
  - hypercalcaemia
  - profound acid–base imbalance.
- Seizures (non-convulsive status epilepticus, post-ictal state).
- Extreme hypothermia or hyperthermia.

DIAGNOSTIC EVALUATION OF COMA

General rules

- Exclude conditions mimicking coma:
  - locked-in syndrome (check for blinking and vertical eye movements)
  - generalised muscle paralysis
  - catatonia
  - extreme abulia
  - psychogenic unresponsiveness.
- Focus first on conditions that demand specific treatment.
- Follow an algorithmic approach that begins by immediately excluding conditions in which recovery depends on the timely institution of a specific acute therapy.

History and physical examination

- The history may hold the most important, and sometimes the only, clues to the correct diagnosis.
- Valuable information may be obtained from family members, paramedics and witnesses of the onset of coma or the preceding events.
- Assign one member of the acute care team to be in charge of collecting information, while others take care of the emergency management of the patient.
- The time following the arrival of the patient to the emergency department may be the only opportunity one has to obtain some vital information.
- Details on medical background, medication or recreational drug use, and exposure to toxic substances should be particularly emphasised.

Initial physical examination should have the following objectives:
- Identify physical signs of focal brain injury or herniation:
  - anisocoria, loss of pupil reactivity to light
  - forced deviation of the eyes (horizontal or vertical)
  - absence of corneal, oculocephalic, oculocaloric reflexes
  - asymmetrical motor response to pain.
- Search for signs of meningeal irritation.
- Carefully inspect the patient for subtle rhythmic movements:
  - nystagmoid jerks or barely noticeable finger or facial repetitive movements may be the only evidence of non-convulsive status epilepticus
  - generalised myoclonus status epilepticus (multifocal, repetitive, unrelenting) may indicate major anoxic injury or intoxication.

- Look for signs of systemic illness on general examination:
  - external signs of trauma
  - fever
  - inspection of the skin, rashes, etc.
  - special attention to the breath odour.

Investigations

- Brain imaging:
  - CT brain scan without contrast is sufficient for initial evaluation in most cases
  - in patients with a normal CT scan, a magnetic resonance imaging (MRI) scan with diffusion-weighted imaging may demonstrate diffuse cortical damage in patients with prolonged status epilepticus or global anoxia/ischaemia, and brainstem ischaemia in patients with acute basilar occlusion
  - MRI can also offer better visualisation of areas of inflammation in encephalitis, plaques of demyelination in acute disseminated encephalomyelitis, multiple small ischaemic lesions in vasculitis and regions of osmotic demyelination
  - magnetic resonance venography may confirm intracranial venous thrombosis.
- Blood analysis:
  - glucose
  - arterial blood gases
  - electrolytes (sodium, calcium)
  - liver function and ammonia (hyperammonaemia can occur with normal levels of transaminases in end-stage cirrhosis and due to a genetic defect alone)
  - renal function
  - serum osmolality (must be measured, since the presence of a gap between measured and calculated osmolality may point to the diagnosis of poisoning with an atypical alcohol)
  - full blood count
  - platelet count, prothrombin time, partial thromboplastin time (prior to lumbar puncture)
  - urine toxicology screen
  - serum alcohol level
  - in selected cases, thyroid function, serum levels of specific drugs, urine keto acids, blood cultures, cortisol.

- Cerebrospinal fluid (CSF) analysis:
  - lumbar puncture should be performed urgently if signs of meningeal irritation or unexplained fever are present, and there are no contraindications (brain lesion with extensive mass effect or profound haemorrhagic diathesis)
  - analysis should include cell count, glucose, protein, microbiological stains and cultures
  - try to preserve some fluid for any additional analyses that may become necessary as the investigation evolves.
- Electroencephalogram (EEG):
  - the only reliable way to exclude non-convulsive status epilepticus
  - certain findings may have prognostic implications (discussed below).
- Cerebral angiography:
  - when acute basilar occlusion is suspected, angiography may confirm the diagnosis and enable thrombolytic therapy.

Assessment of severity and clinical monitoring

The Glasgow Coma Scale (GCS) (Box 8.1) is used to assess initial clinical severity and to monitor the neurological status of patients with altered consciousness. Designed for the evaluation of head-trauma patients, its application has become expanded to other acute neurological diseases. Its great practical value is mainly its simplicity and good interrater reliability. However, it should *never* replace a more comprehensive neurological examination (e.g. the GCS offers no information on asymmetry of reflexes or motor function) (Table 8.1).

TREATMENT OF COMA
General supportive care

It is important to minimise secondary injury to the brain in all comatose patients: any hypoxaemia, hypotension, hyperthermia and hyperglycaemia should all be aggressively prevented.

Specific treatments

See Table 8.1.

PROGNOSIS OF COMA

- Daily clinical examination is the most valuable prognostic tool.
- Confounding factors, such as sedatives and paralytic drugs, should be avoided as much as possible.

Table 8.1   Treatments for specific causes of coma

Diagnosis	Treatment
Focal intra- or extra-axial mass lesion with incipient signs of herniation	Osmotherapy, corticosteroids (if vasogenic oedema), hyperventilation, surgical resection, evacuation or decompression
Hydrocephalus	Ventricular drainage
Recent basilar artery thrombosis	Thrombolysis (intravenous, intra-arterial, mechanical)
Intracranial venous thrombosis	Heparin
Hypertensive encephalopathy	Vasodilators
Meningitis, encephalitis	Antimicrobials
Brain abscess	Antimicrobials, surgical evacuation
Intoxications, poisonings	Antidotes when available,* dialysis when necessary
Carbon monoxide poisoning	100% oxygen, or hyperbaric oxygen chamber if available
Cyanide poisoning	Amyl nitrate, sodium thiosulphate, 100% oxygen, hyperbaric oxygen chamber if refractory
Acute renal failure	Dialysis
Portosystemic encephalopathy	Lactulose, liver transplantation
Hypoglycaemia	Dextrose
Diabetic ketoacidosis	Hydration, insulin
Non-ketotic hyperosmolality	Hydration
Pituitary apoplexy	Corticosteroids
Addisonian crisis	Corticosteroids
Myxoedema	Thyroid hormone
Thyrotoxicosis	Antithyroid drugs, Lugol's solution, beta-blockers
Wernicke's encephalopathy	Thiamine

Continued

Table 8.1 *Continued*

Diagnosis	Treatment
Sepsis	Antimicrobials
Extreme hypothermia	Rewarming

*Flumazenil may be effective in reversing benzodiazepine toxicity but can produce arousal in patients with portosystemic encephalopathy. Its effects are short lasting and it may precipitate seizures. This drug should be used with caution.

Box 8.1   Glasgow Coma Scale

Activity/response	Score
Eye opening (E)	
Spontaneous	4
After verbal stimulus	3
After painful stimulus	2
None	1
Verbal response (V)	
Oriented	5
Confused	4
Inappropriate but recognizable words	3
Incomprehensible sounds	2
None	1
Best motor response (M)	
Obeys verbal commands	6
Localizes painful stimulus	5
Withdraws to painful stimulus	4
Abnormal flexion posturing	3
Abnormal extensor posturing	2
None	1

Caveats in the use of the GCS include:

- The sum score is less informative than the scores of each of the three individual components.
- The value is more limited in ventilated patients (a letter T should be added to the sum score in these patients to denote this limitation).
- The same sum score can be seen in patients with markedly different degrees of unresponsiveness.
- Serial scores are more useful than any isolated, single assessment.

- The underlying cause of the coma is the most important determinant of outcome.
- Outcome is poorest among patients with anoxic–ischaemic coma:
  - chances of awakening decrease rapidly (from 34% in patients comatose at day 1, to at best 13% after 14 days)
  - recovery of independence is very unlikely (approximately 6%) among patients who remain unconscious at 24 hours
  - absent pupillary light reflex at day 1 and withdrawal to pain at day 3 predict lack of recovery beyond severe functional disability
  - other prognosticators of poor outcome are myoclonic status epilepticus, sustained upward gaze, absent cortical scalp somatosensory evoked potentials, burst-suppression electroencephalographic pattern, and evidence of extensive cortical damage on MRI.
- Among patients with toxic–metabolic coma, the outcome is more variable and depends largely on the reversibility of the primary disorder and the presence of secondary brain insults (mainly ischaemia or hypoxia).
- Traumatic coma has a far more favourable prognosis in certain circumstances:
  - patients in coma for more than 6 hours after injury still have a 40% chance of achieving good functional recovery
  - meaningful recovery may continue for 1 year or longer, especially in young patients
  - poor prognostic indicators are older age, GCS sum score of 3 after resuscitation, profound hypoxia or hypotension at the time of first aid, and refractory intracranial hypertension.
- Structural causes of coma (apart from trauma) are generally associated with extremely limited chances of meaningful recovery (although with exceptions such as cerebellar haematoma after evacuation).

Persistent vegetative state

- Some comatose patients evolve to recover sleep–wake cycles but remain totally unaware of themselves and their environment.
- When this condition has been present for longer than 1 month, it is conventionally called the persistent vegetative state.
- This state of chronic wakefulness without awareness is very uncommon.
- However, it has been the subject of endless ethical and legal debate because patients can survive without neurological improvement for many years as long as supportive care is provided.

- The term *permanent vegetative state* has been coined to emphasise the irreversible nature of the condition when many months or years have elapsed and the patient remains unchanged.
- More recently the functional category of *minimally conscious state* was coined for those patients who demonstrate inconsistent but discernible evidence of conscious awareness. Although this condition is often transient, it may become permanent in some cases. The condition remains poorly defined, possibly ambiguous, and requires prospective follow-up studies.

Brain death

Definition

Brain death implies the irreversible cessation of all brainstem function. Its definition requires the unequivocal documentation of complete loss of consciousness, absent motor response to pain, absent brainstem reflexes, and apnoea. Ideally it also requires the exclusion of possible confounding factors and the establishment of the cause of the coma, with demonstration of a structural central nervous system abnormality commensurate with the clinical findings.

Clinical criteria

There must be no:
- pupillary response to bright light; the pupils are typically midsize, but may be dilated
- ocular movements, including oculocephalic and oculocaloric reflexes
- corneal reflexes
- cough reflex despite deep stimulation (suction catheter at the level of the carina) and no gag reflex
- motor response to strong painful stimulation
- ventilatory effort (due to lack of respiratory drive) formally demonstrated with the apnoea test (Fig. 8.1).

Confirmatory tests

- Cerebral angiography shows no intracerebral filling with contrast.
- EEG demonstrates total electrical silence and no reactivity to intense somatosensory or auditory or visual stimuli. Technical requirements: 8 or more scalp electrodes, interelectrode distance ≥ 10 cm, sensitivity ≥ 2 microvolt, recording for ≥ 30 minutes, high-frequency filter > 30 Hz, low-frequency filter < 1 Hz.

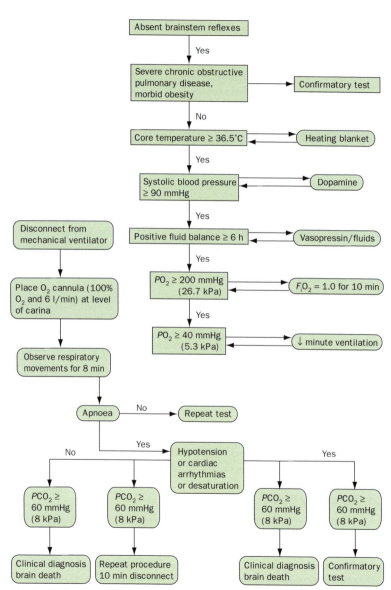

Fig. 8.1   The apnoea test.

- Transcranial Doppler ultrasonography shows no diastolic or reverberating flow and small systolic peaks in early systole.
- Cerebral scintigraphy ([technetium-99m]hexametazime) shows no intracranial radionuclide uptake.

Caveats in the determination of brain death

- Criteria and legal requirements differ in different countries. Thus, the practitioner must be familiar with local regulations.
- Hypothermia and drug intoxication can mimic brain death. Therefore, these factors must be excluded prior to the diagnosis of brain death. Before proceeding with testing for brain death:
  - core body temperature must be > 32°C
  - the patient must not be hypotensive (systolic blood pressure < 90 mmHg (12 kPa))
  - major medical complications that may confound clinical assessment must be excluded or corrected (especially severe electrolyte, acid–base or endocrine disturbances)
  - no evidence of drug intoxication, poisoning or pharmacological neuromuscular paralysis.
- Spinal cord reflexes may generate spontaneous movements of the limbs or the trunk that are not incompatible with the diagnosis of brain death.

Raised intracranial pressure

This is the pathological condition resulting from increased intracranial volume. In practice, it is defined as an intracranial pressure (ICP) exceeding 20 cmH$_2$O or 15 mmHg (2 kPa).

Causes

- Intracranial mass:
  - intra-axial
  - extra-axial.
- Cerebral oedema:
  - cytotoxic
  - vasogenic.
- Increased CSF volume:
  - decreased CSF absorption
  - venous drainage obstruction
  - CSF overproduction.

■ Increased intracranial blood volume:
  – vasodilatation
  – venous drainage obstruction.

Intracranial pressure monitoring (Table 8.2)

Indications

■ Traumatic brain injury with a GCS sum score of 3–8 and:
  – abnormal CT scan
  – normal CT scan but 2 or more of: age > 40 years, unilateral or bilateral limb posturing, systolic blood pressure < 90 mmHg (12 kPa).
■ Acute hydrocephalus of any cause (use ventricular catheter for drainage).
■ Lobar or ganglionic haemorrhage with coma and brain tissue shift (optional).

Table 8.2 Options for monitoring intracranial pressure		
Monitoring type	**Advantages**	**Disadvantages**
Intraparenchymal	Low maintenance	Expensive
	Reliable waveforms	Fragile
	No major drift	No possibility of drainage
	Simple insertion technique	
	May be combined with temperature and oxygen sensors	
	Lower risk of ventriculitis	
Intraventricular	Allows CSF drainage	Higher risk of ventriculitis
	Less expensive	Dampening of waveform (due to blockage by blood or apposition of catheter tip against ventricular wall, air bubble)
	Less fragile	
		Requires daily calibration
		More complex and riskier insertion procedure
Epidural and subdural	Lower risk of bleeding in coagulopathic patients	Less reliable readings

■ Massive hemispheric infarction with coma and brain tissue shift (optional).

Treatment

■ The approach to the treatment of raised ICP is in a stepwise fashion (Fig. 8.2).
■ Whenever possible, surgical removal of an intracranial mass lesion should be pursued.

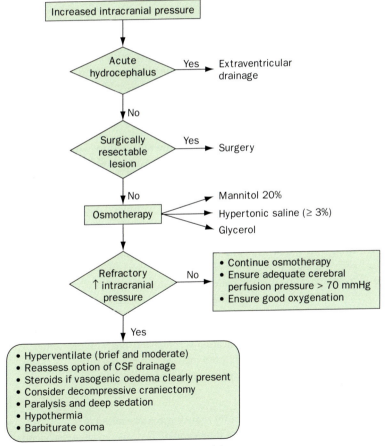

Fig. 8.2 Measures to control raised intracranial pressure.

- CSF drainage through a ventriculostomy catheter is indispensable and urgent in cases of acute hydrocephalus.

Other general and specific measures to control raised ICP are discussed below.

General measures

- Ensure adequate oxygenation and cerebral perfusion.
- Maintain normovolaemia.
- Keep head in neutral position and head of bed elevated at 30° (except when shock, orthostatic fall of blood pressure or pneumocephalus).
- Treat fever aggressively.
- Avoid or treat agitation and pain.

Osmotic therapy

- Very effective in achieving sustained reduction in ICP, and the mainstay of therapy in most cases of acute intracranial hypertension.
- Mannitol (20% solution) is the most commonly used agent:
  - It is given in boluses of 0.5–1.5 g/kg as needed according to ICP or clinical response, or as scheduled doses of 0.25–0.75 g/kg every 4–6 hours.
  - The main potential complication is acute renal failure, which can be averted by carefully avoiding volume contraction. Keeping serum osmolality at < 320 mOsm/l also helps, but higher osmolalities can be tolerated as long as the patient remains normovolaemic. Renal function usually recovers once mannitol is stopped and adequate hydration provided.
  - Although it is a theoretical concern, there is no proof that mannitol worsens ICP gradients in patients with focal brain lesions by preferentially dehydrating normal brain.
- Hypertonic saline is a good alternative osmotic agent:
  - It can be used as repeated boluses of 3–10% solution (e.g. 1–2 ml/kg at 20 ml/minute) or, in recalcitrant cases, as a bolus of 30 ml of 23.4% solution over 15–20 minutes.
  - The main potential complication is congestive heart failure. Other adverse effects to be monitored include hypernatraemia, hypokalaemia and hyperchloraemic acidaemia.

Hyperventilation

- Very effective means of rapidly reducing acutely raised ICP.
- Prolonged use and profound hypocapnia/alkalosis can cause ischaemia due to cerebral vasoconstriction.

- Effect decreases over time due to metabolic buffering of alkalotic CSF.
- Recommend using for periods < 30 minutes and with a PCO_2 target of 30–34 mmHg (4–4.5 kPa).
- Best used as a 'bridge' to other interventions with longer term efficacy.

Corticosteroids

- Useful only for patients with documented vasogenic oedema, such as infections and tumours.
- Detrimental in patients with head trauma, ischaemic stroke or intracerebral haemorrhage.
- Dexamethasone is most commonly used. Doses range between 4 and 10 mg iv every 6 hours.
- Main risks include hyperglycaemia, hypertension, gastrointestinal bleeding and sepsis.

Decompressive craniectomy

- This has been performed with good effect in patients with cerebellar infarction or haematoma (suboccipital craniectomy), large hemispheric infarcts (hemicraniectomy) or severe head trauma (hemi- or holocraniectomy).
- Patient selection and timing are crucial. Good candidates are those with potential for recovery and rehabilitation. Best timing is before clinical signs of herniation are present.
- Hemicraniectomy should be offered only to acute stroke patients who have a chance of achieving meaningful functional recovery. Although often life-saving, it very rarely leads to functional independence among older patients with comorbid conditions.

Hypothermia

- Hypothermia may be effective in cases refractory to other measures. However, evidence is limited.
- Target core temperature should be 32–34°C:
  - induction of hypothermia may be achieved with cooling blankets, ice packs, gastric lavage with iced water, cooling vests or intravascular cooling catheters (the latter two being the most effective)
  - antishivering drugs are required (meperidine, buspirone) and often deep sedation (with propofol) and, less frequently, neuromuscular paralysis may be necessary
  - rewarming may be initiated after 24–48 hours and must be very gradual.

- There are many potential complications, but these are much less frequent when hypothermia is moderate (not below 32°C) and rewarming is carefully controlled:
  - increased risk of infection
  - cardiac arrhythmias
  - thrombocytopenia
  - electrolyte imbalance
  - rebound increase of ICP after rewarming.

Barbiturates

- Reserved for patients with uncontrollable intracranial hypertension despite institution of all the previous measures.
- Requires EEG monitoring. Aim for 20% burst activity and 80% suppression.
- Many potential complications, which may be very severe:
  - increased susceptibility to infections, particularly pneumonia
  - hypotension (often profound and refractory)
  - myocardial depression
  - liver failure.
- Barbiturates complicate brain death determination (clearance of pentobarbital may take several days after discontinuation of the infusion).

Idiopathic intracranial hypertension

This condition is characterised by increased ICP without localising signs, except for papilloedema, but no evidence of any structural brain disorder or CSF abnormalities.

Pathophysiology

- Uncertain cause and mechanism.
- Raised intracranial venous sinus pressure appears to be a consequence rather than the cause of the disease.
- Identifiable causes of raised ICP must be excluded before the diagnosis of idiopathic intracranial hypertension can be made.
- Obesity or pronounced weight gain, especially in young women, is often associated with this disorder.

Management

The aim is to ameliorate the symptoms (particularly headache) and to prevent visual loss.

Medical treatment

- There are no randomised trials for any medical or other treatment options.
- Weight loss through dietary counselling and a structured aerobic exercise programme should be the mainstay of treatment for obese patients and those who have recently gained weight.
- Acetazolamide may be effective by reducing CSF production and intraocular pressure. Recommended doses range from 1 to 4 g/day oral in 2–4 divided doses.
- Frusemide 40–160 mg/day oral may be helpful, especially when used in combination with acetazolamide.
- Chlorthalidone or other thiazides may be preferable in pregnancy because they are less teratogenic.
- Oral glycerol 0.5–1 g/kg of body weight 3–4 times daily may successfully lower ICP, but its use is hampered by its high caloric content and frequent adverse effects (hyperglycaemia, gastric irritation).
- Although frequently used, corticosteroids should be reserved for acute severe cases since they may increase intraocular pressure and promote additional weight gain. High-dose methylprednisolone 250 mg iv four times daily may be administered for 3–5 days in an attempt to avoid surgery.
- Frequent lumbar punctures with removal of large volumes of CSF (30–50 ml) may be a helpful temporising measure, but are rarely effective over time when not combined with other therapeutic alternatives.

Surgical treatments

- These should be considered in patients with progressive visual loss despite medical therapy, or with severe visual deficits on presentation.
- Lumboperitoneal shunting is often effective, but shunt failure may precipitate sudden visual loss and re-operation for malfunction is often needed.
- Optic nerve sheath decompression offers high rates of success in preserving visual function when timely performed. It is generally well tolerated and has a low risk of complications. Headaches also improve in 50–90% of cases.

Hydrocephalus

ACUTE HYDROCEPHALUS

Acute hydrocephalus is traditionally classified as:
- Obstructive or non-communicating, caused by obstruction in the passage of CSF within the ventricular system.

- Communicating, caused by decreased reabsorption or, rarely, increased production of CSF with normal ventricular fluid transit.

Regardless of the underlying cause, the treatment of acute symptomatic hydrocephalus is external ventricular drainage with a ventriculostomy catheter in most cases.

Endoscopic surgery for direct drainage of the third ventricle is needed in cases of obstruction at the level of the fourth ventricle.

In cases of persistent symptomatic hydrocephalus preventing removal of the ventriculostomy catheter (i.e. recurrence of symptoms when the pressure level of drainage is raised or the catheter is clamped), a ventriculoperitoneal shunt is indicated.

NORMAL PRESSURE HYDROCEPHALUS

Normal pressure hydrocephalus is a form of chronic communicating hydrocephalus, either idiopathic or secondary to subarachnoid haemorrhage, meningitis or head trauma. Abnormalities in the CSF formation and reabsorption lead to intermittent rises in CSF pressure with distension of the ventricles and damage to the adjacent subcortical white matter of the brain. This leads to gait disturbance, urinary incontinence and a subcortical dementia. CT or MRI imaging of the brain reveals dilated ventricles and normal cerebrocortical sulci.

Ventriculoperitoneal or lumboperitoneal shunting may be effective, at least in improving the gait if not any dementia, but only when performed early in the course of the disease and in properly selected patients.

Patient selection for shunting

The issue of patient selection remains highly controversial. Practical factors predicting favourable response to shunting include:
- younger age
- known cause of communicating hydrocephalus
- clear improvement after trial of CSF removal (large volume lumbar puncture or temporary continuous lumbar drainage)
- no advanced dementia
- no other explanation for the neurological symptoms (e.g. subcortical ischaemia, severe brain atrophy)
- no systemic conditions increasing the risk of surgical or postsurgical complications.

Complications of shunting

Overall, complications of ventriculoperitoneal shunting are relatively common, occurring in 20–40% of cases at different time points:

■ Intraoperative:
  – intracranial haemorrhage
  – complications related to general anaesthesia
  – intra-abdominal injury (rare).
■ Perioperative:
  – shunt infection
  – CSF overdrainage causing subdural haematomas or hygromas, and the intracranial hypotension syndrome
  – systemic complications (due to immobility, infections, thrombosis, etc.).
■ Medium- and long-term:
  – shunt occlusion (proximal or distal)
  – catheter breakage or dislocation.

Valve selection

■ Different types of shunt valves have been designed to optimise drainage while minimising the risk of overdrainage.
■ Conventional fixed low-pressure valves offer the best rates of improvement of the original neurological symptoms but are associated with the highest risk of excessive drainage.
■ The hydrostatic dual-pressure valve (Miethke dual-switch valve) is designed to avoid overdrainage when the patient is in the upright position and has been associated with fewer complications from overdrainage.
■ Programmable differential pressure valves (Codman–Hakim) have the advantage of allowing postoperative non-invasive adjustment of pressure drainage. Reprogramming has been shown to improve patients with no meaningful initial clinical improvement due to inadequate drainage, and to reverse complications from overdrainage.
■ Lessening effect 2–3 years after shunt placement is not uncommon, and so adjustment of valve resistance over time may be helpful.

Further reading

Manno EM. When to use hyperventilation, mannitol, or corticosteroids to reduce increased intracranial pressure from cerebral edema. In: Tough calls in acute neurology (Rabinstein AA, Wijdicks EFM, eds). Elsevier, Philadelphia, 2004.

Vanneste JAL. Diagnosis and management of normal pressure hydrocephalus. J Neurol 2000; 247: 5–14.

Wijdicks EFM. The diagnosis of brain death. N Engl J Med 2001; 344: 1215–1221.

Wijdicks EFM. Brain death worldwide. Accepted fact but no global consensus in diagnostic criteria. Neurology 2002; 58: 20–25.

Wijdicks EFM. Catastrophic neurological disorders in the emergency department, 2nd edn. Oxford University Press, Oxford, 2004.

Zandbergen EG, de Haan RJ, Stoutenbeek CP, Koelman JH, Hijdra A. Systematic review of early prediction of poor outcome in anoxic-ischaemic coma. Lancet 1998; 352: 1808–1812.

9 MULTIPLE SCLEROSIS AND OTHER INFLAMMATORY CNS DISORDERS

Jackie Palace

Chapter contents

Multiple sclerosis (MS) is an acquired chronic relapsing or progressive inflammatory CNS disorder characterised pathologically by demyelinating white matter plaques. Acutely these lesions are associated with an inflammatory infiltrate which resolves to leave a chronic astrocyte and oligodendrocyte depleted plaque. Neuronal and axonal, non-lesional white matter and grey matter involvement are also recognised features of the pathology.

The *clinical* definition requires objective evidence of symptomatic lesions and for them to be disseminated in time and space. Additionally there should be no better alternative diagnosis.

DIAGNOSIS

When the typical clinical features occur in a young adult and are associated with positive investigations (brain MRI and CSF) the diagnosis of MS is straightforward.

Red flags for other diagnoses include:

- Atypical brain MRI appearances, or CSF findings.
- Onset in childhood or old age.
- Ethnic origin (e.g. MS is unusual in black Africans).
- Abrupt onset or unusual symptoms.
- Involvement outside the CNS (either peripheral nervous system or systemic).
- Chronic symptoms that respond to steroids.

- Relapse symptoms that rebound when steroids are withdrawn.
- Isolated optic nerve and/or spinal cord disease.

TYPES OF MS

MS is conventionally divided into two main clinical types:
- A relapsing–remitting/secondary progressive group.
- A primary progressive group.

Because relapses can be superimposed on the progressive phase, stability between relapses is a key feature of relapsing–remitting MS. Relapsing–remitting MS is referred to as 'benign' if disability is mild many years after onset. Malignant MS can be relapsing or progressive.

THE BURDEN OF MS

- MS incidence is about 1:200,000 population per annum (in the UK).
- MS prevalence is about 1:800 population (in the UK).
- MS is the commonest cause of progressive disability in young adults in the UK.
- Fifteen years from diagnosis about half of patients have significant trouble walking, requiring an aid or wheelchair.
- Considering the mean age of onset is in the third or fourth decade, MS has a serious impact on child care and financial status (unemployment is high: 50–80%).
- Life expectancy is not greatly reduced.
- Favourable prognostic factors include:
  - the relapsing–remitting type of disease
  - younger age at onset
  - female gender
  - initial sensory or optic nerve episode.
- However, these are not strong predictors. The number of relapses in the first year (small), the interval between the first and second relapse (long) and MRI activity may be better predictors of a good prognosis.
- It is not clear if the increased frequency of MS reported in recent studies is due to improved healthcare surveillance and advances in investigational techniques, or is real.

There is marked geographical variation in the frequency of MS. It is rare in equatorial regions and generally increases as one moves towards higher latitudes. It is most common in northern and central Europe, Canada and the northern USA, New Zealand and south-eastern Australia. These variations are likely to be influenced by (or a product of) both genetic and environmental factors.

GENERAL MANAGEMENT

The key features of MS that need to be considered when assessing management are:

- The emotional reaction to the diagnosis and the MS symptoms (exacerbated by uncertainty due to the variable and unpredictable nature of MS).
- Its chronic and progressive/relapsing–remitting nature requiring continual adaptation and changes in management due to new symptoms and increasing disability.
- The financial and family implications, considering that most patients are young/middle-aged adults.
- The complexity and range of symptoms requiring the input of many different experts.
- Individual variation making no two patients quite the same.

A multidisciplinary MS service and rehabilitation

Management requires coordinated multidisciplinary input (including doctors, nurses, physiotherapists, occupational and speech therapists, psychologists, counsellors, social workers, continence advisors, orthotic and wheelchair services), which is individually tailored and has the flexibility to reassess and adapt to changing patient needs. This defines the philosophy of rehabilitation. In many specialist MS units this approach has extended to include services for the early diagnostic and acute care of MS.

Counselling and education

Conveying reliable information, which is timed appropriately, usually requires a number of contacts with a knowledgeable professional such as an MS nurse who can also provide advice about where to get any more information that the patient may want.

- A common concern among patients is the risk of passing MS to their offspring – their lifetime risk is about 2%, a 20-fold increase above background.
- The risk of developing the disease in a monozygotic twin of an affected twin is about 25%.
- The risk of developing the disease in a dizygotic twin of an affected twin is about 4%, the same as in a non-twin sibling.

- Variability in the disease phenotype (i.e. severity and relapsing–remitting versus primary progressive disease) is seen between affected family members.

TREATMENT OF SYMPTOMS

Sensory and paroxysmal symptoms

- Reassurance:
  - when associated with a relapse that the symptoms are likely to resolve
  - with longer lasting but stable symptoms that they are residual and do not represent new pathology (or a relapse).
- Drug treatment:
  - dysaesthetic symptoms occurring as part of short-duration relapses may not need any pharmaceutical treatment
  - the treatment of longer lasting or severe dysaesthesias and trigeminal neuralgia is covered in Chapters 18 and 7 respectively
  - typical paroxysmal attacks, including Lhermittes's symptom, tend to be remarkably responsive to carbamazepine at low doses (i.e. 100 mg twice daily) (see also Chapter 2).

Sphincter and sexual problems

The treatment of these conditions is covered in detail in Chapter 17.

- Many patients resist intermittent self-catheterisation despite large postmicturition urinary volumes. This is usually due to their negative image of the technique itself, or to the implication that this procedure means significant MS disability. However, the technique may offer immediate symptomatic benefit and possibly longer term benefits on the bladder and kidney. In addition, because urinary tract infections may precipitate relapses and make background MS symptoms (such as spasticity) worse, intermittent self-catheterisation may have specific benefits in MS treatment.
- Faecal incontinence can be helped by regular toileting with or without pharmacological intervention (see also Chapter 17).

Depression and fatigue

- The symptoms of depression and fatigue are similar and may be difficult to disentangle; sometimes a trial of antidepressants (see Chapter 13) may be necessary (Fig. 9.1).

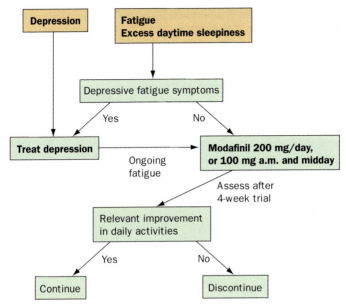

Fig. 9.1 The relationship between fatigue, depression and their treatment in MS.

- Features that suggest fatigue is MS related and not depressive include:
  - worsening as the day goes on
  - improvement with rest
  - worsening of specific physical MS symptoms
  - absence of depressive symptoms.
- Tricyclic antidepressants are favoured by many neurologists because they help multiple and commonly co-existing symptoms such as detrusor hyperreflexia and dysaesthesia.
- Counselling and emotional support are also helpful.
- Modafinil 200 mg/day (divided in one or two doses, see Table 9.1 and Chapter 3) improves fatigue in some MS patients, possibly by reducing excessive daytime sleepiness.
- Amantidine is rarely useful for fatigue at recommended safe doses (up to 400 mg/day in two divided doses).
- Practical advice should be offered, such as reducing unnecessary physical activity, moving physical tasks to the morning when fatigue is less troublesome, and taking a midday nap.

Table 9.1   Drugs for the treatment of fatigue and spasticity

Drug	Regimen	Adverse effects	Licence
Fatigue (MS specific), excessive daytime sleepiness			
Modafinil	200 mg orally daily (1–2 divided doses)	Insomnia, agitation, confusion, headache, gastrointestinal disturbance, cardiac problems Contraindicated with significant cardiac disease, pregnancy and breast-feeding	Treatment of excessive sleepiness in patients with chronic pathological conditions
Spasticity			
Baclofen	5 mg/day to 20 mg 4 times daily, orally	Drowsiness, gastrointestinal symptoms, headache, dizziness, insomnia, weakness, fatigue, confusional state, rarely asthma Contraindicated in peptic ulceration Avoid abrupt withdrawal	Spasticity
Tizanidine	Slow increase from 2 to 24–36 mg/day, orally (3–4 divided doses)	Drowsiness, gastrointestinal symptoms, dizziness, insomnia, fatigue, weakness, hallucinations, hepatotoxicity (monitor liver function every 4 months or if symptomatic), cardiac problems	Spasticity
Dantrolene	Slow increase from 25 mg once daily orally, to maximum 100 mg 4 times daily; usual daily dose 100–200 mg	Drowsiness, fatigue, gastrointestinal symptoms, allergy, weakness, hepatotoxicity (regular monitoring required)	Spasticity
Diazepam	Usual dose: 2 mg orally to 5 mg 3 times daily; maximum 60 mg/day	Drowsiness, fatigue, unsteadiness, confusion, withdrawal symptoms unless reduced slowly, gastrointestinal symptoms	Spasticity

Table 9.1	*Continued*		
Drug	**Regimen**	**Adverse effects**	**Licence**
Gabapentin	Up to 400 mg 3 times daily, orally	Positive effect seen in small studies only	Not for spasticity
		Drowsiness, oedema, gastrointestinal symptoms	
		Avoid abrupt withdrawal	
Botulinum toxin	Equivalent to Dysport 100–1500 units	Weakness	Not for general spasticity
		Contraindicated in myasthenia and breast-feeding	

Spasticity

Spasticity is a complex problem and may require a combination of:

- Physiotherapy.
- Reduction in exacerbating factors (poor posture, pain, infections and bladder distension).
- Pharmacological treatment (see Table 9.1).
- Oral baclofen is the most useful first-line agent due to its efficacy, reasonable adverse-effect profile and ease of dose titration.
- Tizanidine, dantrolene and benzodiazepines are reserved as second-line agents, and are often most useful in combination with baclofen.
- Removing spastic tone in patients with critical lower limb weakness can worsen mobility. It is not clear if there is a separate effect of these antispastic drugs on muscle power.
- Many patients take cannabis for spasticity (as well as pain and bladder irritability). However, the cannabinoid effect on spasticity has not been definitely proven in formal trials. *Sativex*, a cannabinoid, has been licensed in Canada, but the application was refused in the UK on the data available.
- Botulinum toxin injection can help focal spasticity.
- Intrathecal baclofen and phenol have a limited role in severe spasticity and should only be used in experienced units.

Ataxia, oscillopsia and MS-related tremor

- No convincingly effective drug treatments for tremor or ataxia.
- Gabapentin, baclofen and clonazepam may be tried for oscillopsia.
- Physiotherapy advice on stability, posture and walking aids for ataxia.
- Weighted arm bands and practical aids may reduce tremor associated with upper-limb disability.
- Stereotactic brain surgery may help the tremor temporarily, but there may be an adverse effect on the underlying MS activity.

Foot drop

- The dropped foot stimulator works by stimulating contraction of inactive muscles, and also may relax the calf muscles and thus be helpful in foot drop associated with weakness or spasticity.

TREATMENT OF RELAPSES

See Figure 9.2 and Table 9.2.

General

- Most relapses need no treatment, or only a short course of symptomatic management.
- Infection may be the precipitant and antibiotics rather than corticosteroids may be indicated.
- Excluding a urinary tract infection prior to corticosteroid treatment is advisable.

Patients appreciate:
- Prior education as to the nature and treatment options for relapses.
- Support during relapses by the MS team (via a nurse phone line or a relapse clinic).

Corticosteroid treatment

Corticosteroids can be used to speed up natural recovery from a relapse, but because of their adverse-effect profile are only recommended for severe relapses, or where activities of daily living are significantly compromised. This caution is because there is no convincing evidence for (or against) any long-term benefit.

The optimal regimen is not clear, but any differences in outcome between the suggested regimens are not large.

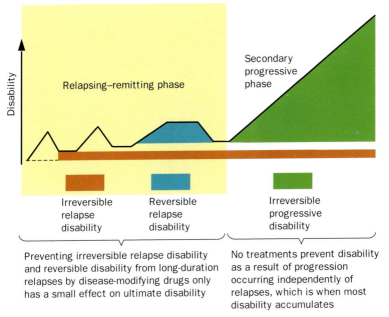

Fig. 9.2   Different ways of influencing disability.

Intravenous immunoglobulin (IVIg) and plasma exchange

When relapses are severe these treatments can be helpful if corticosteroids are contraindicated. Additionally, dramatic responses have been reported in steroid-resistant relapses, but these tend to be in atypical MS patients.

DISEASE-MODIFYING THERAPIES

See Table 9.3.

Immunomodulation

It appears relatively easy to reduce inflammatory activity as measured by the appearance of new MRI brain lesions and relapse frequency, but the effect of the present treatments on disability is disappointing. However, any effect on progressive disability may have been missed by the short-term trials and so it is conceivable that neuroaxonal damage will be prevented by reducing earlier inflammation. This unproven theory is behind the trend to treat early before the damage has been 'pre-programmed'.

Table 9.2   Drugs for the treatment of relapse in MS

Drug	Recommended indication	Regimen	Monitoring safety and response	Adverse effects	License
Corticosteroids	Acute and significantly disabling relapse	Methylprednisolone 1 g/day for 3 days, or 500 mg/day for 5 days, iv or oral, ± oral prednisolone, taper by 60–80 mg/day over 3 weeks	Infection screen prior to starting (even if asymptomatic do urine culture)	Mood change, insomnia, diabetes, infection, aseptic bone necrosis	Not for MS
	Initial therapy in Behçet's disease, systemic lupus erythematosus, Sjogren's syndrome, vasculitis, etc.	Methylprednisolone 1 g/day for 3 days, or 500 mg/day for 5 days, iv or oral, followed by oral maintenance prednisolone (up to 50 mg/day)			

		Daily for 5 days	Relative contraindications: anticoagulation and cardiac disease	Infection risk and allergy associated with human albumin, thrombosis, infection, minor systemic symptoms	Not for MS
Plasma exchange	Acute significantly disabling opticospinal relapse not responding to corticosteroids, acute disseminated encephalomyelitis	Daily for 5 days	Relative contraindications: anticoagulation and cardiac disease	Infection risk and allergy associated with human albumin, thrombosis, infection, minor systemic symptoms	Not for MS
Intravenous immunoglobulin	Acute significantly disabling relapse and inadequate response to corticosteroid, post-partum relapse prevention	0.4 mg/kg daily for 5 days	Contraindicated in IgA deficiency	Systemic adverse effects and allergy, infection risk associated with human blood product, sterile meningitis, renal failure	Not for MS

Table 9.3 Disease-modifying drugs for MS and other immunological disorders

Drug	Recommended indication*	Regimen	Monitoring safety and response	Adverse effects	Licence
Interferon-beta 1b (Betaferon/ Betaseron)	Relapsing disease (≥ 2 relapses in last 2 years) and the relapses are the main cause of disability	250 µg sc on alternate days, not premixed; store at room temperature	Full blood count and liver function tests. Monoclonal gammopathy a contraindication (single case report of fatal capillary leak syndrome)	Bone marrow suppression, hepatotoxic, flu-like symptoms, injection-site reactions (Rebif and Betaferon), made with human albumin, menstrual irregularity, depression (probable)	Relapsing– remitting and secondary progressive MS
Interferon-beta 1a (Avonex)		30 µg im once weekly, premixed; store at 4°C	Stop if disabling relapse frequency increases or ≥ 2 relapses per year, or unable to walk, or secondary progressive MS on Rebif or Avonex	Neutralising antibodies (attenuate response)	Relapsing– remitting MS, 2 relapses in 3 years. Clinically isolated syndrome + abnormal MRI
Interferon beta 1a (Rebif)		22 or 44 µg sc twice weekly, premixed; store at room temperature for < 30 days			Relapsing MS
Glatiramer acetate (Copaxone)		20 µg sc daily, premixed; store at 4°C	Stopping criteria as with Rebif or Avonex	Post-injection shortness of	Relapsing– remitting MS

	Indication	Dose	Monitoring	Side effects	Notes
				breath/chest pain, injection-site reactions, lipoatrophy	
Azathioprine	Interferon/glatiramer not appropriate and frequent relapsing disease, or aggressive progressive disease, or as a steroid sparer in Sjögren's syndrome, SLE, vasculitis, Behçet's disease, etc.	Increase weekly by 50 mg to 2.5 mg/kg orally (divided twice daily dosage)	Where available check TPMT status and withhold where homozygous mutant alleles. Weekly full blood count and liver function tests for 8 weeks, then 3 monthly	Bone marrow suppression, hepatotoxic, cancer in long-term, allergy, gastrointestinal symptoms	Not for MS
Mitoxantrone	Aggressive relapsing disease	10–20 mg iv monthly for 6 months, or every 3 months for 2 years	Urine culture, full blood count, liver function tests 1 week prior to next dose. Echocardiogram before and every 6 months for 5 years. Do not use if left ventricular function is < 50%	Bone marrow suppression, cardiomyopathy, amenorrhoea, nausea/vomiting, leukaemia	MS, only in the USA

Continued

Table 9.3 *Continued*

Drug	Recommended indication*	Regimen	Monitoring safety and response	Adverse effects	Licence
Cyclophosphamide	Vasculitis/SLE/Sjogren's syndrome	1–2.0 mg/kg orally daily, or 5–15 mg/kg pulsed iv with Mesna	Weekly full blood count and liver function tests for 8 weeks, then every 3 months	Bone marrow suppression, haemorrhagic cystitis, bladder cancer, malignancy, infertility in females, cardiotoxicity, pulmonary fibrosis	Not for inflammatory neurological diseases
Methotrexate	Sarcoidosis	7.5–20 mg orally weekly	Weekly full blood count and liver function tests for 8 weeks, then every 3 months. Caution with non-steroidal anti-inflammatory drugs	Bone marrow suppression, hepatotoxicity, pulmonary disease, menstrual disturbances, allergy	Not for inflammatory neurological diseases

'Relapsing MS' refers to relapsing–remitting MS and secondary progressive MS with relapses, and is the term used in the product licence to cover both categories.

*Note indications are recommendations, not necessarily licensed indications.

im, intramuscular; iv, intravenous; sc, subcutaneous.

Interferon-beta (IF-β) and glatiramer acetate

General points

- In relapsing–remitting and relapsing secondary progressive MS these disease-modifying drugs reduce the relapse rate by about 30%, reduce the brain MRI activity dramatically, and perhaps have a small effect on short-term disability.
- The drugs are all very expensive (£5000 to £10,000 per annum).
- The advantages of one product over another are much debated.

Interferon-beta

- There are one 1b (*Betaferon/Betaseron*) and two 1a (*Avonex and Rebif*) formulations of interferon-beta.
- 1b differs from the natural human form by minor amino-acid changes and lack of glycosylation.
- 1a is identical to the natural product and has a higher specific activity than 1b.
- All three products are given at different doses and frequencies by the subcutaneous or intramuscular route. Any differences in effect may be due to the formulation itself, the dosage, or the frequency with which it is given, and the presence of neutralising antibodies.
- All three products can be given using an auto-injector.
- Premixed versions are convenient but generally require storage at 4°C.
- Interferon-beta 1a (*Avonex*) is convenient as a once weekly preparation and induces neutralising antibodies in only 2–4% of patients. Its licence also covers patients with clinically isolated syndromes when the brain MRI is abnormal.
- Interferon-beta 1a (*Rebif*) is available in two doses, and as a premixed version which can be stored at room temperature for up to 30 days. The higher dose of 44 µg/week has a greater effect on relapses over the short-term than interferon-beta 1a (*Avonex*) 30 µg/week. *Rebif* induces antibodies in about 12–23% of patients. Its licence covers secondary progressive patients with relapses.
- Interferon-beta 1b (*Betaferon/Betaseron*) probably has a greater effect on relapses than weekly interferon-beta 1a (*Avonex*) and induces neutralising antibodies earlier and more frequently than the other preparations, but these reduce over time (a feature which is less apparent with the other products). Its licence covers secondary progressive MS. It is not available as a premixed version.

Child-bearing potential and pregnancy

- Prior discussion in women of child-bearing age on the importance of taking adequate contraception and planning pregnancy is important.
- Until more information is available about human safety, glatiramer acetate, mitoxantrone, interferon-beta 1a and 1b, and natalizumab should be discontinued before an anticipated pregnancy.
- Methotrexate and cyclophosphamide are known to be teratogenic.
- Azathioprine is considered safe in pregnancy.
- There is a risk of intrauterine growth retardation with prolonged or repeated corticosteroid treatments, but short-course intravenous steroids may be used with relative safety.

In fact, there is rarely a good reason to continue any MS treatment during pregnancy due to the lack of long-term evidence of treatment benefit, and the reduced risk of relapse during pregnancy. There is an increased risk of relapse during the post-partum period. IVIg during pregnancy or post-partum reduces relapse frequency and has been used in those with active disease.

Aggressive MS

- Severe relapses that do not respond to corticosteroids may respond to IVIg or plasma exchange.
- Aggressive disease generally refers to marked disability relative to a short disease duration, but may also include a clinical course involving unusually severe relapses. Frequent relapses early in the course of the disease and high MRI disease activity are being increasingly used as indicators for more aggressive management:
  - mitoxantrone (and, if licensed, Tysabri) is a reasonable treatment for aggressive relapsing MS
  - azathioprine may be tried in rapidly progressive disease
  - there is no evidence that bone marrow transplantation improves long-term disability, and it carries a high mortality.

OTHER INFLAMMATORY CONDITIONS
Systemic immune diseases

These may be jointly managed with a rheumatologist. They tend to be dependent on and more responsive to immunosuppression than MS, and include:
- Systemic lupus erythematosus (SLE).

- Sjogren's syndrome.
- Sarcoidosis.
- Behçet's disease.
- Systemic vasculitides.

Difficulties distinguishing from MS arise when:
- Patients present with isolated CNS involvement.
- MS patients have associated antinuclear or anticardiolipin antibodies.

CNS-specific inflammatory syndromes

These include:
- Recurrent optic neuritis.
- Monophasic and recurrent transverse myelitis.
- Neuromyelitis optica (Devic's disease).
- MS associated with Leber's optic neuropathy.
- Acute monophasic or recurrent disseminated encephalomyelitis.
- Isolated cerebral vasculitis.

The opticospinal syndromes may require follow-up over long periods to establish whether the clinical picture continues to be anatomically limited.

Treatment

Optic neuritis and transverse myelitis

Where isolated and severe, a high-dose short course of corticosteroids is useful in hastening recovery (see Table 9.3). Where recurrent episodes occur, classification of the underlying disease process is important (e.g. MS versus Devic's versus Sjogren's) to decide on the optimum treatment regimen.

Acute disseminated encephalomyelitis (ADEM)

- ADEM is usually treated with high dose intravenous methylprednisolone (as in Table 9.3).
- In severe cases plasma exchange is an additional option.

Devic's/neuromyelitis optica

- Recent work suggests this is associated with a specific serum antibody, which appears to bind to the blood–brain barrier.
- Treatment is empirical. Patients may respond to corticosteroids or plasma exchange. Other immunomodulatory MS treatments may be tried in severe cases, although the evidence is anecdotal.

Behçet's disease

- High dose intravenous methylprednisolone followed by prednisolone 1 mg/kg orally. This can be reduced to a maintenance level, depending on clinical response, with or without azathioprine as a steroid sparing agent.
- Other options include methotrexate, cyclophosphamide (see Table 9.3) and anti-TNF-α therapy.
- Treatment for any associated intracranial venous thrombosis may be necessary (see Chapter 4).

Neurosarcoidosis

- No randomised studies are available in this condition.
- Corticosteroids (initial high dose intravenously, followed by oral maintenance) with or without oral methotrexate (see Table 9.3) are the mainstay of treatment.
- Hydroxychloroquine, cyclosporin, cyclophosphamide, chlorambucil and cranial radiotherapy have also been used.

Cerebral vasculitis, Sjogren's syndrome and SLE

- Although formal studies have not been performed, initial corticosteroids (high dose intravenously, followed by oral prednisolone) with cyclophosphamide (oral or pulsed intravenous) followed by azathioprine maintenance is commonly used.
- Aspirin or warfarin may be used as antithrombotic agents in SLE if associated with anticardolipin antibodies.

Giant cell arteritis

- If this presents with blindness or stroke it is important to start oral prednisolone 60 mg/day at once, without waiting for a temporal artery biopsy (polymyalgia alone only requires prednisolone 5–10 mg/day).
- Any headache and systemic symptoms should resolve in 24–48 hours and the raised erythrocyte sedimentation ratio (ESR) within a month.
- The prednisolone should be gradually reduced to 20 mg/day over about 2 months, depending on any relapse of the symptoms or a rising ESR.
- Thereafter, reduction of prednisolone should be very cautious over several months, to about 10 mg/day.
- Every 6 months attempts should be made to gradually wean the patient off steroids completely, watching for recurrent symptoms and/or a rising ESR. Eventually the patient will be in remission, but this may not be for a number of years.

Adverse effects of corticosteroids

The adverse-effect profile of corticosteroids is a major limiting factor in long-term or high-dose prescribing.

■ High-dose, short-term treatment is mainly limited by insomnia and psychiatric symptoms (euphoria, anxiety or, rarely, acute psychosis).

■ May unmask diabetes mellitus in those with reduced glucose tolerance. Acute bone necrosis is a serious but rare idiosyncratic complication. It is unclear whether the corticosteroid treatment itself, or the underlying disease associated stress response, is a risk for peptic ulceration.

■ Longer term courses carry additional risks, including cataracts, osteoporosis, increased appetite, weight gain, proximal myopathy, Cushingoid appearance, hypertension, diabetes, bruising and thinning of the skin, dyspepsia and, less commonly, mucosal ulceration and pancreatitis. Immunosuppression-associated infection is in practice rarely a problem, although patients are advised against live vaccination.

■ Ulcer protection with a proton pump inhibitor is prudent in acutely ill patients and in those on longer term corticosteroid treatment.

■ Bone protection: phosphonates (weekly formulations are best tolerated) with adequate vitamin D and calcium intake are advised to reduce the risk of osteoporosis for those on longer term corticosteroid treatment. Particular risk categories include:
  – > 65 years old, > 6 months treatment, > 10–20 mg/day prednisolone
  – maintenance dose > 5–7.5 mg/day
  – bone density 1–1.5 standard deviations below the mean
  – postmenopausal women
  DXA scans every 1–3 years are advised.

Adverse effects of azathioprine

Most adverse effects occur early on when initiating azathioprine.

■ Gastrointestinal symptoms are not uncommon and may be helped by slowly increasing the dose and dividing it into a twice daily regimen.

■ Allergic reactions occur in about 2%.

■ Bone marrow suppression and hepatic dysfunction appear to be dose related. Weekly monitoring of full blood count and liver function for the first 8 weeks followed by 3-monthly blood tests is advised. When abnormalities are identified the azathioprine should be stopped until normality returns and then restarted at a 50 mg lower dose.

■ Low TPMT activity is a risk factor for myelosuppression, but it is less clear if there is an association with the other adverse effects.

■ There is probably a slightly increased risk of cancer when azathioprine is taken over the longer term (5–10 years). Studies differ in the type of cancers implicated, but include skin cancers, non-Hodgkin's lymphoma and an increase in common cancers generally.

Further reading

Association of British Neurologists. Guidelines for the use of beta interferons and glatiramer acetate in multiple sclerosis. Available at: http://www.theabn.org/downloads/msdoc.pdf

Hawkins CP, Wolinsky JS. Principles of treatments in multiple sclerosis. Butterworth Heinemann, Oxford, 2000.

National Institute of Clinical Excellence. Multiple sclerosis – beta interferon and glatiramer acetate. NICE Guideline No. 32. Available at: http://www.nice.org.uk/page.aspx?o=27588

Noseworthy JH. Neurological therapeutics – principles and practice. Martin Dunitz, London, 2003.

Scolding NJ. Immunological and inflammatory disorders of the central nervous system. Butterworth Heinemann, Oxford, 1999.

10 MOTOR NEURON DISEASE, DISORDERS OF THE SPINE AND SPINAL CORD

Andrew M. Chancellor and Harry K. McNaughton

Chapter contents

MOTOR NEURON DISEASE

The terms 'motor neuron *disease*' (MND) and 'amyotrophic lateral sclerosis' (ALS) describe the same condition, whereas the term 'motor neuron *disorders*' is a generic, less specific description of a range of pathologies affecting the motor system. Progressive bulbar palsy, primary lateral sclerosis, adult-onset progressive muscular atrophy and monomelic presentations are restricted forms of MND, which may remain 'pure' but often overlap with the more fully developed MND/ALS.

Arguably the most tragic of human diseases, MND usually develops by inexorable deterioration, due to combined upper and lower motor neuron attrition, affecting corticobulbar function, respiratory muscles and the limbs.

- Annual incidence is about 2–3 new cases per 100,000 population, similar in all parts of the world, with a mean age of onset of 64 years.
- Median survival is just over 2 years from symptom onset.
- Prevalence is around 10 per 100,000 population.
- There has been no improvement in survival as a result of modern care.

General care issues

Media attention is often focused on controversial treatments and assisted dying, whereas MND care teams advocate promoting the remaining quality of life and assisting a peaceful, comfortable and 'natural' death. Treatments are few, management is complex, often challenging, and there are very few randomised trials testing treatment effectiveness.

The management of MND demands a very practical approach. Obstacles faced by the lead clinician, whether neurologist or other, include:

- personal nihilism, a sense of frustration and/or lack of willingness to remain involved with care
- the need for coordination of many health and social services
- the burden of psychological impact on patient and carer
- severe multifaceted disablement, generally with rapid progression
- anticipating changing needs and avoiding crisis response management
- a dying patient
- lack of highly effective therapies.

Despite this, patient satisfaction and quality of life will be improved by:

- a multidisciplinary care team model, similar to management of other complex neurological disorders
- a designated allied health professional, such as an occupational therapist, social worker, or speech and language therapist, to coordinate hospital and community services and to whom the patient and next of kin can turn, as a first contact for help
- good liaison with the family doctor, who will be most familiar with essential community-based support services and palliative care, with help and guidance from the neurologist to maintain the family doctor's participation in care
- involvement of the local MND patient support groups (see http://www.alsmndalliance.org).

Breaking bad news

Establishing a good early rapport and maintaining patient and physician mood is essential, particularly with a terminal disorder. When the disease is particularly aggressive the diagnosis is usually obvious and a prompt explanation is expected. More often, incompletely developed disease allows a 'graduated process of discovery'. In the course of the diagnostic work-up, it is best to introduce the initial concept of 'motor nerve' loss. Later, the patient's realisation that he or she is deteriorating leads to the discussion of neurodegeneration and then the specific term 'MND' and its implications.

When approaching the formal interview to introduce the diagnosis consider:

- The physical context of the appointment, setting time aside in an appropriate environment with family and other professional support.
- Asking the patient what he or she understands to be the problem – the manner of response, as much as the answer, is revealing and a helpful introduction to the consultation.

- An honest, sensitive and empathetic but not sentimental approach.
- Being the *listener* as well as the talker, acknowledge emotions and explore fears, allow time for questions.
- Maintaining optimism, even when life-expectancy may be measured in 1 or 2 years, be cautious about prognosis, allow for hope, emphasising that:
  - other than the discomfort of immobility, which can be managed, MND does not cause painful sensory symptoms, neuralgia or incontinence
  - MND does not affect cardiac muscle or special senses, and cognitive difficulties are not usually a major problem
  - the survival curve has a long tail with 8–10% of patients surviving more than 8 years, which can be optimistically emphasised to the newly diagnosed individual.
- A strategy, at least in outline, before the meeting, to give the patient a plan, usually including:
  - the offer of a second opinion (in part this comes with electrophysiological investigations)
  - the evidence for riluzole treatment
  - symptomatic treatments, including palliative services (not equivalent to terminal care)
  - an introduction to the work of the MND associations
  - the offer of a follow-up consultation within a few weeks of the first, to allow the patient and carer to return with questions
  - discussion of advance directives.

Genetic counselling

- 5–10% of patients with MND have a family history, usually autosomal dominant with variable penetrance.
- As in any neurogenetic disorder, understanding the pedigree at large will assist with counselling the index case.
- Unfortunately, for a few, especially the familial forms, important frontotemporal dementia emerges, with lack of insight, apathy and/or changes in social conduct or behaviour, which may prove very difficult to manage (see Chapter 5).
- Only 20% of patients with familial MND have a mutation in the gene for copper/zinc superoxide dismutase (SOD1). Different mutations within this gene (there are many) have variable phenotypes and prognosis.
- SOD1 gene testing is not recommended for apparently sporadic cases, and predictive testing for relatives is of no use if the index case does not have a SOD1 mutation. The issue is further complicated by variable penetrance of some, but not all, mutations.

- Several other different chromosomal loci for familial forms with different patterns of inheritance are now recognised. All are rare.
- Refer to a neurogenetics clinic; but general genetic clinics usually do not add to informed neurological opinion.

Riluzole

There have been many trials of agents that might, on theoretical grounds, modify disease progression, but the literature is awash with failures. Only riluzole has been approved for the treatment of MND, but not the other motor neuron disorders, in many but not all developed countries.

- The Cochrane Review (amended July 2003) included a total of 876 riluzole treated patients and 406 controls in three trials that studied tracheostomy-free survival.
- Riluzole 100 mg/day probably prolongs survival by about 2 months, perhaps with the effect in the earlier part of the treatment period.
- There are no data on quality of life; this is important as patients value psychosocial well-being more highly than longevity or better strength.
- Some patients report nausea or asthenia and withdraw.
- Testing serum transaminases monthly for 3 months then every 3 months is recommended.
- The price of riluzole in New Zealand is of the order of £250/month equivalent.
- Questions persist about riluzole's utility because of its high cost and modest efficacy. However, the National Institute for Health and Clinical Excellence (NICE) in the UK has declared the drug cost-effective and should be made available.
- Forthcoming treatment trials may need to have riluzole as the best available medical treatment, adding considerable cost to any future developments.

Symptomatic drug and other therapeutic interventions for common symptoms

Salivation and drooling

- Anticholinergics:
    - atropine, eye drops prn or 0.25–0.75 mg oral
    - orphenadrine 50–100 mg oral tds
    - hyoscine hydrobromide 0.4 mg sc or transdermal patches (scopolamine).
    Anticholinergic adverse effects may complicate any constipation associated with immobility. The dose very much depends on response.

Hyoscine may exacerbate muscle stiffness. Dry mouth and blurred vision may be problematic.

- Amitryptiline 10–25 mg/day oral.
- Glycopyrrolate (Robinul) liquid sc/im 0.1 mg prn.
- Propranolol 20–80 mg/day oral in 2 or 3 divided doses.
- Botulinum toxin into submandibular glands, or alternate parotid glands (may adversely affect swallowing via spread to skeletal muscles).
- Low-dose irradiation of salivary glands.
- Laryngectomy (if anarthric and aspirating).
- Possibly surgical redirection of submandibular duct orifices.

All interventions may make the mouth too dry and saliva even more difficult to swallow.

Tenacious secretions

- May be drug induced and exacerbated by mouth breathing.
- Hydration, oral hygiene, reduced dairy intake.

Table 10.1 Equipment and environmental modifications to assist physical challenges in MND	
Indication	**Aids**
Eating	Modified cups, non-slip mats, cup holders
Drooling	Suction machine
Pressure skin care	Cushions, variable pressure mattresses
Comfort	Reclining, electrically operated chairs
Dropped head	Not very satisfactory, collars and wheelchair head extension devices
Environmental controls	Personal alarms, remote operation of lights/equipment, book rest and page turner, talking books
Aids for carers	Turntables, lifting belts, hoists
Mobility aids	Electrically operated wheelchairs using viable muscle groups
Communication	Hands-free telephone, call bells, computerised communication aids (e.g. lightwriter, magic slates, amplifiers)
Bathroom aids	Grab rails, shower chairs, elevated commode

- Carbocisteine 750 mg oral tds is a mucolytic, but may cause occasional gastrointestinal irritation and rashes.

Pain/spasticity/cramp

- Comfort measures, especially Roho seat cushioning.
- Quinine sulphate 200 mg bd or nocte for cramp.
- Baclofen 5–80 mg/day; tizanidine 2–36 mg/day; dantrolene 25–400 mg/day (all given in three or four divided doses) for spasticity (see Chapter 9).

Pseudobulbar palsy, affect/emotionality/depression

- In the early stages pyridostigmine (Mestinon) may provide modest improvements in bulbar symptoms and limb strength (for dose and adverse effects see myasthenia gravis, Chapter 12).
- Counselling.
- Serotonin reuptake inhibitors (e.g. citalopram 20–40 mg/day oral) (see Chapter 13).
- Amitryptiline 25–100 mg oral in the evening (see Chapter 13).

Anxiety (see Chapter 13)

- Lorazepam 1–2 mg sublingual daily or prn.
- Diazepam (stesolid) suppository prn.
- Chlorpromazine 12.5–25 mg im prn.
- Midazolam 5–10 mg iv as part of daily syringe-driver drugs.

Dyspnoea

- Morphine 2.5–5 mg oral qds initially, later as subcutaneous infusion.

Constipation

- Hydration, regular bowel programme including enemas, laxatives (see Chapter 17).

Terminal care

- Syringe driver, primed every 24 hours (e.g. with diamorphine, midazolam, hyoscine as above).

Feeding and gastrostomy

- Undernutrition is common, not only because of the laborious process of eating for a dysphagic patient, but also the embarrassment and hence

reluctance to eat in public. Upper limb motor deficits make eating physically difficult.
- The first step is to change the consistency of food, usually towards a uniform purée or softness (patients generally work out what is best for themselves).
- Head positioning, such as the chin tuck manoeuvre (flexing the neck forward on swallowing to protect the airway) and double swallow, taught by a therapist.
- Most neurologists who worked prior to the widespread use of percutaneous endoscopic gastrostomy (PEG) agree that this has been a helpful development. A Cochrane Review of PEG placement and other tube-feeding regimens on survival, nutritional status, quality of life and patient and caregiver satisfaction is anticipated.
- Patients need to be aware that artificial feeding does not mean an abrupt end to oral intake; the concept of artificial feeding needs early introduction to allow the patient to accept the idea.
- When to start artificial feeding is uncertain; weight loss and loss of enjoyment for meals is as good a guide as anything, and there is no need to wait until the patient is in desperate straits.
- PEG has enormous benefits in the terminal stages of the illness, when it can be used for comfort fluids and medication.
- Endoscopes are generally well tolerated and the procedure may be done in a semi-recumbent position, with an overnight hospital stay.
- Complications of PEG in MND patients include:
  - transient laryngeal spasm (7%)
  - localised infections (7%)
  - gastric haemorrhage (1–4%)
  - failure to place the PEG due to technical difficulties (1–9%)
  - aspiration pneumonia
  - death due to respiratory arrest (1–9%).
- Radiologically inserted gastrostomy (RIG) offers potential advantages over PEG in that it usually avoids sedation; there is no need to swallow a tube; it may be performed in the semi-upright position; and it can be used in patients on non-invasive ventilation.
- Patients whose survival is thought to be less than a few months may be managed with a fine bore nasogastric tube.

Communication
- As speech intelligibility deteriorates, other means of communication become essential.

- A speech and language therapist's regular review is needed in assessing the most appropriate system for the individual, which becomes more complex and technology dependent as the disease progresses.
- The usual first step, after writing becomes too difficult, is a lightwriter, provided the patient can press the keys.
- Dysphasia and other cognitive problems may contribute to communication failure in a few patients.

Respiratory failure and non-invasive ventilation (NIV)

Occasionally the neurologist is confronted with a patient who is already ventilated, as an emergency measure, prior to the diagnosis of MND. The prospects for effective weaning are poor and attempts at long-term domiciliary ventilator support in this circumstance unlikely to be acceptable. More commonly patients die gradually of respiratory muscle failure, rather than aspiration pneumonia or in a choking bout – a common fear.

- Loss of respiratory reserve is not apparent in the early stages, when most attention is directed towards speech and swallowing and/or the patient loses their ability to exercise due to limb weakness.
- Forced vital capacity declines linearly and predicts survival, but it may be difficult to get accurate measurements due to facial weakness or apraxia of facial movement – a feature of pseudobulbar palsy.
- The optimum proportion of MND sufferers who would benefit from NIV is unknown. Involvement of a respiratory physician or technician will be needed.
- No randomised trial of the efficacy and tolerability of NIV for MND has been completed and the literature is contradictory regarding quality-of-life improvements for patient and carer.
- It makes sense to consider NIV when there is some combination of dyspnoea, orthopnoea, disturbed sleep, morning headache, poor concentration, anorexia or excessive daytime sleepiness (Epworth score > 9), especially if combined with significant nocturnal desaturation on overnight oximetry.
- For some patients NIV usefully improves nocturnal and daytime well-being.
- Only a small proportion of patients are offered NIV, even in developed countries, in part due to resource limitations.
- NIV devices are available that deliver intermittent inspiratory positive pressure, or different levels of positive pressure during inspiration and expiration (BIPAP).

- NIV probably increases the risk of aspiration, particularly in patients with conspicuous bulbar symptoms, and some patients with pronounced bulbar symptoms cannot tolerate this technique.
- Cultural influences mean that in some places, particularly Japan, tracheostomy-based ventilation leads to a locked-in state, the patient being unable to communicate and carers making all decisions on their behalf.

Other therapies

- As in other circumstances, some patients choose, at least in the initial to middle phases of the disease, to seek experimental or fringe treatments, which can present ethical dilemmas when neurologists are asked to administer patient-directed treatment.
- Assisted dying may be sought.

PAIN IN THE NECK, ARM AND BACK
General treatment principles

Pain in the neck, arm and back is so common that it can reasonably be considered part of normal adult life. Approximate prevalence figures for the adult population are: neck pain 10%, back pain up to 20% and arm pain 5–10%. Most adults will have an episode of back pain resulting in activity limitation for 48 hours or more sometime in their life. Neurologists tend to see the people with regional pain associated with neurological features, such as sensory and motor deficits. Although this is a very small proportion of the total pain population (perhaps 5% or less), it is still a large number. The broad principles of investigations and treatment are:

- Pain and any neurological features tend to remit, although recurrences of pain are common.
- Chronic pain (defined as lasting 3 months or more) in the neck, arm and back is associated with much misery, work loss, compensation and litigation.
- It is very difficult (or impossible) to make a reliable specific diagnosis when pain is the primary complaint, even when there are neurological features.
- A myriad of practitioners has evolved in western society to attract sufferers for treatments based on diagnoses that are not reliable and imply a particular causation or need for a particular treatment (e.g. 'injury', 'malalignment/vertebrae out', 'cervical strain', 'whiplash', 'overuse syndrome', 'facet joint dysfunction').

- The evidence that low level, repetitive work practices cause acute and chronic pain syndromes is weak or absent.
- Because of the tendency to remission, most treatments appear to be effective to the practitioners that use them.
- Those treatments that have been tested in randomised trials have been shown to be ineffective or, at best, to have only a small, clinically insignificant effect.
- The term 'sciatica', although widely used, has little otherwise to commend it. 'Leg pain, with [or without] back pain' is the terminology recommended. The presence of leg pain in association with back pain increases the chance of a herniated lumbar disc being present. Pain tends to settle more slowly in people with leg pain, although symptoms at 12 months are no different for people with back pain, with or without leg pain. In the absence of neurological features, particularly motor deficit, the general approach and management for people with back and leg pain is no different to that for someone without leg pain.
- The only randomised trial of surgical treatment (in patients with sciatica and radiologically verified herniated lumbar disc) showed no benefit in long-term follow-up compared to conservative therapy.
- Radiological investigations are often misleading. Around 30% of people with no previous history of back or neck complaints, currently asymptomatic, have bulging or herniated lumbar or cervical discs on magnetic resonance imaging (MRI).
- Rarely, MRI may expose unusual disorders, such as idiopathic, inflammatory pachymeningitis, which may progress to compressive myelopathy.
- Arachnoiditis as the basis of pain should be considered if there is a history of spinal surgery, chemical injury (myodil), or recent meningitis, particularly tuberculosis. However, MRI abnormalities have a poor correlation with symptoms; predominately constant low back pain with leg radiation, mimicking other pathologies. The approach to treatment is the same as that for other causes of back pain.

Management

- Careful examination (listening to the patient, examining the part that hurts), including identifying 'red flags' that indicate a higher likelihood of serious underlying disease (Box 10.1).
- Not using diagnostic labels that imply we know more about the condition than we usually do.
- Using descriptive labels for the pain (e.g. neck pain with sensory

---

Box 10.1   'Red flags' indicating a possible underlying disease

- Age > 55 years for people with back pain.
- History of cancer.
- Fever.
- Weight loss.
- Use of corticosteroids.
- Features of cauda equina syndrome (saddle anaesthesia, sphincter dysfunction, bilateral leg weakness).
- Neurological signs in the territory of more than one spinal root.

---

symptoms in left arm, back pain with radiation into left leg) except where examination and electrophysiological findings have convincingly localised a specific nerve, plexus or root problem.

- Investigations only for patients with 'red flags', or who fail conservative management, or who are being prepared for surgery.
- Reassurance of the absence of serious underlying disease in those without 'red flags' and reassurance that the pain will decline with time.
- Reducing any work stress, or psychological, social and emotional issues that might be exacerbating the pain.
- Giving advice that it is alright to keep moving and that prolonged rest (particularly bed rest) is unhelpful.
- Concentrating on improving activity rather than diminishing pain as the primary object of the treatment plan.
- Judicious use of symptomatic measures to reduce pain, particularly in the acute phase (see below).
- Not prescribing passive therapies (e.g. heat, cold, TENS) or devices that restrict movement or encourage the idea of 'protecting' the sore part of the body (e.g. soft cervical collars, back supports).

Medication

- Paracetamol, given regularly (1 g oral qds), is the most useful medication for relief of pain.
- Non-steroidal anti-inflammatory drugs (NSAIDs) are of similar efficacy to paracetamol but have more adverse effects, particularly dyspepsia and gastrointestinal bleeding.
- Narcotic-containing medications should be avoided, except for very short-term intervention, particularly with severe leg pain.

- Benzodiazepines (e.g. oxazepam 10–20 mg) can sometimes be useful at night during exacerbations of pain.
- Tricyclics for subacute or chronic pain, particularly with sleep disturbance. A trial of amitriptyline for a minimum 3 weeks starting with 10 mg at night increasing to 75–100 mg as tolerated helps around 30% of people improve their activity levels, usually with a reduction in overall pain scores.
- Antidepressants: a small group of patients with chronic neck, arm or back pain benefit from a trial of full-dose antidepressant treatment, but it is hard to predict who will benefit (tricyclics are a reasonable first choice especially if sleep is a problem). (See also Chapter 13.)
- Other medications: the evidence for benefit with antiepileptic and antiarrhythmic drugs in chronic musculoskeletal pain is anecdotal. Working through a list of possible medications searching for a 'fix' probably contributes to worse outcomes.
- Medication withdrawal: just as with 'medication overuse headache' (see Chapter 1) there is a syndrome of chronic 'musculoskeletal' pain that responds to withdrawal of regular medication, especially when large amounts of codeine-containing compounds are being consumed. Most patients acknowledge that they are getting little relief from these medications and will agree to a reduction or cessation.

Physiotherapy

- Commonly used, but best estimates suggest a very modest, clinically insignificant benefit for people with acute pain syndromes. However, the best physiotherapists can achieve remarkable results. The trick is to find one.
- Physiotherapy does not benefit people with chronic neck, arm or back pain unless it is delivered as part of a multidisciplinary package of treatment.

Manipulation

- Commonly used, but best estimates suggest a very modest, clinically insignificant benefit for people with acute pain syndromes, similar in degree to physiotherapy.
- The risks of manipulation in people with low back pain are low, but manipulation should be avoided for people with neck pain, especially with any neurological features or known instability (e.g. rheumatoid arthritis).

Multidisciplinary rehabilitation

■ For people with chronic back pain, best results are with a team approach focusing on graded activity, attention to any psychosocial issues, including work stress, and avoiding overconcentration on pain relief in itself. The evidence for positive results from multidisciplinary rehabilitation for people with neck and arm pain, or people with back combined with leg pain, is less convincing but is a reasonable strategy.
■ Monodisciplinary approaches (including multiple specialist opinions) probably contribute to poor outcomes.

Epidural corticosteroids

■ The benefits for back pain, with or without leg pain, remain uncertain despite several trials. This intervention can be a useful way of delaying surgery in patients determined to proceed with surgery and the risks are low in experienced hands.

Surgery

■ There is no convincing evidence that surgery improves long-term outcomes for people with low back or neck pain, with or without radicular symptoms or signs.
■ It is possible that surgery hastens recovery in patients with radicular symptoms and a radiologically proven herniated disc at an appropriate level in the first year following surgery.
■ There is no convincing evidence that surgery helps people with arm pain with or without radicular signs.
■ 'Thoracic outlet syndrome' is overdiagnosed and too frequently operated on.
■ Surgery is inappropriate for most people with 'epicondylitis'.
■ Refer for a surgical opinion if:
  – there is significant underlying pathology (e.g. possible tumour, infection, central disc prolapse) and symptoms or signs of cord compromise
  – there are radicular symptoms/signs and MRI shows a herniated disc at an appropriate level for the clinical signs, there is failure of conservative management of at least 3 months, and the patient is prepared to accept the risks of anaesthesia and surgery in return for a possible improvement in short-term recovery time
  – there is progressive cervical myelopathy (see below).

CERVICAL SPONDYLOTIC MYELOPATHY

Cervical spondylosis is very common. Myelopathy secondary to cervical spondylosis is much less common but may be significantly disabling. Management options are often complicated in older people by comorbid conditions. The natural history of cervical spondylotic myelopathy is not necessarily one of a progressive deterioration, and trials of conservative management should almost always be tried prior to consideration of surgery.

Treatment

Treatment options include:

- Attention to mobility and continence issues, generally with help from a rehabilitation team.
- Pain (regular paracetamol) and spasticity (baclofen 10–80 mg/day in 3–4 divided doses) management is important in some patients. (See also Chapter 9.)
- Surgical intervention has not been shown to improve long-term outcomes and is associated with significant short-term risks. Surgery is often entertained as a way of halting progression, although there is no clear evidence to support this as an effective intervention. A good relationship with a competent surgeon probably leads to best decision-making for the patient. Patients should be fully informed of the risks of surgery and all discussions and decisions documented.

LUMBAR SPINAL STENOSIS

Mild lumbar canal stenosis is radiologically common, even in asymptomatic individuals. The natural history is uncertain and not all patients deteriorate. Pain is the main complaint; neurogenic claudication is much less common.

Treatment

- Attention to mobility and continence issues, generally with help from a rehabilitation team is first-line therapy.
- Pain management (regular paracetamol, supplemented by amitripyline 10–100 mg nocte, especially if there is sleep disturbance) is often difficult, but the main focus should be on maintaining mobility and independence.
- Surgical intervention has not been shown to improve long-term outcomes and is associated with significant short-term risks. A badly claudicating patient should derive symptom relief with decompression. A good relationship with a competent surgeon probably leads to best

decision-making for the patient. Patients should be fully informed of the risks of surgery and all discussions and decisions documented.

RHEUMATOID ARTHRITIS AFFECTING THE NECK

- Neurological complications are not uncommon in patients with significant rheumatoid disease of the cervical spine.
- Decisions about the best management should be made in conjunction with the treating rheumatologist, a surgeon with experience with this patient group, and, preferably, a multidisciplinary rehabilitation team.
- Atlantoaxial subluxation and/or dislocation with neurological signs indicating cord dysfunction is an indication for surgical stabilisation of the neck.

ANKYLOSING SPONDYLITIS WITH NEUROLOGICAL COMPLICATIONS

- Neurological complications are relatively uncommon. Traumatic spinal cord injury is 10 times more common compared with the normal population and can occur with much less trauma (e.g. slips and falls).
- Decisions about best management should be made in conjunction with the treating rheumatologist, a surgeon with experience with this patient group, and, preferably, a multidisciplinary rehabilitation team.
- Inflammatory lesions involving the spinal roots and/or cauda equina should be treated by conventional agents initially (NSAIDs for most patients), sometimes supplemented by short courses of systemic corticosteroids or local steroid injection if appropriate. Further intensification of treatment should be in conjunction with a rheumatologist.
- Although rare, atlantoaxial subluxation and/or dislocation with cord dysfunction is an indication for surgical stabilisation of the neck.
- Spinal fracture may need stabilisation.
- The consequences of spinal cord injury need to be managed by a rehabilitation team experienced in this area (preferably a spinal injury unit).

SPINAL EPIDURAL ABSCESS
Diagnosis

Spinal epidural abscess is uncommon, accounting for around one per 10,000 hospital admissions, principally in the 6th and 7th decades of life. A combination of back pain, tenderness, fever and compressive myelopathy or radiculopathy should ring alarm bells. Systemic symptoms may be relatively inconspicuous. As in all spinal disorders MRI is the initial imaging of choice. An abscess may arise from:

- Haematogenous spread of bacteria, usually from a cutaneous or mucosal source, resulting in an abscess over the posterior aspect of the cord.
- Direct spread into the epidural space from an infective source adjacent to the spine, such as vertebral osteomyelitis. In such cases the abscesses are usually located in the anterior part of the spinal canal.
- Direct spread from a paraspinal abscess.
- As an infective complication of spinal surgery and/or epidural anaesthesia.
- Bacteraemia; *Staphylococcus aureus* is most common but also tuberculosis, *Streptococci*, *Brucella*, anaerobes and fungi.

Treatment

- High-dose systemic bactericidal therapy, pending culture of blood or surgical material. Empirical antibiotic coverage should include antistaphylococcal drugs. If the infection follows a neurosurgical procedure, an antistaphylococcal penicillin, a third-generation cephalosporin and an aminoglycoside are prescribed in combination (see Chapter 14). Culture results guide definitive therapy.
- If a methicillin-sensitive *Staphylococcus aureus* is isolated, successful treatment is possible with a cephalosporin, a penicillinase-resistant penicillin, combination of vancomycin plus aminoglycoside, or trimethoprim sulphamethoxazole (see Chapter 14).
- Treatment should continue for at least 4 weeks, 6–8 weeks if vertebral osteomyelitis is suspected.
- Any delay to decompressive surgery in the presence of significant neurological compromise is likely to result in a poor outcome; the patient who is paralysed preoperatively for more than 24 hours generally does not recover function.
- There are no randomised trials of antibiotics versus antibiotics plus surgery in neurologically intact cases. This is particularly pertinent as MRI is very sensitive in detecting small non-compressive inflammatory lesions that may not yet be a true abscess. The decision to manage with antibiotics alone is difficult and practice varies.

VASCULAR DISEASE OF THE SPINAL CORD
Interruption of spinal cord arterial blood supply

- The most common cause is occlusion of the anterior spinal artery, radicular arteries or, caudally, the great radicular artery of Adamkiewicz, in the setting of aortic disease and its surgery.

- Infarction may also occur in a wide range of other circumstances, such as systemic hypotension, vasculitis (formerly syphilitic aortitis), decompression sickness, coagulopathy and a range of iatrogenic causes such as thoracolumbar sympathectomy.
- In many cases acute infarction is followed by progressive cord atrophy, with irreversible myelopathy and conspicuous autonomic problems.
- For a few causes listed above, identifying the pathology may lead to specific treatments such as corticosteroids and immunosuppression.

Spinal vascular malformations

- Spinal dural arteriovenous fistulae are usually supplied by branches of the intercostal arteries, rarely vertebral, subclavian or lumbar-sacral arteries. Chronic venous hypertension develops (necrotising myelopathy of Alajouanine) as spinal pial veins, which drain the fistula, become engorged.
- Cord arteriovenous malformations and cavernous angiomas also occur.
- Unlike most vascular disorders, myelopathy develops insidiously and may be mistaken for chronic myelitis or a spinal cord tumour, even with MRI.
- Treatment of dural fistulae is either by means of embolisation using IBCA ('glue') or particulate material.

Epidural haematoma

- This can be spontaneous, iatrogenic (e.g. perioperative epidural catheter for anaesthesia, anticoagulants) or result from a bleeding dural vascular malformation.
- It is a neurosurgical emergency to consider evacuation, although some patients recover spontaneously.

SYRINGOMYELIA

Syringomyelia (or hydromyelia) and syringobulbia are cystic cavitations of the cervicothoracic cord and medulla, respectively. MRI has led to earlier recognition, in advance of the classical clinical signs. Syringomyelia may be idiopathic or associated with:

- congenital foramen magnum level anomalies, especially Arnold–Chiari
- basal or spinal arachnoiditis
- cord trauma
- spinal tumours.

Treatment

- No drug treatment is available.
- Progressive myelopathy, sometimes developing over a lifetime, needs symptomatic and supportive care.
- Lack of trial data means the impression that neurosurgical approaches slow or delay the progressive nature of this disorder is impossible to rely on.
- Surgery is generally limited to cavitations associated with an Arnold–Chiari I malformation, and is intended to correct the anatomical distortions, restoring cerebrospinal fluid circulation. A number of procedures have been advocated:
  - decompression of the descended cerebellar tonsils at the foramen magnum by removing the occipital bone and the arch of C1 and C2, with or without:
  - opening the dura, separating the cerebellar tonsils, lysis of adhesions, opening the fourth ventricular outlet and plugging the obex.
  - Where the syrinx is not associated with a Chiari malformation or if ventriculomegaly and raised pressure are thought to contribute, then draining the syrinx with a syringosubarachnoid or syringoperitoneal shunt may be recommended.

Further reading

Hankey GJ, Wardlaw JM. Clinical neurology. Manson, **London**, 2002.
Leigh PN, Abrahams S, Al-Chalabi A et al. The management of motor neurone disease. J Neurol Neurosurg Psychiatry 2003; 74s(Suppl IV): iv32–iv47.

11 PERIPHERAL NERVE DISORDERS

Michael Donaghy

PATHOPHYSIOLOGICAL TYPES OF PERIPHERAL NEUROPATHY

Peripheral neuropathies may affect all, some, or just a single peripheral nerve or root.

Polyneuropathy

- Affects all nerve fibres according to a particular parameter (e.g. by length or whether myelinated).
- Primary pathologies: axonal degeneration, demyelination, conduction block.
- Nerve conduction in demyelination:
  - motor conduction velocity ≤ 80% lower limit of normal (i.e. arm 38 m/s or less (normal ≥ 48 m/s), leg 32 m/s or less (normal ≥ 42 m/s))
  - distal motor latency and/or F waves ≥ 125% upper limit of normal.
- Nerve conduction in motor conduction block:
  - 50% smaller compound muscle action potential amplitude from proximal stimulation compared to distal stimulation.
- Sensory nerve action potentials lost equally in axonal degeneration and demyelination involving sensory nerve fibres.

Focal neuropathy

- Affects a single nerve trunk (mononeuropathy) or multiple individual nerves (mononeuritis multiplex).
- Compression or trauma produce axonal degeneration and/or focal conduction block.
- Vasculitis or diabetes produce axonal degeneration.

GENERAL PRINCIPLES OF TREATMENT

- Treat any specific cause (e.g. diabetes, leprosy).
- Prevent muscle contractures and preserve joint mobility by physiotherapy and/or splinting.
- Control neuropathic pain (see Chapter 18):
  - systemic drugs (carbamazepine, gabapentin or amitriptyline)
  - local measures (cold sprays, protective garments, capsaicin).
- Assist use of weak limb (e.g. footdrop orthosis).
- Acromutilation occurs principally in diabetes, leprosy and hereditary sensory neuropathies. Painless puncture injuries and burns are followed by skin ulceration. Autonomic denervation causes loss of sweating with dry cracked skin. Lack of pain protection leads to joint disruption (Charcot joints). Vulnerable patients should be advised to:
  - wear sensible protective footwear
  - avoid potential heat or puncture injuries
  - rub moisturising oils into any dry foot skin
  - have regular chiropody.

RECOVERY OF FUNCTION

The potential for recovery varies in different types of neuropathy:
- Focal compression if acute, self-limited and without axonal degeneration (neurapraxia) recovers in 8–12 weeks.
- Axonal degeneration recovers more slowly and usually incompletely. Prospects for significant recovery are poor when regeneration is required over long distances, in the elderly, when the gross structure of the nerve has been disrupted, and in those with systemic disease (e.g. diabetes).
- Acquired demyelinating neuropathies (e.g. Guillain–Barré syndrome and chronic inflammatory demyelinating polyneuropathy) and neuropathies with conduction block (e.g. multifocal motor neuropathy) can recover well with treatment, particularly if there is little or no associated axonal degeneration.

Measuring recovery

Assessing useful recovery is important for determining the overall risk–benefit of potentially harmful drugs (e.g. immunosuppressants) in routine clinical practice:

- Nerve conduction studies and electromyography (EMG) do not provide adequate quantification of recovery, or of severity.
- Clinical quantification of muscle power (e.g. Medical research Council (MRC) scale) is not very repeatable.
- Measurable improvements in *functional* ability are valuable (e.g. walking times, stair climbing speeds, grip strength).
- Improved everyday functioning (specific abilities lost by the patient that can be reassessed after treatment) determines whether any treatment response is useful.
- Valuable objective clinical tests include ability to heel–toe walk, stand on tiptoe, Romberg's test and finger extension against gravity.
- Overall quantification of motor function (e.g. for the Guillain-Barré syndrome):
  - Disability Grade 0:   Healthy, no signs or symptoms.
  - Disability Grade 1:   Minor symptoms or signs and able to run.
  - Disability Grade 2:   Able to walk 5 metres without assistance.
  - Disability Grade 3:   Able to walk 5 metres with assistance or sticks.
  - Disability Grade 4:   Chair or bed bound.
  - Disability Grade 5:   Requiring assisted ventilation.

IMMUNOMODULATORY THERAPIES

These are used extensively in various neuropathies including the Guillain–Barré syndrome, chronic inflammatory demyelinating polyneuropathy, neuropathies associated with lymphoproliferative disorders, vasculitic neuropathy and multifocal motor neuropathy.

Corticosteroids

- Oral prednisolone for chronic maintenance therapy:
  - Start at 60 mg/day (adults) for 2–5 weeks depending on treatment response.
  - Then 45 mg/day for 3 weeks.
  - Then transfer slowly to 45 mg on alternate days using schedule:
    Week 1: 45 mg and 40 mg on alternate days
    Week 2: 45 and 35 mg on alternate days
    And so on until 45 mg and 0 mg on alternate days.

- Long-term maintenance usually 15–35 mg on alternate days.
■ Adverse effects, see Chapter 9.

Azathioprine

■ Often used as steroid sparing treatment when long-term immuno-suppression is required.
■ Start with 2.5 mg/kg/day oral until clinical benefit, then maintenance on lower dose (e.g. 1mg/kg/day).
■ Any clinical benefit usually does not occur for some months.
■ Pancytopenia and liver hypersensitivity reactions are not uncommon. Monitor full blood count and liver function weekly for the first 8 weeks of therapy, every 3 months thereafter (see Chapter 9).

Cyclophosphamide

■ Used mainly in vasculitic neuropathy.
■ Given orally: 2 mg/kg/day for 3 months.
■ Bone marrow suppression is the chief early adverse effect: monitor full blood count daily for the first 10 days of treatment, then weekly for 8 weeks, and then every 3 months.
■ Susceptibility to infections can be a problem.
■ Haemorrhagic cystitis, and long-term bladder cancer are risks – administer cyclophosphamide in the morning, and consider administering Mesna too.

Plasma exchange

The rationale of plasma exchange is the removal of pathogenic antibodies from the plasma fraction. It is usually given as:
■ 5-day courses using femoral or other venous access.
■ 50 ml of plasma per kg of body weight exchanged at each daily exchange.
■ Replacement fluid usually human albumin or gelatine solutions.
■ Low-dose heparinisation prevents thrombosis and embolisation from the indwelling venous catheter between exchanges.

Intravenous immunoglobulin (IVIg)

IVIg is derived from pooled human immunoglobulin fraction. Screening and purification methods make transmission of viral infection (hepatitis, human immunodeficiency virus (HIV)) extremely unlikely. It is usually given as:
■ 0.4 g/kg of body weight per day for 5 days.
■ Effect wears off after 6–10 weeks, requiring regular retreatment of chronic neuropathies.

- Long-term maintenance with a single daily dose (~0.5 g/kg) once a fortnight.
- Or domiciliary administration may be feasible and more convenient if training for self-administration is available.
- Minor adverse effects: 5% experience mild, self-limiting reactions such as headache, myalgia, fever, rash or vasomotor reactions (flushing, hypertension). These are generally controllable by reducing the infusion rate or with antihistamines.
- Serious adverse reactions are rare: aseptic meningitis, thromboembolic events, oliguric renal failure and haemolytic anaemia.
- Check immunoglobulin A (IgA) levels before treatment because IgA deficient patients can develop anaphylactic reactions.

IVIg is generally preferred to plasma exchange because:
- it can be administered promptly
- it does not require a specialist operator
- large-vein cannulation and low-dose anticoagulation are not required.

THE GUILLAIN–BARRÉ SYNDROME

There is a spectrum of acute idiopathic polyneuropathies:
- Acute idiopathic demyelinating polyneuropathy (typical Guillain–Barré syndrome (GBS)):
  - predominantly motor ascending paralysis
  - respiratory or bulbar paralysis can cause death if untreated
  - sensory symptoms usually minor.
- Acute motor axonal neuropathy:
  - distinct subtype of GBS with axonal degeneration or conduction block of motor fibres alone.
- The Miller–Fisher syndrome:
  - external ophthalmoplegia, severe ataxia and widespread tendon areflexia.
- Acute sensory or autonomic neuropathies are rare.

General treatment measures

Survival in acute GBS depends on the quality of intensive and nursing care:
- Respiratory muscle failure requires endotracheal intubation and ventilation, generally when the vital capacity has fallen to 15 ml/kg of body weight (i.e. ~1 litre for a 65 kg adult).
- Bulbar muscle failure can lead to aspiration pneumonia or death by choking and also requires endotracheal intubation.
- Nasogastric tube feeding if swallowing compromised.

- Subcutaneous heparin and compression-stocking prophylaxis against deep venous thrombosis and pulmonary embolism.
- Electrocardiographic (ECG) monitoring for cardiac arrhythmias.
- Hypertensive crises may require beta-blockers or other hypotensive drugs.
- Nursing care and physiotherapy will prevent pressure sores and muscle contractures.

Specific treatments

- Plasma exchange or, more conveniently, IVIg have equal benefit in reducing the duration of ventilation, and promoting return of functions such as walking.
- IVIg or plasma exchange should be given within the first 2 weeks of neurological symptoms causing, or progressing towards, significant disability.
- Treatment trials have been conducted only for GBS. However IVIg or plasma exchange is recommended for all the acute idiopathic polyneuropathies.
- No benefit from corticosteroids either orally or intravenously.
- If IVIg or plasma exchange is ineffective, it is unclear whether to repeat the same treatment or switch to the other.

Prognosis

- Although IVIg and plasma exchange promote early recovery, their benefit for survival and 1-year disability is less certain.
- Significant disability (about 16%) and death (about 5%) occur at 1 year even with optimal intensive care and IVIg or plasma exchange.

CHRONIC IDIOPATHIC DEMYELINATING POLYNEUROPATHY
Clinical features and occurrence

- Prevalence approximately 2 per 100,000 population.
- Progresses over > 8 weeks.
- A sensorimotor, symmetrical, demyelinating polyneuropathy.
- Significant bulbar or respiratory muscle involvement is rare.
- Main cause of disability varies in different patients:
  - limb muscle weakness
  - sensory ataxia with Rombergism

- coarse action tremor is rare and associated with extremely slow nerve conduction velocities.
- Without treatment many suffer protracted and serious disability, and the condition may be fatal in up to 10%.
- Can have spontaneously relapsing and remitting course.
- Relapses in women associated with third trimester of pregnancy or immediately post-partum.
- Monoclonal paraproteinaemia can be associated with chronic idiopathic demyelinating polyneuropathy (CIDP):
  - this needs investigation and treatment in its own right in collaboration with a haematological oncologist
  - standard CIDP treatment should be given, although patients are less likely to respond than most with 'ordinary CIDP'.

Treatment

- CIDP has an excellent prospect for significant recovery of disability using immunosuppressant therapy.
- Mild forms of CIDP, without significant disability, may not require treatment, given the potential adverse effects.
- Oral corticosteroids are the mainstay of treatment, with benefit often evident within 3 weeks.
- After high-dose steroid induction, maintenance dose varies between 15 and 45 mg on alternate days, titrated against clinical benefit.
- Withdrawal of prednisolone often leads to relapse within the subsequent months; low-dose, alternate-day steroid therapy needs to be continued for years – few patients make permanent spontaneous recovery.
- IVIg or plasma exchange are effective in 80% of CIDP patients and are recommended:
  - if steroid response is inadequate
  - when steroids are contraindicated
  - to 'kick start' improvement in the elderly, who respond slowly to steroids
  - in severe disability at the outset
  - to reverse relapses promptly and avoid reinstating high-dose steroids
  - in diabetics where steroids may be problematic.
- Treatment-unresponsive patients do occur:
  - many have a significant degree of associated chronic axonal degeneration
  - underlying paraproteinaemia, lymphoproliferative disorders and carcinoma should be sought as an explanation and treated on their respective merits
  - the POEMS syndrome is a particular cause of unresponsive CIDP.

POEMS syndrome

The clinical features of the POEMS syndrome (**P**olyneuropathy, **O**rgano-megaly, **E**dema, **M**-band (paraprotein) and **S**kin changes (diffuse cyanosis or hair growth changes)) include:

- Polyneuropathy, which can be axonal degeneration or demyelinating, or most usually a mixture, sometimes presenting as treatment-unresponsive CIDP.
- Underlying Castleman's disease (angiofollicular lymph node hyperplasia) or, less frequently, osteosclerotic myeloma.
- Treatment:
  - advice should be sought from a haematological oncologist
  - approximately half show a good neurological response to melphalan or cyclophosphamide and prednisolone, the remainder are unresponsive
  - remorseless downhill progression occurs in a minority, with eventual death despite chemotherapy.

The CANOMAD syndrome

This syndrome is a combination, often incomplete at presentation, of **C**hronic **A**taxic **N**europathy with **O**phthalmoplegia, **M**-proteins, cold **A**gglutinins and anti-**D**isialated ganglioside antibodies. The ataxia is generally out of proportion to other signs of neuropathy, which can be mild. It responds moderately well to long-term IVIg but often poorly to steroids.

MULTIFOCAL MOTOR NEUROPATHY WITH CONDUCTION BLOCK

In past years this was often diagnosed as a benign form of motor neuron disease. The clinical features include:

- chronic, slowly progressive, asymmetrical weakness of the arms, or sometimes legs
- the clinical feature of conduction block is significant weakness in a muscle that is not obviously wasted
- differential finger drop is a common early symptom
- there are no sensory features
- motor conduction block is demonstrable electrophysiologically in most
- anti-GM1 ganglioside antibodies are present in 30%.

Treatment

- IVIg is the treatment of choice, with a clear clinical response, often within days. Maximal effect occurs in 10–14 days. Wearing off occurs by

about 6–12 weeks, so regular repeated therapy is required. Self-infused home therapy at 2–3 week intervals is effective and convenient. Background progression is prevented or greatly slowed by regular IVIg.
- Corticosteroids cause deterioration, or are ineffective.
- Cyclophosphamide is effective but not advised as primary treatment because of the severe adverse-effect profile.
- A rare syndrome of symmetrical pure motor demyelinating neuropathy also responds to IVIg, and deteriorates with steroids.

VASCULITIC NEUROPATHY

Vasculitic neuropathy is generally a medical emergency requiring prompt recognition and treatment to avoid progressive, severe and permanent nerve damage. The ischaemic damage to individual nerves is due to inflammatory vasculitis. It presents as a mononeuropathy, or mononeuritis multiplex, and individual nerves are usually affected in a sequential, stepwise manner with sensory and motor loss in the territory of involved nerve(s), and neuropathic pain is common in affected nerve territories. Rarely, an isolated nerve-specific form occurs, but vasculitic neuropathy is usually associated with systemic vasculitis:
- Churg–Strauss syndrome (eosinophilia and asthma)
- Wegener's granulomatosis (respiratory tract granulomas and glomerulonephritis)
- microscopic polyarteritis
- antineutrophil cytoplasmic antibody may be positive.

Histological evidence of vasculitis is generally required before treatment with curative, but potentially toxic, cyclophosphamide. Therefore, if there is no non-neurological histological evidence of vasculitis:
- full-thickness sural nerve biopsy if sural sensory nerve action potential abnormal
- otherwise, muscle biopsy.

There have been no randomised trials of systemic treatments but:
- corticosteroids alone are often effective in Churg–Strauss vasculitis, and vasculitis restricted to the peripheral nervous system
- relapse may occur when the steroid dose is reduced or withdrawn
- cyclophosphamide can produce dramatic remissions and cures, but beware adverse effects with considerable morbidity and mortality
- relapse of vasculitic neuropathy is rare after cyclophosphamide
- patients resistant to steroids or cyclophosphamide should be investigated for cryoglobulinaemia.

DIABETIC NEUROPATHIES

In diabetes there is a wide spectrum of neuropathy:

- Symmetrical, sensory, axonal polyneuropathy, so-called 'diabetic polyneuropathy', causes numb or painful feet, but is often mild or asymptomatic:
  - no known treatment for established axonal degeneration
  - progress of neuropathy minimised by tight control of glycaemia with insulin or by pancreas transplantation
  - protective measures reduce acromutilation as a result of loss of pain sensation, and so diabetic foot ulcers
  - neuropathic pain may require carbamazepine etc (see Chapter 18)
  - acute neuropathic pain, lasting months, may be precipitated by initiation of insulin therapy.
- Autonomic neuropathy produces postural hypotension, impotence, nocturnal diarrhoea, sweating abnormalities, predisposes patients to sudden death during anaesthesia, and reduces awareness of hypoglycaemia:
  - symptomatic postural hypotension requires compressive stockings, sleeping with head-up tilt, and promotion of fluid retention by fludrocortisone (see Chapter 6)
  - nocturnal diarrhoea may respond to codeine phosphate, clonidine or one or two doses of tetracycline
  - gastroparesis causing serious vomiting can improve with oral erythromycin
  - erectile failure may require sildenafil (see Chapter 17).
- CIDP is about 10 times commoner in diabetics than non-diabetics:
  - initial trial of therapy with IVIg to identify those responding to immunomodulation and to avoid the problems posed by steroids in managing hyperglycaemia
  - once IVIg treatment response established, general principles of treatment as for CIDP
  - liaison with diabetologist about managing hyperglycaemia during administration of high-dose and alternate-day steroid therapy, and in patients with visual or physical difficulties that make insulin injections difficult.
- Diabetic microvascular disease renders nerves vulnerable to compression, which should be managed by normal measures (see below). The prognosis for recovery of function is poorer due to underlying axonal degeneration in diabetes.

- Diabetic truncal and proximal neuropathy tends to develop over weeks or months in non-insulin-dependent diabetics and is associated with weight loss. It usually causes unilateral or asymmetrical anterior thigh pain and quadriceps muscle weakness. Truncal neuropathy causes patches of painful sensory disturbance. It generally recovers with neurological improvement after some months, but residual low-grade pain may persist and recurrence occurs in one-fifth. Glycaemic control should be reviewed, but there is no evidence that hypoglycaemic therapy is curative. A trial of corticosteroids should be considered in relentlessly progressive or unresolving forms.

CRITICAL ILLNESS POLYNEUROPATHY

- Sensorimotor polyneuropathy can develop in patients being ventilated and who develop multiorgan failure or sepsis.
- The neuropathy usually comes to light when patients fail to wean from the ventilator.
- The principal differential diagnosis in the intensive-care setting is critical illness myopathy, usually occurring in association with an acute respiratory disorder, such as asthma treated with non-depolarising neuromuscular blocking agents or high-dose steroids.
- Those who recover neurologically do so over 3–6 months; there is no treatment known to accelerate recovery.

NEUROPATHY DUE TO INFECTIONS

Leprosy

There is a spectrum of neuropathy, from tuberculoid leprosy with loss of sensation in the territory of a single peripheral nerve, to lepromatous leprosy with progressive and extensive involvement of multiple skin nerves, and nerve thickening. Early diagnosis is crucial because antibiotics prevent further irreversible nerve damage.

- Treatment of lepromatous and borderline leprosy:
  - daily self-administration of dapsone 100 mg oral and clofazimine 50 mg oral plus supervised once monthly clofazimine 300 mg oral and rifampicin 600 mg oral
  - for a minimum of 2 years, and until skin scrapings and biopsies are negative for bacilli.
- Treatment of tuberculoid leprosy:
  - daily dapsone 100 mg oral with supervised monthly rifampicin 600 mg oral
  - 6 months treatment required.

■ Corticosteroids are recommended to prevent treatment reactions in patients with erythema nodosum, iritis, and for those who develop worsening of neuropathy after initiation of antibiotics.

HIV-associated neuropathies

These may cause:

■ Typical GBS, where underlying HIV is suggested by cerebrospinal fluid (CSF) pleocytosis – treat as for normal GBS.
■ CIDP – treat as for CIDP.
■ Cytomegalovirus polyradiculopathy is rare, with sacral sensory loss, urinary retention and flaccid paraparesis over a few weeks – early therapy with gancyclovir or cidofovir is necessary.
■ Sensory polyneuropathy affects up to 30% by the acquired immune deficiency syndrome (AIDS) stage of HIV infection. Differential diagnosis is the painful sensory neuropathy caused by antiretroviral drugs (e.g. didanosine).

Borrelia burgdorferii

Also known as Lyme disease, this causes varying combinations of facial palsy, painful polyradiculopathy, peripheral neuropathy including mononeuritis multiplex and acute brachial plexus neuropathy, and chronic central nervous system involvement. Immunological proof of diagnosis can be difficult, blood enzyme-linked immunosorbent assay (ELISA) for *Borrelia* antibody is the best screening test. CSF pleocytosis is typical but can be absent in isolated facial palsy or peripheral neuropathy.

Treatment of peripheral neuropathy or radiculopathy is with benzylpenicillin 2.4 g iv 6-hourly for 10 days, or cephtriaxone 2 g/day iv infusion for 14 days, or doxycycline 100–200 mg oral bd for 14–21 days.

Diphtheria

■ Polyneuropathy is the most common complication of diphtheria.
■ Severe early bulbar and/or respiratory muscle failure may require:
  – ventilation and intubation as for the Guillain–Barré syndrome
  – nasogastric tube feeding to preserve nutrition.
■ Immediate antibiotic therapy is required:
  – benzylpenicillin 2.4 g iv 6-hourly for 14 days
  – or erythromycin 50 mg/kg/day iv for 10–14 days for patients with penicillin allergy.

- Diphtheria antitoxin intravenously or intramuscularly:
  - potential benefit falls after first few days of throat infection
  - serum sickness may occur in 10%.

Herpes zoster

- Reactivation of latent varicella zoster virus in sensory ganglia causes shingles:
  - initially tingling or lancinating pain in a dermatomal distribution
  - visible vesicular skin lesions accumulating by 3–5 days
  - associated segmental motor involvement can occur
  - conjunctivitis and keratitis can occur when ophthalmic division of the trigeminal nerve is affected.
- Treatment of acute attack:
  - analgesics
  - antiviral drugs (acyclovir, valaciclovir, famciclovir) speed resolution of the acute eruption, and are particularly indicated in immunocompromised hosts (see Chapter 14).
- Postherpetic neuralgia may require systemic or local pain relieving measures (see Chapter 18).

TOXIC POLYNEUROPATHIES

Therapeutic drugs (Box 11.1) and less often heavy metals (Box 11.2) and industrial toxins (Box 11.3) cause a slowly progressive axonal and predominantly sensory polyneuropathy. Management consists of removing

Box 11.1 Drugs that induce polyneuropathy		
Alcohol	Disulfiram	Phenytoin
Almitrine	Ethambutol	Pyridoxine
Amiodarone	Gold	Sodium cyanate
Chloroquine	Isoniazid	Statins
Cisplatin	Lithium	Suramin
Clioquinol	Metronidazole	Tacrolimus
Colchicine	Misonidazole	Taxol
Dapsone	Nitrofuranotoin	Thalidomide
Didanosine and other antiretroviral drugs	Perhexiline	Vinca alkaloids

> ## Box 11.2   Metal-poisoning polyneuropathy
>
> Arsenic
> Lead
> Mercury
> Thallium

> ## Box 11.3   Industrial and agricultural chemicals that cause polyneuropathy
>
> Acrylamide
> Carbon disulphide
> Dimethylaminopropionitrile
> Ethylene oxide
> Herbicides
>
> Hexacarbons
> Methylbromide
> Pesticides
> Trichloroethylene

the suspected drug or toxin, but if the neuropathy is mild, and any drug is of major therapeutic importance (e.g. statins or antiretrovirals), continued treatment may be judged in the patient's best interest, despite the neuropathy.

ACUTE BRACHIAL NEURITIS

- Acute pain in one shoulder followed by weakness of shoulder girdle muscles noted 1 or 2 weeks later, as the pain subsides.
- Spontaneous recovery is good in most, occurring over 12–18 months.
- Poorer prognosis for recovery in those with diabetes, or the elderly.
- No treatment known to affect the long-term outcome. Some consider that corticosteroids or ACTH diminish the severity of the pain in the early stages.

ENTRAPMENT AND COMPRESSIVE FOCAL NEUROPATHIES
General principles

- External compression produces a focal area of demyelination in a nerve, with block of conduction, known as 'neurapraxia'. If the compression is relieved neurapraxia recovers spontaneously over 8–12 weeks.
- Severe or prolonged compression severs axons as well, with the development of muscle wasting. Then any recovery will be slow and depends on axonal regeneration.

- Patients who develop repeated compressive mononeuropathies, often after relatively mild compression, may have the autosomal-dominant condition of hereditary liability to pressure palsies.
- To differentiate between a temporary compressive and an entrapment neuropathy, for instance affecting the ulnar nerve at the elbow, wait 12 weeks to allow spontaneous recovery after *compression* before considering surgical exploration for *entrapment*.

Carpal tunnel syndrome

Entrapment of the median nerve under the transverse carpal ligament at the wrist causes painful tingling in the fingers at night, or when using the hand, as the main symptom. It can be secondary to hypothyroidism, acromegaly, rheumatoid arthritis and pregnancy.

- Symptoms interfering with sleep, or causing significant interference with manual tasks, merit treatment.
- Definitive treatment is by surgical decompression of the nerve at the wrist.
- Local corticosteroid injection is an alternative but does not provide permanent cure.

Ulnar nerve lesions at the elbow

Ulnar neuropathy is due to entrapment within the cubital tunnel, external compression of a nerve which dislocates from the condylar groove, or by bony abnormalities at the elbow joint/condylar groove.

- Surgery is most likely to be successful if there is local conduction block or electrophysiological slowing along the ulnar nerve at the elbow, rather than axonal degeneration with muscle wasting.
- Choice of operation lies between simple decompression of the cubital tunnel, anterior transposition of the ulnar nerve or medial epicondylectomy.

Thoracic outlet syndrome

This syndrome is due to compression of the lower brachial plexus as it passes over a cervical rib, or less often a radiologically invisible fibrous band. Patients present with either painless wasting of the small muscles of the hand and the forearm flexor compartment, or pain in the ulnar side of the arm and hand provoked by using the arm and carrying.

- Diagnosis of severe and established thoracic outlet syndrome is relatively easy, but surgical treatment will not restore power to wasted muscles.

■ Diagnosis of early and incomplete forms of thoracic outlet syndrome is difficult, but surgical treatment at this stage offers the prospect of curing pain and preventing further denervation of hand and forearm muscles.

Meralgia paraesthetica

■ Pain in the anterolateral thigh usually provoked by walking.
■ Lesion of the lateral cutaneous nerve of the thigh, thought to be due to entrapment and/or kinking where the nerve passes through the inguinal ligament.
■ Most common in obese or pregnant patients and may improve with dieting or delivery.
■ Meralgia paraesthetica often resolves spontaneously.
■ If troublesome, local anaesthetic infiltration around the lateral half of the inguinal ligament may relieve symptoms. If this is unsuccessful, operative decompression of the nerve just medial to the anterior superior iliac spine may be indicated.

Common peroneal nerve lesions

■ Cause foot drop and loss of sensation on the outer aspect of the leg, below the knee, and over the dorsum of the foot.
■ Various causes: external compression (e.g. tight plaster or sitting with crossed legs), upper fibular fracture, penetrating wound around the knee joint, arthroscopic knee surgery, popliteal bursa, cyst or tumour.
■ Entrapment by a fibrous band in the fibula tunnel is rare and hard to diagnose, but is an indication for surgical decompression.
■ If a spontaneously occurring common peroneal nerve palsy does not recover within 3 months with avoidance of leg crossing or kneeling, surgical inspection of the nerve at the fibula neck is required in those for whom there is no convincing explanation for the neuropathy.

Further reading

Donaghy M. Polyneuropathy. In: Brain's diseases of the nervous system (ed Donaghy M), 11th edn. Oxford University Press, Oxford, 2001, pp 337–403.
Donaghy M. Focal peripheral neuropathy. In: Brain's diseases of the nervous system (ed Donaghy M), 11th edn. Oxford University Press, Oxford, 2001, pp 405–442.

12 DISORDERS OF SKELETAL MUSCLE AND THE NEUROMUSCULAR JUNCTION

David Hilton-Jones

Chapter contents

Disorders of skeletal muscle (myopathies) and the neuromuscular junction are rare (Table 12.1). Therefore, general neurologists are unlikely to be looking after more than a handful of patients with these conditions, and will see a new case no more than once or twice a year. As a rough guide, a new case of myasthenia gravis might be encountered once a year, of myotonic dystrophy every couple of years, of facioscapulohumeral muscular dystrophy, myositis or limb-girdle muscular dystrophy every 3 or 4 years, and of any of the many metabolic myopathies every 5–10 years. Because of such inevitably limited familiarity, the lack of a firm evidence base for many of the treatment options, specific management issues (e.g. cardiorespiratory complications in the dystrophies, thymectomy for myasthenia), and the complexities of genetic counselling issues for many of the inherited disorders, consideration should always be given to referring the patient for more specialised advice.

ACQUIRED VERSUS INHERITED NEUROMUSCULAR DISORDERS

- Most acquired conditions respond, or even resolve completely, when the cause is removed (e.g. drug-induced myopathy) or treated (e.g. endocrinopathy, autoimmune myositis, neuromuscular junction disorder), an important exception being inclusion body myositis.

■ Conversely, no curative treatment is yet available for any of the inherited neuromuscular disorders, although symptomatic treatments can be highly effective (e.g. for periodic paralysis and myotonia congenita) or life-saving (e.g. cardiac pacemaker, non-invasive ventilation).

■ Genetic counselling is a major management issue with inherited conditions.

■ Whether a condition is treatable or not, patient-led groups can provide invaluable support and information for patients and their relatives – and also for healthcare professionals. Local information must be sought, and there are useful websites, many of which also provide useful information for healthcare workers (Box 12.1).

Table 12.1   Approximate prevalence of some of the more common myopathies and neuromuscular junction disorders

Condition	Prevalence/100,000 population
Myasthenia gravis	10
Myotonic dystrophy	12
Dermatomyositis	5*
Facioscapulohumeral muscular dystrophy	3
Duchenne muscular dystrophy	3
Becker muscular dystrophy	2
Inclusion body myositis	1
McArdle's disease	1†
Oculopharyngeal muscular dystrophy	1
Periodic paralysis	1
Myotonia congenita	1
Limb-girdle muscular dystrophy	<1
Lambert–Eaton syndrome	0.5

*Not all patients have significant muscle involvement.
†Those with a special interest in McArdle's disease estimate the prevalence to be > 1:100,000, with many cases being undiagnosed. In the UK (population 60 million) only ~60 cases are known to the relevant patient support groups – a 10-fold discrepancy.

Box 12.1   Reliable websites

Muscular Dystrophy Association USA	http://www.mdausa.org
Muscular Dystrophy Campaign UK	http://www.muscular-dystrophy.org
Duchenne Support Group UK	http://www.ppuk.org
Myasthenia Gravis Association UK	http://www.mgauk.org
Myasthenia Gravis Foundation USA	http://www.myasthenia.org
Glycogen storage disease association UK	http://www.agsd.org.uk/home
Myotonic Dystrophy Support Group UK	http://www.mdsguk.org

Myopathies

These can be divided into several major categories of both inherited and acquired disorders:

- Inherited myopathies:
  - muscular dystrophies
  - myotonic dystrophy
  - congenital myopathies
  - metabolic myopathies
  - ion channelopathies.
- Acquired myopathies:
  - idiopathic inflammatory myopathies (myositis)
  - endocrinopathies
  - drug- and toxin-induced myopathies
  - metabolic myopathies.

Numerically, drug-induced and endocrine myopathies are amongst the commonest of these conditions, but are less likely to appear in a neurology clinic than some of the considerably less common 'primary' myopathies. Drug-induced myopathies are probably underdiagnosed and mild weakness associated with endocrinopathy is often not sought or identified.

MUSCULAR DYSTROPHIES

The severity of the muscular dystrophies ranges from profound disability in early childhood (e.g. some sarcoglycanopathies) to undetectable weakness in late life (e.g. some cases of facioscapulohumeral muscular dystrophy). Furthermore, the range of severity, as well as the pattern of muscle involvement, in the same disease can vary markedly, even sometimes within the same family. Thus, in facioscapulohumeral muscular dystrophy severity in different families can range from presentation with severe facial weakness in the first year of life, to an asymptomatic condition in the elderly. The same caveolin mutation may present within one family with asymptomatic elevation of the serum creatine kinase, limb-girdle weakness, distal myopathy or rippling muscles. However, certain general management approaches can be applied:

- Genetic counselling.
- Psychosocial support.
- Physiotherapy:
  - gait
  - exercise advice
  - joints
  - ligaments
  - chest.
- Occupational therapy:
  - specific aids
  - home adaptations.
- Orthotics:
  - single joint orthosis
  - walking aids.
- Surgery:
  - tendons
  - spinal
  - ptosis correction.
- Speech and language therapy:
  - speech
  - swallowing.
- Dietician.
- Cardiorespiratory management.

Prednisolone has been shown to prolong ambulation in boys with Duchenne muscular dystrophy and is now widely used, although questions remain about the best regimen as well as the treatment and prevention of complications such as osteoporosis. Neither steroids nor indeed any other drugs have been shown to be helpful in any of the other dystrophies.

Cardiac management

- For those dystrophies with cardiac complications (Table 12.2), patients should be advised to report relevant symptoms (e.g. palpitations, syncope, breathlessness), and to have an annual electrocardiogram

Table 12.2   The likelihood of cardiac and respiratory complications in the muscular dystrophies

Inheritance Protein		Cardiac complications		Ventilatory failure*	
		Conduction	Cardio-myopathy	Early	Late
X-linked					
Duchenne	Dystrophin	+	++		+
Becker	Dystrophin	+	++		+
EDMD	Emerin	++	+		+
Autosomal recessive					
LGMD 2A	Calpain	−	−		+
2B	Dysferlin	−	−		+
2C	γ-Sarcoglycan	+	+		+
2D	δ-Sarcoglycan	+	+		+
2E	α-Sarcoglycan	+	+		+
2F	β-Sarcoglycan	+	+		+
2G	Telethonin	−	−		?
2H	TRIM-32	−	−		?
2I	FKRP	+	+	+	+
2J	Titin	−	−		?
Autosomal dominant					
LGMD 1A	Myotilin	−	−		?
1B	Lamin A/C	++	+		?
1C	Caveolin	−	−		?
EDMD	Lamin A/C	++	+		+
FSH	Unknown	−	−	−	+
OPMD	PABPN2	−	−	−	−

EDMD, Emery–Dreifuss muscular dystrophy; FSH, facioscapulohumeral muscular dystrophy; LGMD, limb-girdle muscular dystrophy; OPMD, oculopharyngeal muscular dystrophy.
*Ventilatory failure sufficient to cause symptoms and/or requiring intervention.
Early: can develop while the patient is still ambulant.
Late: develops after the patient has become wheelchair-bound.
? Either not reported or too few cases to make useful comment, periodic measurement of forced vital capacity advised.

(ECG) and, for those associated with cardiomyopathy, echocardiography as frequently as advised by the cardiologist.

- Cardiac arrhythmias are a common cause of morbidity and mortality in the lamin A/C disorders, and ECG abnormalities are inevitable in all forms of Emery–Dreifuss syndrome by early adult life where presymptomatic insertion of an implantable defibrillator may be considered, because of the high risk of sudden death.
- Cardiomyopathy is inevitable in Duchenne muscular dystrophy and is an occasional cause of death (respiratory failure is a commoner cause). Particularly with longer survival as the result of the introduction of non-invasive ventilation, cardiomyopathy management is currently being reviewed. Presymptomatic introduction of angiotensin-converting enzyme (ACE) inhibitors and other cardiac-related drugs (e.g. beta-blockers, diuretics, digoxin, anticoagulants) is increasingly common and gaining an evidence base.
- In Becker muscular dystrophy cardiomyopathy does not always parallel the skeletal muscle involvement. Patients with profound weakness may have no significant cardiac involvement, whereas in others severe cardiomyopathy, requiring cardiac transplantation, may develop without any significant limb weakness.

Respiratory management

- Most myopathies that cause severe weakness leading to immobility can be associated with respiratory insufficiency (Table 12.2). Symptoms include:
  - excessive daytime sleepiness
  - poor appetite and weight loss
  - poor night-time sleep and early morning headache
  - breathlessness is relatively uncommon, in part due to limited mobility and exertion.
- In some dystrophies, notably LGMD 2I, respiratory failure can develop when the patient is still walking.
- The presence of significant spinal deformity (e.g. in some cases of autosomal dominant Emery–Dreifuss syndrome) increases the risk of ventilatory insufficiency.
- First awareness of any respiratory insufficiency may be respiratory failure precipitated by intercurrent infection or general anaesthesia.
- Routine assessment should include forced vital capacity. When significantly reduced (e.g. < 1.5 litres in an adult), or when the patient has suggestive symptoms, more detailed investigations, including sleep and arterial gas studies, are required.
- Treatment is by non-invasive, facial mask, positive pressure ventilation which, at least initially, will probably be required only at night. In

Duchenne muscular dystrophy this has increased the age of death from about 20 years to more than 30 years, with improved quality of life.

MYOTONIC DYSTROPHY

Many management issues are the same as those discussed for the muscular dystrophies in general, but a few points merit specific comment.

Genetic counselling

- Even within a family there may be considerable variation in severity.
- It is inappropriate, and potentially very misleading, to use the term 'carrier' for a person with the abnormal gene, even if they are asymptomatic. They often have signs, however minor, and are at risk of complications of the disease, particularly cardiorespiratory.
- A major concern is the young woman with the abnormal gene who is unaware of the diagnosis until she gives birth to a child with the severe congenital form of the disease.
- Anticipation is also seen when the father is the transmitting parent, but not leading to such severe disease in the offspring as when the mother is the transmitting parent.
- Genetic counselling issues are particularly complex and include cascade screening for other family members. An appropriate neurogenetics referral must be made.

Cataracts

- Although common, their management does not differ from other cataracts. Surgery is indicated when vision is significantly affected.

Excessive daytime sleepiness

- This symptom, which is common and sometimes a major practical problem, can be due to respiratory insufficiency and fragmented night-time sleep (which must be excluded, see below), but is more frequently 'central' and a manifestation of cerebral involvement in the condition.
- It may respond to oral modafinil, initially 200 mg in the morning, adding in 200 mg at lunchtime if needed. If after 1 month on 400 mg/day there has been no improvement, the drug should be discontinued (see Chapter 3).

Cardiac involvement

- Conduction abnormalities are extremely common, but cardiomyopathy and impaired contractility are rare.

- From the teenage years patients should have an annual ECG and be advised to report symptoms such as palpitations, dizzy spells and syncope.
- Most patients develop a prolonged PR interval. Other common changes include:
  - intraventricular conduction delay
  - partial and complete bundle branch block
  - atrial flutter and fibrillation
  - complete heart block.

Sudden death can be due to bradyarrhythmia or tachyarrhythmia. The optimal timing of pacemaker insertion is unclear, but is usually either after symptoms develop or if the ECG has shown substantial change. Implantable defibrillators have not been evaluated, but some patients have died from ventricular tachycardia/fibrillation. Conduction abnormalities may become more evident, or symptomatic, during the stress of infection, surgery or anaesthesia.

- Routine echocardiography is not required.

Respiratory involvement

- Most patients with limb weakness, even when relatively mild, have reduced forced vital capacity.
- There are many examples of the diagnosis of myotonic dystrophy first being made after a patient develops respiratory failure during an intercurrent chest infection, or following general anaesthesia.
- The most common mode of death in patients with myotonic dystrophy is chest infection.
- Respiratory insufficiency worsens in sleep, and fragmentation of sleep by arousals can contribute to excessive daytime sleepiness, although as noted above it is more often due to primary cerebral involvement from the disease.
- Overnight sleep studies are useful in assessing respiratory function. However, even in those with undoubted respiratory insufficiency, long-term treatment with nocturnal non-invasive positive pressure ventilation is often poorly tolerated, and rarely seems to help any excessive daytime sleepiness.

Dysphagia

- This is common in the later stages of the disease and aspiration increases the risk of chest infection.

- Speech therapy and specialist ear, nose and throat assessment, usually with videofluoroscopy, are helpful, but treatment options are limited. Cricopharyngeal myotomy and balloon dilatation may be beneficial.

Diabetes

- Although laboratory demonstrable insulin resistance is common, frank diabetes is not much more common than in the general population, and the management is the same.

Pregnancy and related issues

- Fertility is reduced in both sexes.
- Females with the disease have an increased risk of spontaneous abortion, probably often due to a non-viable fetus carrying a large gene expansion.
- Although uterine (smooth muscle) contractility is reduced, it is rarely a major problem during labour.
- The cardiorespiratory complications relating to general anaesthesia, and the issues around generalised weakness when carrying a pregnancy, are all more troublesome in practice.

CONGENITAL MYOPATHIES

This term is used for a number of conditions that can indeed be evident at birth, but which can also present in later life, sometimes not until adulthood (Table 12.3). Initially defined on the basis of histological or ultrastructural

Table 12.3   The congenital myopathies and their inheritance patterns

Disease	Inheritance*	Protein	Gene
Nemaline myopathy	AR	Nebulin	NEM2
	AR	Slow troponin T	TNNT1
	AD/AR	α-Actin	ACTA1
	AD/AR	α-Tropomyosin	TPM3
	AD	β-Tropomyosin	TPM2
Central core disease	AD/(AR)	Ryanodine receptor	RYR1
Multiminicore disease	AR	Selenoprotein N1	SEPN1
Myotubular myopathy	XR	Myotubularin	MTM1

*AD, autosomal dominant; AR, autosomal recessive; XR, X-linked recessive.

abnormalities, they are now being reclassified at a molecular level. There is considerable phenotypic and genetic heterogeneity.

There are no specific therapies, and management issues overlap with those of the muscular dystrophies. Cardiac involvement has been reported rarely in nemaline myopathy, but not in the other conditions listed. There are two important potential complications for which specific management may be required:

- There may be disproportionate respiratory muscle involvement in nemaline myopathy and multiminicore disease, resulting in ventilatory failure in patients who are still walking. There should be regular monitoring of forced vital capacity and introduction of non-invasive ventilation when required. Myotubular myopathy is often fatal in early life, but of those who survive most are ventilator dependent.
- There is a strong association between central core disease and malignant hyperthermia (described below). There is a more dubious association with multiminicore disease.

METABOLIC MYOPATHIES

Muscle derives most of its adenosine triphosphate (ATP), which provides the energy to drive contraction as well as general metabolic processes, from two sources:

- Glucose derived from the circulation is stored in muscle as the polymer glycogen. During early exercise, before adaptive processes lead to increased muscle blood flow and the delivery of free fatty acids and oxygen, ATP is derived from the anaerobic breakdown of glycogen.
- Free fatty acids which are derived from stored intramuscular triglycerides and from circulating free fatty acids. They are transported into mitochondria through the carnitine system and then undergo β-oxidation. The reducing equivalents generated are converted to ATP via the mitochondrial respiratory chain, the process being aerobic. With sustained exercise, free fatty acid metabolism becomes the main source of ATP.

Although it is an oversimplification, metabolic myopathies become symptomatic when the demand for ATP exceeds its supply (acid maltase deficiency is an exception and is discussed separately). Therefore, the main clinical features are exercise-induced muscle pain and weakness, stiffness (contracture), muscle fibre necrosis (rhabdomyolysis), myoglobinuria and the risk of acute renal failure. On this basis it can readily be seen why disorders of glycogen metabolism (Table 12.4) present with symptoms during early exercise, particularly intense exercise, whereas disorders of

Table 12.4   Glycogenoses affecting skeletal muscle

Disease	Defective enzyme	Exercise intolerance
McArdle's	Myophosphorylase	+++
Cori-Forbes	Debrancher enzyme	+
Tarui	Phosphofructokinase	+
Other rarities	Phosphorylase b kinase	+
	Phosphoglycerate kinase	+
	Phosphoglycerate mutase	+
	Lactate dehydrogenase	+
	Branching enzyme	−
Pompe's	α-Glucosidase (acid maltase)	−

fatty acid transport and metabolism (Box 12.2), including mitochondrial disorders, present with exercise intolerance during sustained activity (e.g. route marches, endurance activities), particularly if combined with relative starvation, which enhances fatty acid metabolism.

Many of the fatty acid transport and metabolism disorders can present with severe systemic features, including metabolic crises, as well as exercise-induced symptoms and progressive myopathy. The limited management

Box 12.2   Disorders of free fatty acid transport and metabolism

Transport
- Primary carnitine deficiency
- Carnitine palmitoyltransferase deficiency

Metabolism
- Very-long-chain acyl-CoA dehydrogenase deficiency
- Medium-chain acyl-CoA dehydrogenase deficiency
- Short-chain acyl-CoA dehydrogenase deficiency
- Electron transfer flavoprotein dehydrogenase deficiency (glutaric aciduria type II)
- Riboflavin-responsive multiple acyl-CoA dehydrogenase deficiency
- Mitochondrial trifunctional protein deficiency

and therapeutic options for the characteristic exercise-induced symptoms can readily be understood:

- Glycogenoses:
  - avoid sudden, particularly intense, activity
  - 'warming up' gradually will allow enhanced ATP generation from free fatty acids, and to some extent from circulating glucose and amino acids as muscle blood flow increases, giving rise to the 'second wind' phenomenon
  - regular aerobic exercise improves exercise tolerance.
- Free fatty acid transport and oxidation disorders:
  - avoid fasting (especially during intercurrent illness/infection)
  - low-fat/high-carbohydrate diet
  - medium-chain triglyceride supplementation in some patients
  - L-carnitine and riboflavin supplementation in some patients
  - intravenous glucose during crises (inhibits lipolysis)
  - alkaline diuresis during crises (to reduce risk of acute tubular necrosis).

Acid maltase deficiency

This lysosomal enzyme breaks down glycogen, but the pathway is separate from ATP-generating processes. Exercise-induced symptoms are not a feature. In infancy the condition presents as a severe multisystem disorder leading to early death (Pompe's disease). Later onset, including adult onset, is with progressive limb-girdle weakness. The diaphragm is selectively involved and ventilatory insufficiency, which in up to one-third of patients can be the presenting feature, is common. Management is with non-invasive positive pressure ventilation. Recent trials have shown that infants with the severe form of the disease respond to intravenous enzyme replacement therapy and trials on the later onset forms are now starting.

CHANNELOPATHIES

The major clinical features of the muscle ion channelopathies (Table 12.5) include periodic paralysis, myotonia and malignant hyperthermia. Management of the periodic paralyses involves treatment of individual attacks to restore strength, and long-term strategies (diet and medication) to try to reduce attack frequency. Some patients develop a progressive proximal myopathy, which can occur even without paralytic attacks, and as yet no useful treatment has been identified.

In hyperkalaemic periodic paralysis the attacks are often mild and require no specific treatment.

Table 12.5   The pattern of inheritance and clinical syndromes of the muscle channelopathies

Ion channel	Inheritance*	Clinical associates
Sodium	AD	Periodic paralysis (hyperkalaemic, normokalaemic, and rarely hypokalaemic)
	AD	Paramyotonia congenita
	AD	Potassium-aggravated myotonia
Calcium	AD	Periodic paralysis (hypokalaemic)
	AD	Malignant hyperthermia
Potassium	AD	Andersen syndrome: – periodic paralysis (hyper- or hypokalaemic) – dysmorphism – cardiac ventricular arrhythmia
Chloride	AD	Myotonia congenita (Thomsen)
	AR	Myotonia congenita (Becker)
Ryanodine receptor	AD	Malignant hyperthermia
	AD/AR	Core diseases

*AD, autosomal dominant; AR, autosomal recessive.

Hyperkalaemic and normokalaemic periodic paralyses

- Acute attacks may respond to:
  - carbohydrate-rich food
  - salbutamol (inhaler).
- Preventive measures:
  - low potassium diet
  - frequent carbohydrate-rich meals
  - thiazide diuretic (to maintain a low to normal serum potassium)
  - acetazolamide 125 mg/day oral, up to 500 mg bd
  - dichlorphenamide 25 mg oral up to 75 mg/day (like acetazolamide, it is a carbonic anhydrase inhibitor with similar adverse effects; it is not available in the UK, but in the USA some clinicians believe it to be more effective than acetazolamide).

Hypokalaemic periodic paralysis

- Acute attacks (may be severe) respond to:
  - oral potassium (unsweetened solution, 2–10 g)
  - **avoid** intravenous potassium.
- Preventive measures:
  - low carbohydrate, low sodium diet
  - acetazolamide 125 mg/day oral, up to 500 mg bd
  - dichlorphenamide 25 mg oral up to 75 mg/day
  - potassium-sparing diuretics (uncertain role).

Myotonia

Mexiletine is the drug of choice for treating chloride-channel myotonia. Start at a low dose (e.g. 50 mg oral once daily) and increase as required up to 200 mg tds. If mexiletine cannot be tolerated, try phenytoin or carbamazepine up to typical antiepileptic doses (see Chapter 2).

Malignant hyperthermia

Although particularly associated with ryanodine-receptor mutations, and thus with central core disease, malignant hyperthermia-like reactions can be seen in patients with other neuromuscular disorders, including periodic paralysis, myotonia congenita, and Duchenne/Becker muscular dystrophy. Unless it has been proved otherwise (which is unlikely), the following patients should be considered to be susceptible – those with:

- central core disease
- ryanodine-receptor mutations
- family history of malignant hyperthermia
- unexplained raised serum creatine kinase
- previous anaesthetic reaction (e.g. masseter spasm, hyperthermia).

The management of a malignant hyperthermia-susceptible patient includes:

- Avoid halogenated volatile anaesthetics (e.g. halothane, see Chapter 19).
- Avoid suxamethonium, curare, phenothiazines.
- If a hyperthermic reaction occurs:
  - stop anaesthesia and hyperventilate with oxygen
  - dantrolene iv 2.5 mg/kg body weight initially, repeated as needed up to total dose of 10 mg/kg
  - cooling (general, and cooled intravenous fluids)
  - sodium bicarbonate for metabolic acidosis.

IDIOPATHIC INFLAMMATORY MYOPATHIES

There is much debate about the classification and aetiology of these conditions, but there are four main groups: dermatomyositis, polymyositis, myositis associated with connective tissue disease ('overlap' syndromes), and inclusion body myositis.

Acute myositis

This is exemplified by dermatomyositis and, even if the typical skin changes are not present, the possibility of an underlying malignancy should be considered. There is no specific associated malignancy and the malignancy may not become apparent for up to several years after the onset of dermatomyositis, so remain vigilant. The patient should be investigated, repeating after 1 year if he or she is in a high-risk group (older people, smokers, family history):

- full blood count, erythrocyte sedimentation rate (ESR), liver function, protein electrophoresis
- serum tumour markers
- faecal occult bloods
- chest, abdomen, and pelvis imaging (techniques are constantly developing and local availability varies, discuss with imaging department)
- endoscopy if suggestive symptoms, positive occult bloods, family history
- mammography.

There is a dearth of controlled trials, but corticosteroids are the mainstay of treatment. Many use second-line ('steroid sparing') immunosuppressant drugs, but none has been adequately evaluated. Monitoring the response to therapy can be difficult. Clinical observation is vitally important and, although the pitfalls are well recognised, the serum creatine kinase (CK) level can be very helpful. Treatment is almost certainly inadequate if CK does not fall to normal. As treatment is tapered, a significantly rising CK is cause for concern as it may precede clinical deterioration. Despite the lack of formal trials, there is evidence for the efficacy of intravenous immunoglobulin (IVIg), but not that this is any more or less effective than corticosteroids. IVIg is used by some as early treatment in patients presenting with severe disease, but by others only at a later stage in 'treatment-resistant' patients.

- Prednisolone (see Chapter 9):
  - initially methylprednisolone 500 mg/day iv for 5 days
  - followed by prednisolone 1 mg/kg body weight oral (maximum 100 mg) once daily until CK is back to normal and patient is improving

- then reduce the alternate-day dose by 5 mg per dose until the patient is taking 1 mg/kg body weight on alternate days
- if CK remains normal and patient is improving, gradually reduce dose (e.g. by 10 mg every 3–4 weeks until down to 40 mg on alternate days, and thereafter more slowly) depending on clinical status – aiming to find the minimum maintenance dose.

■ Azathioprine (see Chapter 9):
  - 2.5 mg/kg body weight oral from outset of treatment
  - can be used in pregnancy (with appropriate counselling).

■ Other immunosuppressants; if the patient is intolerant of azathioprine, other drugs may be considered (Table 12.6). There are specific issues for women of childbearing age as none of the other immunosuppressants are recommended in pregnancy, although this is often more to do with lack of evidence of safety than specific evidence of hazard. Some specialists would not use a second-line agent, either at all, or after azathioprine has 'failed', unless the disease is severe and not responding adequately to moderate doses of prednisolone.
  - Methotrexate: many specialists (especially rheumatologists) use this from the outset in preference to azathioprine. There are problems with fertility in men and women. Typical dose is up to 25 mg weekly, usually oral but subcutaneous administration may reduce adverse effects (particularly gastrointestinal) and some authorities think it may be more effective (see also Chapter 9).
  - Ciclosporin A: typical dose 2.5 mg/kg body weight per day oral. Adverse effects include hypertension, renal impairment and hypercholesterolaemia.
  - Mycophenolate mofetil: 1 g oral bd. Relatively new for treating myositis and shows promise.

Table 12.6   Alternative (to azathioprine) immunosuppressant drugs

Drug	Typical oral dose
Methotrexate	Up to 25 mg weekly (can also be given subcutaneously, which may reduce adverse effects, particularly nausea/vomiting)
Ciclosporin A	2.5 mg/kg body weight per day oral
Mycophenolate mofetil	1 gm bd oral

- Osteoporosis prophylaxis is constantly changing, and there is sometimes conflicting advice from specialist organisations (see Chapter 9).
- Stomach protection:
  - proton-pump inhibitor.
- General advice:
  - recommend appropriate exercise/physiotherapy
  - avoid excess sun exposure (use ultraviolet blocking cream) as the rash is photosensitive.

Chronic myositis

The management of patients with chronic myositis causing very slowly progressive proximal weakness is more difficult than the acute situation noted above, but fortunately it is less common. Pure polymyositis is a very rare disease.

- When associated with connective tissue disease, the management of that will often also deal with the myositis.
- In this chronic situation treatment may prevent progression of the myopathy, but may not reverse it, so a clear clinical response may be difficult to judge, at least over a relatively short period of time.
- CK levels tend to be lower than in the acute situation, and sometimes within the normal range, so they are less useful for monitoring therapy.
- The 'second-line' immunosuppressants may be particularly helpful as their dosage is relatively fixed (see above), unlike prednisolone, the dose of which is varied according to clinical response and CK.
- One approach is to use an initial combination of prednisolone and a second-line agent, such as azathioprine or methotrexate, and then to withdraw the prednisolone over 6–12 months depending on clinical response and CK.
- IVIg is not effective in this group of patients.

Inclusion body myositis

The general consensus is that there is little response to immunosuppression and that any benefits are outweighed by the complications of treatment. Early encouraging reports from uncontrolled trials of IVIg have not been substantiated. In older patients, with typical slowly progressive disease, many muscle experts do *not* recommend a trial of immunosuppression, but would always discuss the options with the patient. Anecdotally, such specialists may be more inclined to make a trial of treatment in younger patients, those with more rapidly progressive disease and those with evidence of particularly active inflammation (e.g. very high CK or extensive inflammatory infiltrates on muscle biopsy).

DRUG-INDUCED MYOPATHIES

There are a huge number of drugs that can cause myopathy. Some invariably cause myopathy if used at an appropriate dose for long enough (e.g. corticosteroids), while with others the response is idiosyncratic (e.g. statins). For many, the pathogenetic mechanisms are unknown. Most are reversible when the offending agent is withdrawn.

Few specific treatments are available.
- Secondary hypokalaemic myopathy responds to potassium repletion.
- Rhabdomyolysis with myoglobinuria and the threat of acute tubular necrosis needs close observation and consideration of alkaline diuresis (with sodium bicarbonate and an osmotic diuretic such as mannitol), and haemodialysis if renal function deteriorates significantly.

Drug-induced myasthenia is a complex area. Many drugs may simply unmask subclinical/presymptomatic autoimmune myasthenia gravis; the myasthenia may persist after drug withdrawal and requires appropriate treatment (see below). D-Penicillamine induces an immune form of myasthenia gravis, with antiacetylcholine receptor antibodies. This usually resolves over a few months after drug withdrawal, but pyridostigmine may be required during that period.

ENDOCRINE MYOPATHIES

Many endocrine disorders can cause myopathy (Table 12.7 and see Chapter 16). The most common feature is proximal weakness, which may be evident on examination but not to the patient, and which invariably resolves when the underlying disorder is corrected.
- Thyrotoxic periodic paralysis resolves once the patient is euthyroid; in the interim propranolol can be used to prevent attacks.
- Osteomalacia due to dietary deficiency responds to small oral doses of vitamin D. If due to malabsorption, higher oral doses or, occasionally, intramuscular treatment are required. When associated with renal failure the preferred treatment is 1-α-hydroxycholecalciferol, which does not require the renal hydroxylation step.

Disorders of the neuromuscular junction

Neuromuscular junction disorders may be inherited or acquired, and affect presynaptic (i.e. motor nerve terminal), synaptic, or postsynaptic (i.e. the acetylcholine receptor and associated proteins) structures (Table 12.8). Although most are associated with weakness, often fatiguable, exceptions

Table 12.7   The myopathic features of endocrine disorders

Endocrinopathy	Myopathic features
Hypothyroidism	Proximal myopathy
Hyperthyroidism	Proximal myopathy Thyrotoxic periodic paralysis
Dysthyroidism	Myasthenia gravis Graves' ophthalmopathy
Cushing's syndrome	Proximal myopathy
Growth hormone excess (pituitary adenoma, ectopic tumour production)	Proximal myopathy
Primary aldosteronism (Conn's syndrome)	Hypokalaemic myopathy
Adrenal insufficiency (Addison's disease)	Proximal myopathy Secondary hyperkalaemic periodic paralysis
Osteomalacia	Proximal myopathy

include neuromyotonia, characterised by muscle twitching and cramps, and episodic ataxia type 1. All respond to treatment.

MYASTHENIA GRAVIS

Seronegative myasthenia (i.e. no detectable antibodies to the acetylcholine receptor (AChR) or to muscle-specific kinase (MuSK)) and anti-MuSK positive myasthenia tend to be less responsive to treatment than myasthenia gravis associated with anti-AChR antibodies (Boxes 12.3 and 12.4). In practice, two important features influence the approach to treatment – whether the myasthenia is generalised or purely ocular, and the presence or absence of a thymoma. Although virtually all patients have a useful response to pyridostigmine, most will also require some form of immunotherapy.

Thymoma

These tumours can be locally invasive and spread within the thoracic cavity, extending into the spine. For this reason, most patients with thymoma, whether their myasthenia is generalised or ocular, should undergo thymectomy. In the elderly and in those with concomitant health problems

Table 12.8   Disorders of the neuromuscular junction and their pathophysiology

Acquired disorders

Disease	Pathophysiology
Myasthenia gravis	Antiacetylcholine receptor (AChR) antibodies – without thymoma – with thymoma Anti-muscle-specific kinase (MuSK) antibodies Seronegative
Lambert–Eaton myasthenic syndrome	Anti-voltage-gated calcium channel (VGCC) antibodies – cancer associated (usually small-cell lung) – non-cancer associated
Neuromyotonia	Anti-voltage-gated potassium channel (VGKC) antibodies

Inherited disorders

Disease	Protein

Congenital myasthenic syndromes:
  Presynaptic
  Synaptic
  Postsynaptic
	
	Choline acetyltransferase
	Acetylcholinesterase
	Acetylcholine receptor subunits
	Rapsyn

Episodic ataxia 1	Nerve terminal voltage-gated potassium channel
Neuromyotonia/myokymia	Nerve terminal voltage-gated potassium channel

it may be appropriate to observe by serial scanning. Management of the myasthenia is outlined below.

Generalised myasthenia gravis

The management is summarised in Fig. 12.1. There is a lack of randomised trial data and so uncertainties about the role of thymectomy and the use of alternative immunosuppressant drugs to azathioprine. Particular points are:

- Azathioprine can be continued in pregnancy but the safety of the other second-line drugs is not known and they are not recommended.
- If the patient is intolerant of azathioprine (about 10% of patients), then it is appropriate to continue with corticosteroids alone, and to consider

Box 12.3   Anticholinesterase therapy

- **Pyridostigmine** (60 mg tablets):
  - initially 15 mg (1/4 tablet) qds
  - after 2 days increase to 30 mg qds
  - if needed, increase after a further 2 days to 60 mg qds
  - maximum dose, 6 tablets daily (360 mg/day)
  - withdraw (over a few weeks) once immunosuppression, when used, has induced remission

- **Propantheline** (15 mg tablets):
  - given if patient develops abdominal cramping/diarrhoea as a result of the pyridostigmine
  - depending upon severity and timing of symptoms use either 15 mg tds or 15 mg taken 30 minutes before each dose of pyridostigmine

Box 12.4   Prednisolone and azathioprine for generalised myasthenia gravis

- **Prednisolone** (patients should usually be admitted to hospital for initiation):
  - given as an alternate-day regimen from outset
  - first dose 10 mg as a single morning dose
  - increase by 10 mg each dose until on 1.5 mg/kg body weight on alternate days, or 100 mg on alternate days, whichever is the lower
  - maintain until patient is in remission (may take many months)
  - then reduce by 10 mg every 3–4 weeks until on 40 mg on alternate days
  - then reduce by 5 mg every 3–4 weeks until on 20 mg on alternate days
  - then reduce by 1 mg every month
  - reinstitute an appropriate higher dose if symptoms relapse

- **Azathioprine:**
  - if available, check thiopurine methyltransferase (TPMT) status (see Chapter 9)
  - start on 25 mg bd
  - increase by 25 mg/day until patient is on a dose of 2.5 mg/kg body weight per day
  - assess full blood count and liver function before starting treatment and after a few days of initiation, then weekly for 8 weeks, then, if all stable, every 3 months

another immunosuppressant drug only if remission cannot be maintained on a reasonable dose of prednisolone (e.g. < 25 mg on alternate days).
- IVIg 0.4 g/day for 5 days and plasma exchange are of equal efficacy, but their beneficial effects last only up to 2 months. They can be used in

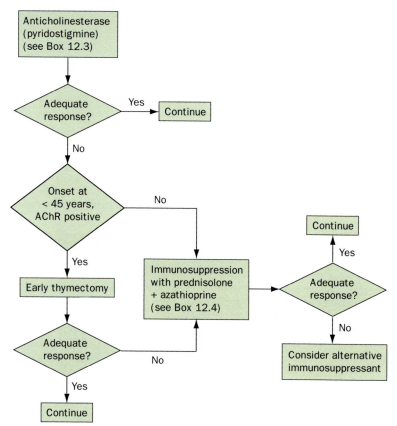

Fig. 12.1   Management of generalised myasthenia gravis.

patients with severe weakness at the initiation of therapy, or during crises (see also Chapter 11).

■ Osteoporosis prophylaxis and stomach protection should be used, as outlined in Chapter 9.

Ocular myasthenia gravis

The management is summarised in Fig. 12.2. In general, the condition responds well to moderate doses of prednisolone, and a second-line immunosuppressant is usually not required. In some patients with a fixed and persisting deficit extraocular muscle surgery may be appropriate.

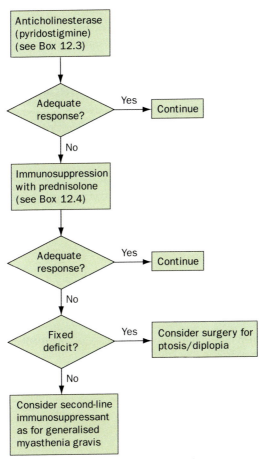

Fig. 12.2 Management of ocular myasthenia gravis.

Managing a relapse ('crisis')

A relapse may be due to too great a reduction of immunosuppressant therapy, introduction of a drug that interferes with neuromuscular transmission (e.g. beta-blocker, certain antibiotics), intercurrent illness, particularly infection, or a combination of these. Management depends on severity, but includes:

- treatment of any precipitating factors
- increasing immunosuppression if appropriate

- reintroduction of pyridostigmine
- for severe weakness, IVIg and plasma exchange
- ventilatory support may be required and forced vital capacity should be monitored.

LAMBERT–EATON MYASTHENIC SYNDROME

Management is similar to myasthenia gravis. When due to an associated malignancy (typically small-cell lung cancer) the myasthenia may improve or resolve after successful treatment of the tumour, and relapse if the tumour recurs.

Symptomatic benefit may be obtained from pyridostigmine, but generally 3,4-diaminopyridine up to 100 mg/day oral is more successful, although it can cause peripheral and perioral paraesthesia (these two drugs may be used together).

The approach to immunosuppressant therapy is very similar to that for generalised myasthenia gravis.
- Prednisolone:
  - can be started, orally, without titration, at a dose of 1.5 mg/kg body weight on alternate days, or 100 mg on alternate days, whichever is the lower
  - titrate down to find the minimum dose required for adequate symptom control.
- Azathioprine:
  - probably best avoided in small-cell cancer associated disease due to its very slow onset of action
  - in non-cancer cases, 2.5 mg/kg body weight per day as for myasthenia gravis.
- Other immunosuppressants:
  - As for myasthenia; other drugs may act more quickly than azathioprine, and thus be preferred in cancer-associated disease.
- IVIg and plasma exchange can be used when there is severe weakness, but tend to be less effective than in myasthenia gravis.

NEUROMYOTONIA

This may be autoimmune in origin, but is also seen in association with inherited peripheral neuropathies and, rarely, with inherited potassium channel disorders. In all circumstances symptomatic relief can be obtained from carbamazepine, lamotrigine, phenytoin, valproate or gabapentin, started at low dose and titrated upwards as required, to typical 'antiepileptic' doses (see Chapter 2). However, some patients fail to benefit.

When autoimmune in origin, immunosuppression will help, but this is not justified unless the symptoms are very severe or there is an associated autoimmune disorder, such as myasthenia gravis.

CONGENITAL MYASTHENIC SYNDROMES

These may be presynaptic (impaired acetylcholine synthesis/storage/release), synaptic (cholinesterase deficiency), or postsynaptic (AChR deficiency, kinetic abnormality of the AChR). Treatments differ for each and specialist assessment is required.

■ Pyridostigmine will help presynaptic disorders, and postsynaptic disorders with AChR deficiency, but not cholinesterase deficiency or the slow-channel syndrome. The latter may respond to quinidine.

■ Steroids and immunosuppressants do not help as there is no immune component to these disorders.

Cramps

True cramps are neurogenic in origin; an overexcitable nerve drives a muscle into sustained, and painful, contraction. Any predisposing factors should be identified and excluded where possible. Symptomatic benefit can be obtained from quinine, carbamazepine, lamotrigine, valproate, phenytoin or gabapentin. Not infrequently, all fail to give adequate relief, or their use is limited by adverse effects.

True cramps must be distinguished from the painful contractures of McArdle's disease and other glycogenoses, the painful cramps sometimes seen in Duchenne/Becker muscular dystrophy, and the extremely rare condition Brody's disease (which may respond to verapamil).

Further reading

Bushby K, Muntoni F, Bourke J. Neuromusc Disord 2003; 13: 166–172.

Engel A, Franzini-Armstrong C (eds). Myology, 3rd edn. McGraw-Hill, New York, 2004.

Hilton-Jones D. Diagnosis and treatment of inflammatory muscle diseases. J Neurol Neurosurg Psychiatry 2003; 74(Suppl 2): ii25–ii31.

Karpati G, Hilton-Jones D, Griggs R (eds). Disorders of voluntary muscle, 7th edn. Cambridge University Press, Cambridge, 2001.

107th ENMC International Workshop: The Management of Cardiac Involvement in Muscular Dystrophy and Myotonic Dystrophy, 7–9 June 2002, Naarden, The Netherlands.

13 EMOTIONAL DISORDERS, FUNCTIONAL SOMATIC DISORDERS AND PSYCHOSES

Michael Sharpe, Jon Stone and Alan J. Carson

Neurology is about much more than neurological 'disease'. Whilst the non-neurologist might imagine that neurologists simply treat disease (objective diagnosable lesions and disorders discernible on examination, scans and other tests), like all clinicians, neurologists actually spend much of their time managing the symptoms, distress and disability that patients – with or without any discernible disease – bring to the consultation. These constitute a far broader problem than that of disease alone. Indeed, about one-third of all new neurology outpatients have somatic symptoms disproportionate to any identifiable disease (functional symptoms), and about one-quarter of all neurology patients can be given a diagnosis of anxiety or depressive disorder (emotional disorders).

Neurologists might ask: is all of this illness really our concern? Are these problems not really 'psychiatric'? Whilst they might refer some patients to psychiatry, and share the management of others, the size of the problem is such that to refer all would clearly not be feasible. The brain is the organ of the mind – psychiatrists and neurologists share the same organ – and so one cannot be a brain specialist without also being concerned with the mind, and vice versa. This chapter covers those 'psychiatric' disorders that neurologists are likely to see and may wish to manage themselves, at least initially.

PSYCHIATRIC TERMINOLOGY

Psychiatric illnesses are referred to as 'disorders' because most do not have an established biological pathology – a disease. Because they are diagnosed predominantly by recognising patterns of symptoms, they should really be considered 'syndromes', but because much is known about their natural history, response to treatment and aetiology, the term 'disorder' is used to reflect a status intermediate between a syndrome and an established disease. Many psychiatric disorders represent extremes of normal phenomena, and 'cases' of disorder are often defined as a significant level of subjective distress or impairment in function. Even when terms seem familiar, it is important to take care in their use. For example, anxiety or depressed mood may be a normal state, a symptom or a diagnosis.

CLASSIFICATION OF PSYCHIATRIC DISORDERS

There are two main psychiatric classifications in current use:

- American Psychiatric Association, Diagnostic and Statistical Manual (4th edition), or DSM-IV
- World Health Organisation International Classification of Disease (10th edition), or ICD-10.

The two systems are very similar, but ICD-10 is more familiar outside the USA and will be used in this chapter (Box 13.1).

DEPRESSION

- Depressed mood, sadness or unhappiness is most commonly transient and caused by loss, such as deterioration in function as a result of disease, or other difficult life circumstances. If severe this may be called an 'adjustment disorder'.
- Depressive disorder describes a collection of symptoms central to which are the core symptoms of persistent low mood and loss of interest and pleasure (anhedonia). This often coexists with an anxiety disorder, and is associated with neurological symptoms including fatigue and unexplained pain.
- Depression may be mild, moderate or severe. Major depression refers to at least moderately severe depressive symptoms (including low mood and/or anhedonia) that have been present for a minimum of 2 weeks.
- Depression may also occur as part of a fluctuating pattern of depressed and then elevated mood (mania), so-called 'bipolar affective disorder'.

Assessment of depression

This requires questioning about the core depressive symptoms, of low mood and anhedonia, as well as other typical symptoms (Box 13.2). Patients are often sensitive to the implication that they may be considered depressed and it can be helpful to ask 'Have your symptoms got you down?' rather

> **Box 13.1   Classification of psychiatric disorders in ICD-10**
>
> - Stress-related disorders:
>   - acute stress disorder
>   - post-traumatic stress disorder
>   - adjustment disorder.
> - Anxiety disorders:
>   - generalised anxiety
>   - panic disorder
>   - phobic anxiety.
> - Obsessive–compulsive disorder.
> - Affective (mood) disorders:
>   - depression disorder
>   - mania and bipolar disorder.
> - Schizophrenia and delusional disorders.
> - Substance misuse:
>   - alcohol
>   - drugs.
> - Organic:
>   - acute (i.e. delirium)
>   - chronic (i.e. dementia).
> - Disorders of adult personality and behaviour:
>   - personality disorder
>   - factitious disorder.
> - Eating disorders:
>   - anorexia nervosa
>   - bulimia nervosa.
> - Somatoform disorders:
>   - somatisation disorder
>   - hypochondriasis
>   - dissociative (conversion) disorder
>   - body dysmorphic disorder
>   - pain disorder
>   - somatoform autonomic dysfunction
>   - neurasthenia.
> - Puerperal mental disorders.

than ask directly 'Are you depressed?'. When a person has depressed mood it is also essential to ask whether they have ideas of suicide: 'Have you ever got to the point where you felt that life wasn't worth living?', 'Have you thought you would be better off dead?' and 'Have you had any concrete plans to kill yourself?'.

A diagnosis of depression should be based on the presence of at least one core symptom; many of the other symptoms in Box 13.2 are also common in those with medical conditions. Persistence or severity beyond normal adjustment to having an unpleasant illness should also be sought.

Treatment of depression

Depressed mood as part of an adjustment to events will usually resolve in time, but may also develop into a depressive disorder. Its progress should therefore be monitored. More persistent or severe depression requires treatment. Even if the depression was precipitated by circumstances, such

> ## Box 13.2   Common symptoms of depression
>
> - Core symptoms:
>   - low mood
>   - loss of interest, motivation and pleasure.
>
> - Other symptoms:
>   - poor memory and concentration*
>   - poor sleep with early morning waking
>   - fatigue*
>   - pain*
>   - loss of appetite and weight
>   - constipation
>   - amenorrhoea.
>
> *These are also common symptoms in organic neurological disease.

as the diagnosis of a serious disease, this is never a reason not to treat, any more than a stab wound is a reason not to treat bleeding.

Treatments for depression include:

- Antidepressant drugs and psychological therapies, especially cognitive–behaviour therapy.
- Electroconvulsive therapy (ECT) is now reserved for severe cases of depression that are either life-threatening or unresponsive to conventional treatments, especially when delusions or hallucinations are present.
- Bipolar disorder is traditionally treated with lithium carbonate, a so-called mood stabiliser, to prevent mood swings.
- Recently, antiepileptic drugs such as carbamazepine (see Chapter 2) have also been widely used as prophylaxis against relapse.
- If a patient describes suicidal ideation it is important to clarify whether he or she has specific plans and if so whether he or she has the means to carry these out. If such a risk assessment reveals both an intention and a clear and practical plan, an urgent psychiatric assessment is required.

Lithium

- Many elderly patients cannot tolerate the adverse effects of lithium, or they are taking other medications that significantly increase the risk of lithium toxicity: diuretics, non-steroidal anti-inflammatory drugs (NSAIDs), aspirin, metronidazole, angiotensin-converting enzyme (ACE) inhibitors and angiotensin II receptor antagonists, calcium channel blockers, and selective serotonin uptake inhibitors (SSRIs).

- The occurrence and severity of adverse reactions are generally directly related to the serum lithium concentration, as well as to individual patient sensitivity to lithium.
- Fine hand tremor, polyuria and mild thirst may occur during initial therapy and persist throughout treatment.
- Transient and mild nausea and general discomfort may also appear during the first few days of lithium administration.
- At therapeutic levels the patient may experience a fine tremor, metallic taste, dry mouth, thirst, mild polyuria, nausea and weight gain.
- Hypothyroidism occurs in 20% of women but is rarer in men.
- Renal impairment may occur after prolonged use, but is rare if toxic levels have been avoided.
- Toxic symptoms occur above a plasma level of about 2.5 mmol/l: coarse tremor, ataxia, giddiness, agitation, tinnitus, blurred vision, twitching, thirst and polyuria.
- Diarrhoea, vomiting, drowsiness, muscular weakness and lack of coordination may be early signs of lithium intoxication, and can even occur at lithium levels < 2.0 mmol/l.
- Serum lithium levels should not be permitted to exceed 2.0 mEq/l during the acute treatment phase. Blood samples should be drawn immediately prior to the next dose, when lithium concentrations are relatively stable.
- Serum lithium levels > 3.0 mmol/l may produce a complex clinical picture, involving multiple organs and organ systems.
- Above 4 mmol/l polyuric renal failure, seizures, coma and death may result.
- Toxic levels can occur as a result of even mild dehydration, or with low salt diets, hence there is a need for education of the patient and carer, and monitoring of plasma levels.
- Fatalities after overdose are not uncommon and survivors may be left with renal failure or brain damage.

Antidepressant drugs (Box 13.3)

- Tricyclic antidepressants (also effective in chronic pain, see Chapter 18):
  - inhibit the reuptake of the amines noradrenaline and 5-hydroxytryptamine (5-HT; serotonin) at synaptic clefts
  - adverse effects can be troublesome, including anticholinergic effects (e.g. dry mouth, constipation, blurred vision), weight gain, postural hypotension, lowering of epileptic seizure threshold and cardiotoxicity
  - may be dangerous in overdose, and in people who have coexisting heart disease, epilepsy, glaucoma or prostatism.

- SSRIs:
  - are less cardiotoxic and less sedative
  - have fewer interactions and anticholinergic effects than tricyclics, but can still cause headache, nausea, anorexia and sexual dysfunction, and are more likely to cause withdrawal symptoms.
- Some newer antidepressants are available – venlafaxine, mirtazepine, reboxetine and duloxetine – with different profiles of action and adverse effects, but none have been shown to be more effective than the more established agents.
- Monoamine oxidase inhibitors (MAOIs) are now rarely used.
- The chance of success is best if the patient is persuaded to take the antidepressants in the first place, which may be difficult because of:
  - the stigma of 'mental disease'
  - a perception that the drugs are addictive; they may have some withdrawal effects in some people, but there is no tendency for dose escalation
  - adverse effects.

Box 13.3	Common antidepressants and their use		
Type	**Example**	**Starting daily dose (mg)**	**Usual effective daily dose (mg)**
Tricyclic	Amitriptyline	50	150–200
	Lofepramine	70	140–210
SSRI	Fluoxetine	20	20–60
	Sertraline	50	150–200
Others	Venlafaxine	75	150
	Mirtazepine	15	30–45

General guidance

- Become familiar with one drug from each category.
- Explain the reason for prescription carefully – warn about, but do not overemphasise, potential increase in symptoms on withdrawal, which should be done gradually.
- Start low, increase slowly if necessary, but monitor progress and titrate dose according to response. Attain a therapeutic dose. A therapeutic response may take up to 4 weeks at full dose. Successful treatment should be continued for at least 6 months to prevent relapse.
- If there is no response it is worth trying an agent from another class and consider referral to psychiatry.

All these issues must be discussed before prescribing, for example saying to the patient 'The so-called antidepressants often help these symptoms even in patients who are not feeling depressed. They have wider actions than treating depression – for example on energy, appetite and sleep – and can reverse the abnormalities in brain function we have talked about'. The patient must be made aware that any therapeutic effect may take 2–4 weeks.

■ Treatment should be continued for at least 6 months to reduce the high risk of relapse, and the dose then tapered off over several weeks to avoid discontinuation symptoms such as headache, nausea, paraesthesiae, dizziness and anxiety. The patient should be advised to consider restarting the drug should the depression or original symptoms return.

Cognitive–behaviour therapy

This non-drug treatment is a way of helping patients to become aware of, examine and, if appropriate, revise the way they cope with, think about and behave in response to their symptoms and other problems. Its use does not imply that the problem is 'all in the mind', or psychoanalysis. It is used to help patients cope with a variety of problems, most commonly depressive and anxiety disorders and functional somatic symptoms, including chronic fatigue (see below).

Patients meet a therapist every 1 or 2 weeks. They are encouraged to examine the evidence for their thinking (e.g. is the prognosis for their neurological condition as bad as they imagine, will they really have no quality of life, is there really nothing they can do to help themselves?) and to try new ways of responding to their symptoms (e.g. be less fearful of them, be more active, use problem-solving, talk to their partner) between these sessions. Cognitive–behaviour therapy may be given by a psychologist, psychiatrist, nurse or other professional who is appropriately trained – and its approach reinforced in visits to the neurologist.

ANXIETY

Anxiety is the name given to a range of symptoms associated with the emotions of fear and apprehension, many of which are similar to those of neurological disease (Box 13.4).

Generalised anxiety disorder may be associated with particular situations leading to avoidance (phobic disorders), or may be severe and episodic (panic disorder). Anxiety can also be associated with recollections of a previous traumatic event (post-traumatic stress disorder). Types of anxiety disorder are shown in Table 13.1.

Anxiety is most commonly transient and associated with threatening situations (e.g. an appointment with the neurologist), but may become chronic and is then often associated with depression, which may be missed.

Assessment of anxiety

- When considering unexplained neurological somatic symptoms, particularly tingling in the peripheries, dizziness and unsteadiness, it is important to consider whether anxiety is the cause.
- It is useful to ask when the symptoms occur, looking both for any association with anxiety-provoking situations (those associated with phobias), and for episodic anxiety of sudden onset with multiple physical symptoms, including breathlessness, palpitations and often a fear of impending doom (panic attacks). Panic attacks are markedly aversive and may lead a person to anxiously avoid going out for fear of having one of these away from home – agoraphobia.

Box 13.4 Common symptoms of anxiety

- Psychological symptoms:
  - anxiety, irritability
  - exaggerated worries and fears
  - avoidance of feared situations.
- Somatic symptoms:
  - tingling in extremities and lips
  - dizziness
  - tight chest
  - shortness of breath
  - palpitations
  - tremor
  - aches and pains
  - poor sleep
  - frequent desire to pass urine and defecate.

Table 13.1 Features distinguishing types of anxiety disorder

	Phobic anxiety	Panic disorder	Generalised
Occurrence	Situational	Paroxysmal	Persistent
Behaviour	Avoidance	Escape	Agitation
Cognitions	Fear of situation	Fear of symptoms	Worry
Somatic symptoms	On exposure	Episodic	Persistent

- Anxiety disorders are often associated with depression, so it is important to look for this in the anxious patient.

Treatment of anxiety

- A variety of psychological treatments are effective, including those aimed at reducing arousal and tension (e.g. relaxation) and those aimed at correcting overthreatening appraisals of situations and their avoidance (e.g. cognitive–behaviour therapy, see above).
- Benzodiazepines, such as diazepam, are markedly effective for anxiety (and night sedation), but if used for more than short periods can produce dependency. They were the main anxiolytic agents in the 1960s and 1970s, but with increasing awareness of their potential for dependency, and withdrawal problems, they have been replaced by antidepressants as the usual drugs for anxiety.
- The so-called antidepressants can also be effective for anxiety and do not lead to dependency, but may cause an initial transient increase in symptoms that the patients should be warned about (especially in patients with panic attacks).
- Propranolol (40 mg oral 1–3 times daily) reduces the somatic symptoms of anxiety (tachycardia, tremor), but has a limited role. It should be avoided in asthmatics because it can cause bronchospasm.
- Buspirone is a non-sedating anxiolytic, useful in generalised anxiety disorder (5 mg tds increasing gradually to a maximum of 30 mg/day in 2–3 divided doses). It is said not to be addictive and takes several days to work.

PATHOLOGICAL EMOTIONALISM

- Pathological emotionalism includes 'emotional lability' and 'emotional incontinence', which describe the outward manifestations of what appear to be, but are not necessarily, strong inner emotions, usually crying but sometimes laughing. It must be distinguished from distress secondary to difficulty in communicating (e.g. in aphasia). It is usually temporary.
- It is excessive or inappropriate to the situation and typically recognised as such by patients, who may report not feeling the emotion in question, and they may be embarrassed by their behaviour.
- It is common after stroke and in multiple sclerosis, and may occur in Parkinson's disease and motor neuron disease.
- Explanation of the nature of the problem and treatment with antidepressant drugs may be strikingly effective.

FUNCTIONAL SOMATIC SYMPTOMS

Around one-third of all new patients presenting to neurologists have symptoms such as dizziness, fatigue, headache, weakness, blackouts and numbness that appear to be genuinely experienced but which are not adequately explained by neurological disease. These are often called 'somatoform' – medically unexplained or functional somatic symptoms. The large number of words to describe such symptoms is a reflection of the diverse concepts that have been applied to understanding them over the years. The term 'functional', meaning a disturbance of brain functioning rather than structure, is arguably more accurate, and certainly more acceptable to patients, than explanations that imply malingering or mental illness.

- Functional symptoms do not necessarily improve spontaneously – about one-third to one-half of patients are unchanged or worse a year after diagnosis.
- Persistence is more likely for those with motor symptoms or pseudoseizures, than for those with only sensory symptoms.
- Some patients (sometimes described as having somatisation disorder) develop, or have a history of, multiple functional symptoms, such as chest pain and bowel complaints, and attend other medical specialities. In these cases iatrogenic harm from overinvestigation, unwarranted surgery and therapeutic drugs is a major problem.
- Many doctors worry that a high proportion of patients presenting with functional symptoms, especially hysterical or dissociative (conversion) symptoms, such as paralysis and non-epileptic attacks, will go on to develop structural disease that, with hindsight, explains their symptoms. In fact, the misdiagnosis rate of only around 5% is no different from that for 'real' diseases such as motor neuron disease and multiple sclerosis. When misdiagnosis does occur, it is most common in gait and movement disorders and where the clinician has placed too much emphasis on a bizarre or 'psychiatric' presentation.

Assessment of functional symptoms

A diagnosis of functional symptoms is made largely, but not entirely, by excluding neurological disease. There are two main presentations: those with predominant worry about the cause of their symptoms (sometimes called hypochondriasis or health anxiety) and those with predominant concern about the discomfort caused by the symptoms themselves (sometimes called somatisation, somatoform pain disorder or somatoform autonomic dysfunction).

Extensive investigation must be reserved for where it is clinically necessary, and not done just to reassure the patient; repeated investigation may actually increase the anxiety of patients who are worried about disease.

When assessing functional symptoms the neurologist must make sure that any depression and anxiety (especially panic in the case of episodic symptoms) are identified and treated.

Treatment of functional somatic symptoms

Most people who develop symptoms want to know what is causing them. Explaining the diagnosis in a clear, logical, transparent and non-offensive way is the key to management by the neurologist:

- Explain what patients *do* have, not just what they do not have: 'You have functional weakness. Your nervous system is not damaged, it is just that it is not working properly'.
- Make it clear that you believe the patient's symptoms are real and disabling: 'I do not think you are mad, imagining or putting on your symptoms – they are as real and worrying as the symptoms of other neurological disorders'.
- Explain what they do not have: 'You do not have multiple sclerosis, epilepsy, etc.'.
- Tell them that functional problems are common: 'I see lots of patients with symptoms like yours'.
- Emphasise reversibility: 'Because there is no damage to your nervous system you can certainly get better'.
- Explain that self-help is a key part of getting better, but avoid blame: 'I know you didn't bring this on but there are things you can do to help get it better'.
- Analogies may be useful: 'The hardware is alright but there's a software problem', 'The clock has stopped not because it has broken but only because it needs a new battery'.

For patients with mild symptoms, explanation and reassurance about the absence of disease with encouragement to resume normal activity may be sufficient. In those with more resistant symptoms, one or more of the following treatments may also be helpful:

- Patients with physical problems often respond to physical treatments, indeed they may expect a physical and not a psychological approach. Experienced physiotherapists who accept the notion of functional symptoms are able to combine hands-on, physical treatments combined with positive suggestion and encouragement.

- Cognitive–behaviour therapy (see above) can often help with functional symptoms, as well as with depression and anxiety.
- Antidepressants (in usual antidepressant doses, but starting low) can be helpful in patients with functional symptoms, even those who are not depressed.

Special management issues in functional somatic symptoms

- Should a patient with functional symptoms receive disability benefits? These can be substantial, even more than previous earnings, and so lead to a situation where patients will lose money if they get better. This dilemma may be usefully discussed openly with the patient. Remember that there is little research to support the idea that secondary gain is a greater factor in causing disability in patients with functional symptoms than in those with disease.
- A similar dilemma arises when thinking about aids such as walking sticks and wheelchairs. These aids can be both helpful, in improving independence and confidence, and harmful, leading to dependence on them and decreased activity. Each case must be evaluated on its merits.
- Some patients with functional symptoms are hard to treat and have a very long history of symptoms, disability and medical consultations. It is therefore important, as with any chronic condition, to have a realistic expectation of recovery. Rather then ending contact on a negative note you may wish to tell patients that they are coping well with a difficult illness and that you are sorry you have not been able to help more.
- If the patient has a history of repeated presentation to secondary care with the associated risk of iatrogenic harm, a positive plan to 'contain' the patient in primary care may help – e.g. by the general practitioner making regular monthly appointments regardless of whether there are new symptoms or not. This may reduce the number of new symptom presentations, but the neurologist may still need to review the patient from time to time. Excessive medical investigation is best avoided in such cases.
- Chronic fatigue syndrome, sometimes referred to as myalgic encephalomyelitis (ME), and also neurasthenia, is characterised by disabling fatigue for at least 6 months in the absence of an alternative explanation. If the patient also has evidence of anxiety and depression this should be treated, which may sometimes lead to resolution of fatigue. Other evidence-based treatments include very carefully graded exercise (usually administered by a physiotherapist or someone else

experienced in the execution and monitoring of such a programme) or cognitive–behaviour therapy (again given by a therapist with specific expertise in this condition and not merely a generic therapist).

■ Malingering is a description of behaviour, not a diagnosis, and refers to the conscious simulation of signs of disease and disability. Patients have motives that are clear to them, but which they usually conceal from doctors. Examples include the avoidance of burdensome responsibilities (work, court appearances) or financial gain (fraudulent claims for benefits or compensation). Malingering can be hard to detect at clinical assessment, but is suggested by evasion or inconsistency in the history. Observation of behaviour that is inconsistent with the reported disability is an indicator, and some law firms commission private detectives to unearth evidence that patients regularly do what they claim they cannot. If malingering is suspected, the best approach is a sympathetic but firm discussion of the observations suggesting this conclusion.

PSYCHOSES

Psychoses are severe psychiatric illnesses characterised by very abnormal mental functions, such as hallucinations and delusions.

Hallucinations and delusions

■ Hallucinations are perceptions with no external stimulus. They may occur in any modality, but are most commonly visual (seeing things) and auditory (hearing voices). They have to be distinguished from illusions, which are misperception of actual stimuli, usually visual, and from normal perceptions (e.g. being aware that one talks to oneself inside one's head).

■ Delusions are fixed false beliefs that persist despite evidence that they are mistaken. They have to be distinguished from overvalued ideas that are strongly held, if unusual views, which are amenable to reason (at least to some degree), and from normal socially sanctioned strong beliefs such as religious convictions.

■ Someone with hallucinations and/or delusions may be described as being psychotic. Psychosis can have its origins in gross disturbance of brain structure or functioning (organic) or more subtle changes (confusingly called functional because historically the brains looked normal). There are many causes of grossly disturbed brain structure and function in neurological practice. These include focal causes such as tumours and focal epilepsy, and more general causes such as drugs and hypoxia – characterised by changes in attention and cognitive function and this is termed 'delirium' (see below).

■ The main functional psychoses are schizophrenia, delusional disorders and bipolar affective disorder (mania or depressive psychosis). Schizophrenia is differentiated from bipolar disorder by the absence of major mood change and by the presence of certain characteristic types of hallucinations and delusions, especially auditory hallucinations of voices commenting on one's actions and the delusion that one's thoughts are being directly interfered with in some way.

Schizophrenia

This is a functional psychosis that occurs in acute (with prominent hallucinations, delusions and associate disturbed behaviour) and chronic forms (with flatness and lack of motivation). The acute treatment is with antipsychotic drugs, often in large doses (e.g. haloperidol 100 mg or more), and specialist psychiatric management is indicated (Box 13.5).

Delusional beliefs can occur without the other features of schizophrenia and may be about disease. The treatment is as for schizophrenia.

Catatonia

This refers to mute or stuporous behaviour and may be associated with the adoption of odd postures for hours on end. It is usually a feature of schizophrenia, but is rare. It must be distinguished from the motor effects of antipsychotic drugs. Referral to psychiatry is indicated (Box 13.5).

Delirium

Delirium is an organic psychosis. It is differentiated from dementia (see Chapter 5) by its transient nature and impaired concious level.

The characteristic features of delirium are a disturbance of attention and cognition, which usually fluctuates and manifests as wandering attention and disorientation that is not chronic as in dementia (although delirium can be superimposed on a background of dementia). Visual hallucinations should always suggest delirium.

Delirium has many causes, in fact almost anything that can disturb brain function. In practice the most common is drugs (most commonly prescribed drugs, but also recreational drugs, including alcohol intoxication and withdrawal).

> ## Box 13.5   When to refer to psychiatry
>
> - **How often?**
>   - Remember that if you send everyone you see with functional or emotional symptoms to a psychiatrist, you will be sending one-third of your neurology clinic to them. Patients with mild symptoms, symptoms that respond positively to initial explanation, or those with a good general practitioner will probably not need (or accept) the complication of another referral.
>
> - **Which patients should be referred?**
>   - Psychosis other than delirium.
>   - Unmanageable behaviour in delirium.
>   - Severe depression or anxiety.
>   - Suicide risk.
>   - Severe functional somatic symptoms unresponsive to neurological management.
>
> - **To whom should patients be referred?**
>   - A liaison or neuropsychiatrist is best, if available.
>   - Psychologists provide cognitive–behaviour therapy.

The management is:

- to contain the behaviour and treat the cause
- antipsychotic drugs may be used, but with caution (they can make things worse), e.g. haloperidol initially 0.5 mg im
- beware Wernicke–Korsakoff syndrome in alcohol withdrawal (see Chapter 16).

Further reading

Alwyn Lishman W. Organic psychiatry: the psychological consequences of cerebral disorder, 3rd edn. Blackwell Science, Oxford, 1998.

Harrison P, Geddes J, Sharpe M. Lecture notes on psychiatry, 9th edn. Blackwell, Oxford, 2005.

Johnstone E, Owens D, Lawrie S, Sharpe M, Freeman C. Companion to psychiatric studies, 7th edn. Churchill Livingstone, Edinburgh, 2005.

Mayou R, Sharpe M, Carson A (eds). ABC of psychological medicine. BMJ Books, London, 2003.

Stone J, Carson A, Sharpe M. Functional symptoms in neurology: assessment and diagnosis. J Neurol Neurosurg Psychiatry 2005; 76(Suppl 1): 2–12.

Stone J, Carson A, Sharpe M. Functional symptoms in neurology: management. J Neurol Neurosurg Psychiatry 2005; 76(Suppl 1): 13–21.

14 INFECTIONS

Jeremy Farrar

Infectious diseases account for about 25% of all deaths worldwide and, as a result of their complications, infectious diseases of the nervous system inflict a disproportionate burden on individuals, their families and their communities – particularly in the developing world. Malaria kills a child every 12 seconds, and human immunodeficiency virus (HIV) and tuberculosis (TB) continue to devastate much of Africa, and increasingly Asia and Latin America. Increased global travel means that many patients with these 'tropical developing world infections' now present to clinicians in the developed world – 4000 patients presented with malaria in the UK during 2004 (Table 14.1). Despite vaccines against many of the common causes of meningitis and encephalitis, patients still die in their thousands of these preventable diseases every year.

In the developed world irrational public fears of vaccination have led to an alarming drop in immunisation rates and a predictable rise in a number of preventable infectious diseases such as diphtheria, mumps and rubella. The recent outbreaks of Nipah virus, severe acute respiratory syndrome (SARS) and avian influenza, the re-emergence of polio in certain parts of the world, and the global spread of drug resistance suggest that we may soon enter a period similar to the pre-antibiotic, pre-vaccine era.

This chapter outlines the management of the most common infectious diseases affecting the nervous system. It is not exhaustive and far from

Table 14.1	Prevalence of infectious diseases			
Organism	Massachusetts General Hospital, Boston, USA, 1962–1988	Queen Elizabeth Centre Hospital, Blantyre, Malawi, 1997–1999	The Netherlands community based study, 1998–2002	Hospital for Tropical Diseases, Ho Chi Minh City, Vietnam, 1998–2001
Streptococcus pneumoniae	38	25	51	8
Streptococcus suis	0	0	1	13
Gram-negative bacilli	4	6	1	2
Neisseria meningitidis	14	18	37	2
Streptococcal species	7	2	3	2
Staphylococcus aureus	5	0	1	1
Listeria monocytogenes	11	0	4	0
Haemophilus influenzae	4	0	2	1
Mixed bacterial species	2	0	0	1
Mycobacterium tuberculosis	Not reported	13	Not reported	51
Other	2	17	1	1
Probable bacterial meningitis, culture	13	19	0	19

complete, as space prevents a comprehensive account of all infectious diseases affecting the nervous system (for leprosy, *Borrelia* and diphtheria, see Chapter 11).

BACTERIAL MENINGITIS

Bacterial meningitis is an inflammation of the leptomeninges caused by infection of the cerebrospinal fluid (CSF) within the subarachnoid space around the brain and spinal cord, and the ventricular system. It can be categorised into:

- spontaneous community-acquired meningitis, which is the most important category
- post-traumatic meningitis following neurosurgery or fracture of the skull
- device-associated meningitis, particularly in association with CSF shunts and drains.

Clinical picture

Early clinical manifestations include non-specific malaise, apprehension or irritability, followed by fever, headache, myalgia and vomiting. Convulsions occur in infants and children – meningitis must always enter into the differential diagnosis of childhood febrile convulsions. Photophobia, drowsiness or more severe impairment of consciousness usually develop later. In older children and adults the symptoms most suggestive of meningitis are irritability, severe headache and vomiting, but in the case of meningococcal infection, diarrhoea is a common non-specific symptom and the vasculitic rash is a crucial sign.

Management

- Any patient with headache and a rash should be *suspected* of having meningococcal meningitis and treated immediately (although most will actually have milder viral illnesses).
- Almost all adults present with at least two of the classic symptoms of bacterial meningitis: headache, fever, neck stiffness and altered consciousness.
- Case fatality remains at 15–30%, with neurological sequelae in a further 15–30% of patients.
- Co-infection with HIV can have a dramatic effect on the clinical presentation, the spectrum of bacterial infection and the patterns of drug resistance (local knowledge is essential in guiding rational therapy).

Table 14.2   Treatment for presumed bacterial meningitis before the organism and sensitivities are known

Type	Drug	Dose	Frequency	Duration
Spontaneous meningitis				
Infants	Ceftriaxone	100 mg/kg/day iv	Once daily	7–14 days
	Ampicillin if *Listeria* is a possibility			
Childhood	Ceftriaxone	100 mg/kg/day iv	Once daily	7–14 days
	or			
	Cefotaxime	200 mg/kg/day iv	6 hourly	7–14 days
Adult	**Intermediate penicillin-resistant organisms low and *Staph. aureus* unlikely**			
	Penicillin	2.4 g iv	4 hourly	7–14 days
	Intermediate penicillin-resistant organisms > 5% and *Staph. aureus* unlikely			
	Ceftriaxone	2 g iv	12 hourly	7–14 days
	or			
	Cefotaxime	2 g iv	4 hourly	7–14 days
	High prevalence of penicillin-resistant pneumococci (MIC > 1 mg/ml)			
	Ceftriaxone	2 g iv	12 hourly	7–14 days
	or			
	Cefotaxime +	2 g iv	4 hourly	7–14 days
	Vancomycin	1 g iv	12 hourly (measure blood levels of vancomycin)	

- Early diagnosis and treatment are essential; if bacterial meningitis is suspected empirical antibiotic treatment should be started immediately (Table 14.2).
- Cultures of blood and CSF should be taken as soon as possible but must not delay treatment.

Type	Drug	Dose	Frequency	Duration
Table 14.2 *Continued*				
	Underlying immunosuppression, pregnancy or age > 65 years			
	Ampicillin	2 g iv	4 hourly	14–21 days
	+ Ceftriaxone	2 g iv	12 hourly	14–21 days
	or Cefotaxime	2 g iv	4 hourly	14–21 days
Post-traumatic meningitis				
Community acquired	Treat as for spontaneous meningitis in adults			14–21 days
Nosocomial	**Probability of *Pseudomonas* spp. high**			
	Ceftazidime	2 g iv	8 hourly	4 weeks
	or Meropenem	2 g iv	8 hourly	4 weeks
	Probability of *Pseudomonas* spp. low			
	Ceftriaxone	2 g iv	12 hourly	14–21 days
	or Cefotaxime	2 g iv	4 hourly	14–21 days
Shunt-associated meningitis				
Insidious	Vancomycin	1 g iv	12 hourly	14–21 days
	+	5–10 g intrathecally	48–72 hourly	2–4 weeks
Acute onset	Treat as for nosocomial post-traumatic meningitis			

Table 14.3 Antibiotics that may be appropriate for various pathogens in bacterial meningitis

Type of infection and drug	Dose	Frequency	Duration
Pneumococcal (choice of drug depends on susceptibility tests)			
Penicillin	2.4 g iv	4 hourly	10–14 days
or			
Ceftriaxone	2 g iv	12 hourly	10–14 days
or			
Cefotaxime	2 g iv	4 hourly	10–14 days
or			
Vancomycin	1 g iv	12 hourly	10–14 days
Meningococcal			
Penicillin	1.4 g iv	4 hourly	7 days
or			
Ceftriaxone	2 g iv	12 hourly	7 days
or			
Cefotaxime	2 g iv	4 hourly	7 days
Haemophilus influenzae			
Ampicillin	2 g iv	4 hourly	10–14 days
or			
Ceftriaxone	2 g iv	12 hourly	10–14 days
or			
Cefotaxime	2 g iv	4 hourly	10–14 days
Gram-negative bacillary (e.g. *Escherichia coli*)			
Ceftriaxone	2 g iv	12 hourly	3–4 weeks
or			
Cefotaxime	2 g iv	4 hourly	3–4 weeks
or			
Meropenem	2 g iv	8 hourly	3–4 weeks
Pseudomonas aeruginosa			
Ceftazidime	2 g iv	8 hourly	3–4 weeks
or			
Meropenem	2 g iv	8 hourly	4 weeks
Listeria monocytogenes			
Ampicillin	2 g iv	4 hourly	3 weeks
or			
Trimethoprim/ sulphamethoxazole*	5 mg/kg trimethoprim iv	12 hourly	3 weeks

Type of infection and drug	Dose	Frequency	Duration
Table 14.3 *Continued*			
Staphylococcus aureus Vancomycin	1 g iv	12 hourly	4 weeks
or Flucloxacillin	2 mg iv	4 hourly	4 weeks
*Trimethoprim/sulphamethoxazole is formulated in a fixed ratio of one part trimethoprim and five parts sulphamethoxazole.			

- It is essential to start treatment as soon as possible and not wait for microbiological confirmation from CSF or blood. There may be clues in the history or on examination as to the likely pathogen, but usually antibiotic treatment needs to be started empirically.
- Once the specific organism and the antibiotic sensitivity are known, change to the appropriate antibiotic (Table 14.3).

Corticosteroids

Corticosteroids are used to reduce the inflammatory response in bacterial meningitis and hence reduce mortality and morbidity.

- All *adults* presenting with suspected or proven bacterial meningitis should be given dexamethasone 0.4 mg/kg body weight per day iv for 4 days, starting before the first dose of antibiotics if possible. If the patient has already started on antibiotics, still administer steroids for 4 days, as above. The exceptions to this are:
  - clear contraindications to short-course steroid use
  - in regions of the world where TB meningitis is common and may be mistaken for bacterial meningitis
  - in patients with HIV infection.
- All *children* with suspected or proven bacterial meningitis should receive dexamethasone 0.4 mg/kg body weight per day iv for 4 days, preferably with the first dose of antibiotics. If the patient has already started on antibiotics, still administer steroids for 4 days, as above. The exceptions to this are:
  - clear contraindications to short-course steroid use
  - children in Africa, where the evidence suggests no benefit (this discrepancy between the developed and developing world may reflect later presentation, frequency of co-infection with HIV, malnutrition, antimicrobial drug resistance, and suboptimal antibiotic use).

Recurrent meningitis

Recurrent bacterial meningitis is rare in the developed world but relatively common in the developing world where post-traumatic meningitis is more common and the underlying CSF leak often not corrected. In any patient with recurrent meningitis a careful history is needed for previous head trauma, congenital occult spina bifida, or fracture of the base of the skull. Rarely, recurrent bacterial meningitis is due to a genetic defect in the complement pathway.

Mollaret's meningitis

This is a benign but recurrent aseptic meningitis that can occur in almost any age group. Most patients make a spontaneous recovery in a few days, although neurological sequelae (cranial nerve lesions, hemiplegia) have been reported. The presentation is similar to that of typical meningitis with a CSF pleocytosis and a predominance of lymphocytes plus large endothelial cells (Mollaret's cells). CSF protein is raised and the CSF glucose low or normal. If a diagnosis is established then treatment is supportive. Indomethacin has been used in isolated case reports.

Other causes of recurrent meningitis include:

- Sarcoidosis
- systemic lupus erythematosus
- Viral meningitis
- Malignant infiltration of the meninges
- Rarely, Behçet's syndrome.

AMOEBIC MENINGITIS

- *Naegleria fowleri* is a parasite found in warm stagnant water and soil. People can be infected after swimming or taking a spa in infected water, usually in the 2 weeks prior to the onset of symptoms. It occurs in temperate climates and most commonly in the summer months.
- The amoebae can cause meningoencephalitis, and patients typically present with headache, fever, convulsions and coma. The CSF is cloudy with a low glucose, high protein and predominantly a high neutrophil count, very similar to bacterial meningitis. No organisms are seen on Gram stain.
- The diagnosis is made by seeing the amoebae in wet specimens using phase-contrast microscopy, or by iron haematoxylin stain of fixed preparations.

- Amphotericin B (1 mg/kg body weight per day iv for 2–4 weeks) is the only available treatment (for adverse effects, see below).

BRAIN ABSCESS AND SUBDURAL EMPYEMA

Whenever an abscess is suspected a detailed search for the primary source of infection is important:

- direct spread of bacteria from contiguous anatomical structures such as middle ear and mastoid cavity, frontal, paranasal, ethmoidal and sphenoidal sinuses
- skull injury or local infection
- metastasis from a distant source such as the heart (endocarditis), the lungs (bronchiectasis, pulmonary arteriovenous malformation), dental abscess, the pelvis or the gastrointestinal tract.

Once diagnosed, surgical drainage remains the treatment of choice in almost all cases. Empirical antibiotic therapy is guided by consideration of the likely primary focus of the infection, but should include a third-generation cephalosporin (cefotaxime or ceftriazone) and metronidazole. For abscess complicating trauma, flucloxacillin or vancomycin should be added. Treatment should continue for a minimum of 6 weeks.

TUBERCULOUS MENINGITIS

Tuberculous meningitis is a difficult disease to diagnose and treat. It accounts for approximately 1% of all clinical presentations of TB, is increasing with the spread of HIV, and has a high case fatality (30%) and morbidity (30% of patients left with neurological sequelae).

Clinical features

It usually presents with a longer history than bacterial or viral meningitis (more than a week) of headache, fever, vomiting and anorexia, with a stiff neck, focal neurological signs (particularly lower cranial nerves), urinary retention and reduced conscious level. Convulsions are rare.

Diagnosis

The diagnosis is made by demonstration of acid-fast bacilli by Zeihl–Neelsen (ZN) stain of the CSF. The sensitivity of this test can be improved by thorough examination of a large volume of CSF (up to 10 ml in adults) and if performed well is more sensitive than a polymerase chain reaction (PCR) based approach. Unfortunately the ZN stain only has a sensitivity (at best) of 40–60% and culture of the CSF can take up to 6 weeks to become positive.

The CSF is classically slightly yellow, lymphocytic, with a low glucose (< 50% of the blood glucose), moderate lactate (4–6 mmol/l) and high protein (Table 14.4). However, in many patients, especially early in the illness or in those with HIV infection, the CSF is often neutrophilic.

Treatment

Treatment should start as early as possible, as with all bacterial meningitis. The idea that this is a subacute or chronic meningitis and a clinician can therefore wait is wrong. Treatment is urgent, with four antibiotics to begin with (Table 14.5).

Table 14.4   A simple clinical algorithm to aid the diagnosis of TB meningitis, particularly in regions with a low prevalence of HIV

Variable	Score
Age (years)	
≥ 36	+2
< 36	0
Blood white cell count (10^3/ml)	
≥ 15,000	+4
< 15,000	0
History of illness (days)	
≥ 6	–5
< 6	0
CSF total white cell count (10^3/ml)	
≥ 750	+3
< 750	0
CSF % neutrophils	
≥ 90	+4
< 90	0
Total score ≤ 4 = tuberculous meningitis	
Total score > 4 = non-tuberculous meningitis	

All patients with TB meningitis (adults and children) with any grade of disease should also receive dexamethasone with their antibiotics (as above) unless there is a very clear contraindication.

There is a major and growing problem with the emergence of multidrug-resistant *Mycobacterium tuberculosis*. If it is possible to culture the bacteria from the CSF then antimicrobial sensitivity testing should be performed and second-line antibiotics introduced (if available) if the bacteria are resistant to the original antibiotics.

Complications

■ The commonest complications are hydrocephalus, stroke-like events, encephalopathy and secondary infections.

Table 14.5   The treatment of tuberculous meningitis

Drug	Daily dose		Route	Duration
	Children	**Adults**		
Isoniazid	5 mg/kg	300 mg	Oral	9–12 months
Rifampicin	10 mg/kg	450 mg (< 50 kg)	Oral	9–12 months
		600 mg (> 50 kg)		
Pyrazinamide	35 mg/kg	1.5 g (< 50 kg)	Oral	2 months
		2.0 g (> 50 kg)		
Ethambutol or	15 mg/kg	15 mg/kg	Oral	2 months
Streptomycin	15 mg/kg	15 mg/kg (max. 1 g)	im	2 months
Dexamethasone	0.4 mg/kg/day		iv	1 week
	0.3 mg/kg/day		iv	1 week
	0.2 mg/kg/day		Oral/iv	1 week
	0.1 mg/kg/day		Oral	1 week
	3 mg/day /total		Oral	1 week
	2 mg/day/total		Oral	1 week

- The anti-TB drugs commonly cause severe hepatitis and also induce liver enzymes, which may interfere with other drugs, including the adjunct dexamethasone.
- There are complicated interactions between anti-TB drugs and antiretroviral drugs.

SYPHILIS

The incidence of syphilis is increasing with the global spread of HIV/AIDS.

- Syphilis is caused by the bacteria *Treponema pallidum* and is a chronic systemic infectious disease usually acquired sexually, although it can also be transmitted in utero.
- The incubation period is 2–4 weeks and at this stage a primary sore develops at the site of infection, usually the genitalia, with surrounding lymphadenopathy.
- This is followed by the secondary bacteraemic phase with an associated symmetrical rash and generalised lymphadenopathy.
- If untreated, there can be a period of prolonged latency (many years) followed by a destructive late stage with skin, central nervous system (CNS), skeletal and vascular involvement. During the late stages there is often a uveitis, choroidoretinitis and optic atrophy.
- Neurosyphilis includes:
  - acute and chronic meningitis
  - myeloradiculopathy
  - space-occupying lesions in the brain or spinal cord
  - an arteritis leading to strokes
  - multiple cranial nerve palsies
  - Argyll–Robertson pupil
  - personality changes and dementia
  - the dorsal roots can be affected leading to tabes dorsalis.

The disease is eminently treatable and to miss the diagnosis is a disaster.

Diagnosis

- The diagnosis relies on serology and examination of the CSF.
- The Venereal Diseases Research Laboratory test (VDRL) and the *Treponema pallidum* haemagglutination test (TPHA) are the most commonly used tests of blood and CSF, but false negatives are seen, especially in late syphilis.
- In patients with neurosyphilis there is usually a lymphocytic pleocytosis in the CSF and an elevated protein.

- The sensitivity of CSF-VDRL is approximately 50%, although it is highly specific.
- A negative CSF-TPHA excludes the diagnosis.

Treatment

- Penicillin G 2–4 mU iv every 4 hours for 14 days.
- If allergic to penicillin, doxycycline 200 mg oral qds for 28 days.

VIRAL MENINGOENCEPHALITIS

There is enormous geographical variation in the cause of viral meningo-encephalitis:

- In the developed world, the commonest causes are herpes simplex type-1 (HSV-1), mumps, enteroviruses, herpes zoster, adenoviruses and Epstein–Barr virus.
- In the USA, St. Louis, West Nile, Eastern and Western equine encephalitis and bunyaviruses, such as California (La Crosse) encephalitis viruses are also relatively common.
- In Central and Eastern Europe, the tick-borne encephalitis virus is endemic and causes encephalitis.
- Herpes simplex type-2 (HSV-2) causes disease mostly in neonates and immunosuppressed patients.
- In Asia, Japanese encephalitis is the commonest cause of encephalitis, while measles, rabies and Nipah also occur.
- Rift Valley fever virus in Africa and the Middle East, and naviruses in Latin America, are other causes in various parts of the world.
- Postinfectious encephalomyelitis can follow almost any viral infection, but has been most commonly associated with measles.
- Guillain–Barré syndrome has been associated with infections by Epstein–Barr virus, cytomegalovirus, Coxsackie B, and herpes zoster virus.
- Immunodeficient patients are particularly vulnerable to certain viral infections:
  - Those with depressed cell-mediated immunity, including patients infected with HIV, may develop encephalitis due to herpes zoster or cytomegalovirus
  - Progressive multifocal leukoencephalopathy is caused by reactivation of a common polyoma virus in patients with AIDS or other causes of immunosuppression. The diagnosis can be made by PCR for JC virus from the CSF or following brain biopsy. Treatment is of the underlying

immunosuppression (i.e. highly active antiretroviral therapy (HAART) in patients with AIDS, see below). It is worth considering adding cidofovir 5 mg/kg iv once weekly.

Clinical features and diagnosis

The history is usually of a few days of fever, headache, a stiff neck, myalgia and vomiting, with altered consciousness and possibly epileptic convulsions if encephalitis as well as meningitis is prominent. Some viral meningo-encephalitides are associated with specific clinical features; temporal lobe changes in HSV-1, skin blisters with the enterovirus, fear of water in rabies, and abnormal movements in Japanese encephalitis, but most present with a non-specific illness.

- A viral cause is usually confirmed in only 30–50% of clinically suspected cases of viral meningoencephalitis, although PCR has revolutionised the sensitivity and speed of diagnosis.
- Electroencephalography (EEG) is helpful as an early indicator of cortical involvement, although the severity of the EEG abnormality is not a good indicator of prognosis.
- Magnetic resonance imaging (MRI) can be helpful in demonstrating predominant temporal lobe and insular changes in HSE-1 and basal ganglia lesions in Japanese encephalitis.

Treatment

- Treatment is supportive in most cases of viral meningitis and encephalitis.
- The only specific treatment is aciclovir 10 mg/kg iv every 8 hours for 10–14 days (or 21 days in patients who are immunocompromised) for HSV infection. It is well tolerated and should be started in all patients with suspected viral encephalitis; renal failure is unusual. It can be stopped if the diagnostic tests are negative and the clinical suspicion of HSV infection is low.
- Aciclovir is also effective against varicella zoster virus.
- There is no proven benefit for corticosteroids, interferons, intrathecal administration of drugs or any other adjuvant therapy in viral encephalitis.

NEUROLOGICAL COMPLICATIONS OF HIV INFECTION

- HIV infection of the brain and meninges may itself cause an acute meningoencephalitis at the time of seroconversion, and later patients with AIDS are at risk of a subacute chronic encephalopathy and dementia.

- The introduction and widespread use of HAART in the developed world have had a dramatic impact on the spectrum of neurological infectious diseases in individuals who are infected with HIV.
- Sadly, neurological opportunistic infections continue to be a major cause of mortality and morbidity in patients with HIV in the developing world where access to HAART remains lamentable.
- Primary CNS lymphoma remains common and must be considered in the assessment of any patient infected with HIV who presents with a meningeal syndrome.

MALARIA

Malaria is the most important parasitic disease of man. On any one day approximately 5% of the world's population are infected and the disease kills somewhere between one and two million people each year. Of the four species of malaria parasites that infect humans, only *Plasmodium falciparum* is lethal. Cerebral involvement causing coma in severe *P. falciparum* malaria is a characteristic development with a 15–20% treated case fatality (Table 14.6). Cerebral malaria is probably the most common cause of coma in tropical areas of the world.

Diagnosis

Malaria must be excluded in any person with a fever who lives in or who has visited an endemic region. The diagnosis is based on a thick and thin malaria blood film, by rapid immunochromatographic tests, or by PCR. Mortality is considerably higher if the diagnosis and start of therapy are delayed.

Treatment

- Patients with cerebral malaria should ideally be admitted to an intensive care unit with accurate fluid balance and monitoring of the haematocrit.
- The blood glucose should be assessed every 4 hours as hypoglycaemia is a common feature of severe malaria even when not using quinine.
- The main options for the treatment of severe malaria are artesunate, quinine, quinidine and artemether and depending on whether the patient is being treated in a health clinic or hospital intensive care unit (Table 14.7).
- Artesunate is the best treatment for severe malaria and can be given by bolus intravenous injection, while artemether is given by intramuscular injection. Artesunate is preferable as the water-soluble drug is instantly

Table 14.6   Laboratory indicators of a poor prognosis in cerebral malaria

Indicator	Value
Haematology	
Leucocytosis	$> 12,000/\mu l$
Severe anaemia	PCV $< 15\%$
Coagulopathy	Platelets $< 50,000/\mu l$
	Prothrombin time prolonged >3 seconds
	Prolonged partial thromboplastin time
	Fibrinogen < 200 mg/dl
Blood film	
Hyperparasitaemia $> 500,000/\mu l$	
$> 20\%$ of parasites are pigment-containing trophozoites and schizonts	
$> 5\%$ of neutrophils contain visible pigment	
Biochemistry	
Hypoglycaemia	< 2.2 mmol/l
Hyperlactataemia	> 5 mmol/l
Acidosis	Arterial pH < 7.3, serum $HCO_3 < 15$ mmol/l
Serum creatinine	$> 265\ \mu mol/l$*
Total bilirubin	$> 50\ \mu mol/l$
Liver enzymes	sGOT (AST) $\times 3$ upper limit of normal
Muscle enzymes	sGPT (ALT) $\times 3$ upper limit of normal
Urate	$>600\ \mu mol/l\ \mu l$
5-Nucleotidase	$\uparrow$
CPK	$\uparrow$
Myoglobin	$\uparrow$

CPK, creatine phosphokinase; PCV, packed cell volume; sGOT (AST), serum glutamic oxaloacetic transferase (aspartate aminotransferase); sGPT (ALT), serum glutamic pyruvic transaminase (alanine aminotransferase).

*This is the criterion for adults. Less elevated values are found in children with severe malaria.

bioavailable, whereas absorption of artemether from intramuscular injection is slow and erratic, especially in patients who have a severe metabolic acidosis.

Table 14.7 The treatment of cerebral malaria

Hospital intensive care unit	Health clinic: no intravenous infusions possible
Artemisinin derivatives	
Artesunate 2.4 mg/kg by iv injection followed 1.2 mg/kg daily for 7 days or until the patient can take oral medication	Artesunate suppositories: 10mg/kg stat, then daily for 7 days
or	
Artemether 3.2 mg/kg by im injection followed by 1.6 mg/kg daily for 7 days	As for hospital: artesunate can also be given by im injection
Quinine	
Quinine dihydrochloride 7 mg salt/kg infused over 30 minutes followed immediately by 10 mg/kg over 4 hours	Quinine dihydrochloride 20 mg salt/kg diluted 1:2 with sterile water given by split injection into both anterior thighs
or	
20 mg salt/kg infused over 4 hours	Maintenance dose: 10 mg/kg 8-hourly* for 7 days
Maintenance dose: 10 mg salt/kg infused over 2–8 hours at 8-hour intervals* for 7 days	
Quinidine	
10 mg base/kg infused over 1–2 hours followed by 1.2 mg base/kg per hour[†] for 7 days	
Electrocardiographic monitoring advisable	

*The preferred dosage interval for parenteral quinine in African children is 12 hours.
[†]Some authorities recommend a lower dose of quinidine: 6.2 mg base/kg initially over 1 hour followed by 0.012 mg base/kg per hour.

Adverse effects of antimalarial drugs

■ Quinine and quinidine commonly cause hypoglycaemia and a number of minor adverse effects (collectively termed 'cinchonism'), evident on recovery of consciousness, which include tinnitus, nausea, dysphoria and high-tone hearing loss.

- Quinidine commonly produces prolongation of the QT interval and hypotension. The infusion should be slowed if the blood pressure falls, the plasma concentration exceeds 7 mg/ml or if the QT interval increases by more than 25%.
- The artemisinin derivatives (Artemether and Artesunate) have no serious adverse effects.

Additional treatments

- Standard antiepileptic drugs if seizures occur (see Chapter 2).
- Small series and anecdotal reports suggest that exchange blood transfusion may be beneficial: if safe supplies of blood are available this can be tried in severe cases. This may work by providing a supply of functional non-parasitised red blood cells.

General points

- Do not use chloroquine as most *P. falciparum* infections are now chloroquine-resistant.
- Infusions can be given in 0.9% saline, or 5% or 10% dextrose/water.
- Infusion rates for quinine or quinidine should be carefully controlled.
- Oral treatment should start as soon as the patient can swallow reliably enough to complete a full course of treatment.

SCHISTOSOMIASIS

- Schistosomiasis is caused by blood flukes transmitted by snails, which invade the circulation, usually via small abrasions in the skin.
- It is a huge global public health problem, with an estimated 200 million people infected, particularly in Africa, Asia and Latin America.
- There is an immune reaction to the eggs, which can lead to focal granulomatous lesions causing diffuse encephalopathy, focal neurological deficits, focal epileptic fits and severe headache. CSF and blood usually show an eosinophilia with a normal CSF glucose but raised CSF protein.
- Schistosomiasis can also present as a myeloradiculopathy with the eggs being deposited in the lower spinal cord. The patient presents with back pain and rapidly developing weakness, sensory loss and bladder dysfunction.
- Patients should be treated with Praziquantel 60 mg/kg body weight per day oral for 3 days plus prednisolone 2 mg/kg body weight per day for 3 weeks and tapered off over 3 weeks. Praziquantel is well tolerated, although it is not recommended during pregnancy.

CYSTICERCOSIS

- Cysticercosis is caused by the larvae of the pork tapeworm *Taenia solium*. Humans ingest diseased pork and the cysticerci invade the gut mucosa where the tapeworm develops and can reach 2–4 m in length.
- Seizures, either generalised or focal, are the commonest presenting feature. It is a very common cause of late-onset seizures in many parts of Africa and South and Central America and is being increasingly recognised in the southern USA. In addition patients may have fever, headache, ataxia, vomiting and confusion or present with stroke.
- Approximately 15% of patients have ventricular cysts at presentation, which can block CSF flow and cause drop attacks, episodic vomiting and sudden death.
- The most important aspect of treatment is the control of seizures with standard antiepileptic drugs (see Chapter 2) and, if needed, management of intracranial hypertension.
- Patients should be treated with Albendazole 15 mg/kg body weight per day oral for 7 days and with dexamethasone 0.4 mg/kg body weight per day oral for 7 days.
- An alternative is Praziquantel, either as a 1-day regimen of 25 mg/kg in 3 doses 2 hours apart, or a 15-day regimen of 100 mg/kg body weight per day oral. The 1-day regimen should only be used for those with a single or low cyst burden.

TOXOPLASMOSIS

- *Toxoplasma gondii* is an intracellular parasite and is a common opportunistic infection in immunocompromised patients, particularly those with AIDS who have a CD4 count less than 100/mm^3.
- Patients usually present with subacute progressive focal neurological deficits, headache, mild fever and contrast-enhancing lesions on brain computed tomography (CT) or MRI.
- Treatment is with sulfadiazine 1–2 g oral qds and pyrimethamine 200 mg oral for 2 days loading dose, then 50–100 mg oral qds plus oral folinic acid 10 mg for 6 weeks. Up to 50% of patients have adverse reactions on this regimen, including bone marrow suppression and drug rashes. Patients should have weekly full blood counts for leukopenia and bone marrow suppression. The addition of folinic acid can help prevent this drug-induced adverse effect.
- Alternatives include trimethoprim–sulfamethoxazole 160 mg/800 mg or pyrimethamine plus azithromycin 1 g/day.

- Treatment is continued for 6 weeks and then patients go onto secondary prophylaxis with pyrimethamine 50 mg/day oral with sulfadiazine 500 mg oral qds.

CRYPTOCOCCAL MENINGITIS

- Most cryptococcal meningitis occurs in patients who are severely immunocompromised either due to HIV infection, long-term steroid use, neutropenia or other chronic immunosuppression.

Table 14.8	Treatment of cryptococcal meningitis			
Drug	**Dose**	**Duration**	**Adverse effects**	**Alternative**
Induction phase				
Liposomal amphotericin	Up to 10 mg/kg/day iv	At least 2 weeks	Dose-dependent nephrotoxicity (usually reversible if total dose does not exceed 4 g), rigors during infusion	Amphotericin B 1 mg/kg/day if liposomal preparation not available
+				
Flucytosine	100 mg/kg/day iv in 4 divided doses	At least 2 weeks	Marrow suppression, vomiting, abdominal pain	
Consolidation phase				
Fluconazole	400 mg/day oral	10 weeks	Raised liver enzymes	Itraconazole 400 mg/day oral
Maintenance phase				
Fluconazole	200 mg/day	Life-long, although consider stopping after immune reconstitution with HAART		

- Cryptococcal meningitis accounts for approximately 20% of all AIDS deaths globally, making it the second commonest cause of death associated with HIV, after tuberculosis.
- The fungus is distributed worldwide, although certain serotypes (B and C) are mostly found in the tropics.
- It is usually a subacute illness with a 2–4 week history of severe headache, mild fever, double vision and vomiting. VI nerve palsies are common. CT and MRI of the brain are abnormal in approximately 70% of cases, with hydrocephalus the commonest abnormality.
- The diagnosis is made by an India Ink stain of the CSF, culture of the CSF and by cryptococcal antigen testing in CSF and in blood.
- Patients may have very high intracranial pressure leading to severe and often intractable headaches, VI nerve palsies and blindness. Frequent lumbar punctures (every other day if needed), external CSF drainage or ventriculoperitoneal shunting may all need to be tried.
- There are no data to support either mannitol or corticosteroids.
- The treatment of cryptococcal meningitis is based on amphotericin, flucytosine and fluconazole (Table 14.8).

Further reading

Day JN, Lalloo DG. Neurological syndromes and the traveller: an approach to differential diagnosis. J Neurol Neurosurg Psychiatry 2004; 75(Suppl 1): i2–i9.

Portegies P, Solod L, Cinque P, Chaudhuri A, Begovac J, Everall I, Weber T, Bojar M, Martinez-Martin P, Kennedy PG. Guidelines for the diagnosis and management of neurological complications of HIV infection. Eur J Neurol 2004; 11(5): 297–304.

Steiner I, Budka H, Chaudhuri A, Koskiniemi M, Sainio K, Salonen O, Kennedy PG. Viral encephalitis: a review of diagnostic methods and guidelines for management. Eur J Neurol 2005; 12(5): 331–343.

Thwaites GE, Nguyen DB, Nguyen HD, Hoang TQ, Do TT, Nguyen TC, Nguyen QH, Nguyen TT, Nguyen NH, Nguyen TN, Nguyen NL, Nguyen HD, Vu NT, Cao HH, Tran TH, Pham PM, Nguyen TD, Stepniewska K, White NJ, Tran TH, Farrar JJ. Dexamethasone for the treatment of tuberculous meningitis in adolescents and adults. N Engl J Med 2004; 351(17): 1741–1751.

van de Beek D, de Gans J, McIntyre P, Prasad K. Corticosteroids in acute bacterial meningitis. Cochrane Database Syst Rev 2003; 3: CD004305.

White N. Cerebral malaria. Practical Neurol 2004; 4(1): 20–29.

15 TUMOURS AND PARANEOPLASTIC SYNDROMES

Robin Grant

Intracranial tumours

Intracranial tumours have an overall incidence of 25 per 100,000 population per year.

- Intracerebral tumours may be:
  - primary (e.g. gliomas, 8 per 100,000 population per year)
  - secondary (metastasis), 12 per 100,000 population per year
  - other (e.g. medulloblastoma, primary central nervous system (CNS) lymphoma).
- Intracranial extracerebral tumours most commonly arise from:
  - meninges (meningioma)
  - pituitary gland (pituitary adenoma)
  - Rathke's pouch cells (craniopharyngioma)
  - cranial nerve sheaths (acoustic neuroma).
- Primary intracerebral tumours are:
  - the most common solid tumour in children
  - the fourth most common tumour under age 40 years
  - the eighth most common under age 65 years
  - there is a slight male predominance (1.2:1).

Diagnosis

- History (frequency at hospital presentation):

- late-onset epilepsy (26%)
- gradual onset unilateral weakness, sensory problems, dysphasia (60%)
- headache plus memory/personality problems (50%)
- raised intracranial pressure (25%).
- Neurological examination:
  - nil (especially when late-onset epilepsy)
  - focal neurological deficit
  - memory/personality problems
  - papilloedema.
- Magnetic resonance imaging (MRI) or computed tomography (CT) brain scan with contrast:
  - intracerebral lesion (? tumour)
  - intracranial extracerebral lesion (? tumour).

Immediate management

Corticosteroids

- Corticosteroids improve symptoms and neurological impairments, and reduce cerebral oedema on imaging. Rarely, tumours disappear on imaging (e.g. primary CNS lymphoma).
- If raised intracranial pressure or significant brain shift/herniation:
  - Dexamethasone 12–16 mg iv, followed by 16 mg oral each day in 2 divided doses until symptoms improve, then dose can be rapidly reduced to 4 mg/day. Avoid after 6 pm because of the common adverse effect of insomnia.
  - Plan to relieve any hydrocephalus if appropriate.
  - Plan to decompress tumour surgically if appropriate.
- If there are neurological deficits, but no signs of raised intracranial pressure, dexamethasone 4 mg/day oral.
- Corticosteroids are not required if epilepsy only.
- Adverse effects of corticosteroids are described in Chapter 9. Caution in: the elderly; past history of tuberculosis, heart, liver or renal failure; diabetes; hypertension; glaucoma; and severe psychosis.

Mannitol and diuretics

Only rarely needed if dexamethasone is ineffective and there is impending transtentorial or cerebellar tonsillar herniation ('coning') while awaiting surgery:

- Mannitol: iv 0.25 g/kg test dose, then 1 g/kg bolus as 20% solution, up to 2 g/kg if necessary, monitoring fluid and electrolyte balance (see Chapter 8).

- Frusemide 40 mg iv bolus is an alternative.
- Acetazolomide 250 mg oral or iv bd is another alternative.

Gut protection
- Proton pump inhibitor (e.g. omeprazole 20 mg once daily oral), or
- H_2 receptor antagonist (e.g. ranitidine 150 mg oral bd).

Antiepileptic drugs
- No need for prophylactic antiepileptic drugs prior to surgery.
- If seizures have occurred, use single agent (e.g. carbamazepine) at the lowest effective dose and build up dose slowly unless the patient is actively seizing or in status epilepticus (see Chapter 2).

Deep venous thrombosis prophylaxis
A multimodality approach is required using:
- Compression stockings before and after surgery.
- Pneumatic intermittent compression boots during surgery.
- Prophylactic perioperative heparin is safe and is recommended in patients at high risk. There is no evidence that low-molecular-weight heparin (enoxaparin 40 mg/day sc) is superior to unfractionated heparin (5000 units sc bd).

Intermediate management
Is it a tumour?
In some circumstances, where the imaging diagnosis is uncertain, further investigation to exclude abscess, inflammation, multiple sclerosis and stroke is indicated.

Is it a primary or secondary tumour?
It can be very difficult to distinguish between high-grade glioma, metastasis and primary CNS lymphoma by imaging alone. When uncertain, investigations should be made to look for multiple lesions/secondary spread (e.g. MRI brain, chest X-ray/CT and abdomen CT (? metastasis), slit lamp of eyes and examine CSF for clonal lymphocytes (? lymphoma)).

Good clinical practice
- Multidisciplinary meeting to discuss management plan.
- Timely, verbal and written communication between the doctor and patient, and between doctors involved in care.

- Discussion with patient about likely diagnosis in a quiet private setting, with a close relative present, with sufficient time to answer questions.
- What has been discussed and the concerns of the patient/relative should be documented.
- Histopathology is the key to appropriate treatment and accurate prognosis.
- Patients must have sufficient time to decide whether they wish to opt for surgery, especially the elderly where any benefits are not clear cut.
- It is wise not to be drawn into the details of treatment before the diagnosis is certain.

Biopsy versus resection

- Biopsy will confirm the histological type and grade of tumour in > 95% of cases.
- General agreement that lobar tumours in patients under 60 years of age who have a good Karnofsky performance score (Table 15.1) should be maximally resected when this can be achieved safely.
- Deep hemisphere lesions and diffuse cerebral tumours cannot be resected safely and biopsy is the simplest method of confirming the diagnosis for the least risk, especially in elderly patients with a poor performance score, where prognosis is usually less than 6 months.

LOW-GRADE GLIOMA (GRADES 1 OR 2)

- Better outcome if:
  - age < 40 years old better than 40–60 years better than > 60 years
  - good Karnofsky performance score (≥ 70)
  - grade of malignancy (grade 1 better than 2)
  - presentation with epilepsy
  - possibly extent of resection
  - tumour size < 6 cm diameter, no midline shift.
- Grade 1: complete resection can lead to cure. Radiation only required following incomplete resection in patients with advancing neurological impairment or radiological progression. Late effects of radiation are common (see below).
- Grade 2: management options for patients with suspected low-grade glioma and tumour-associated epilepsy alone are:
  - 'watchful waiting' and antiepileptic drugs with interval scans at 3 and 6 months and then annually, and surgical intervention only if there is tumour progression
  - surgical intervention, biopsy or resection at diagnosis to confirm grade.

Table 15.1   Karnofsky performance status scale

Performance	Score	Ability
Able to carry on normal activity and to work; no special care needed	100	Normal with no complaints; no evidence of disease
	90	Able to carry on normal activities; but minor signs or symptoms of disease
	80	Normal activity with effort; some signs or symptoms of disease
Unable to work but able to live at home and care for most personal needs; varying amount of assistance needed	70	Cares for self but unable to carry on normal activity or to do active work
	60	Requires occasional assistance, but is able to care for most personal needs
	50	Requires considerable assistance and frequent medical care
Unable to care for self requiring the equivalent of institutional or hospital care; disease may be progressing rapidly	40	Disabled and requiring special care and assistance
	30	Severely disabled; hospital admission is indicated although death not imminent
	20	Very sick; hospital admission necessary; active supportive treatment necessary
	10	Moribund, fatal processes, progressing rapidly
	0	Dead

Radiotherapy

- 'Early' after histological diagnosis or 'late' at radiological or clinical progression. Total dose delivered should be 45–50 Gy in 5 weeks (25 fractions).
- Early radiotherapy may increase time to progression but does not extend survival.
- Early radiotherapy may cause radiation induced leukoencephalopathy and pituitary insufficiency (see below).

Chemotherapy

- Chemotherapy may delay the need for radiotherapy in patients with oligodendroglioma (e.g. in children).
- No evidence that it is superior to radiotherapy, or radiotherapy followed by chemotherapy at recurrence.

HIGH-GRADE GLIOMA (GRADES 3 OR 4)

- Better outcome if:
  - age < 40 years better than 40–60 years better than >60 years
  - Karnofsky performance score ≥ 70
  - grade of malignancy (grade 3 better than 4)
  - tumour type (oligodendroglioma better than astrocytoma)
  - possibly extent of resection.

Surgery

- No good evidence that extent of resection improves survival.
- Morbidity is related to tumour site (eloquent versus non-eloquent) and extent of resection.

Radiotherapy

- Postoperative external beam radiotherapy recommended as standard practice.
- Radiation field should incorporate the enhancing tumour and a surrounding margin of 2–3 cm for the planning target volume.
- Total dose should be 60 Gy in 30 fractions, 2 Gy given on weekdays over a 6-week period.
- Radiation dose intensification is ineffective and highly toxic.
- Stereotactic radiotherapy and interstitial brachytherapy offer no greater survival than conformal beam radiation using a linear accelerator, and they have more adverse effects.
- Radiation sensitisers are ineffective.

- For Karnofsky performance score < 70 and age ≥ 60 years, similar survival benefit may be achieved with less morbidity using a shorter course of radiation with larger fraction sizes (30 Gy in 10 fractions).
- For Karnofsky performance score < 60 and age > 70 years, supportive care without radiotherapy is the norm.

Chemotherapy

- One-third of patients < 65 years old have a partial response (50% reduction in tumour size), but only 5–10% of those > 65 years old.
- Median survival advantage (2 months) in patients < 65 years old with a good performance score.
- There is a 5–15% increase in 2-year survival with chemotherapy.
- No evidence that 'neoadjuvant' chemotherapy (prior to radiotherapy) has any advantage over radiotherapy alone.
- Chemotherapy can be:
  - PCV: procarbazine 60 mg/m² oral on days 8 –21 plus CCNU 110 mg/m² on day 1 plus vincristine 1.4 mg/m² iv days 8–29 (maximum 2 mg/dose)
  - carmustine (BCNU) 200 mg/m² iv every 6 weeks
  - temozolomide, oral, concomitantly 75 mg/m² per day 7 days per week with radiation therapy, and then adjuvantly at a dose of 150–200 mg/m² on days 1–5, repeated every 28 days
  - for adverse effects, see below.
- Intraoperative chemotherapy using BCNU impregnated wafers (Gliadel) placed in the tumour cavity, followed by radiation, gives a survival advantage of 1–2 months over surgery and radiotherapy alone.

BRAIN METASTASES

The most common primary cancer sites are lung (39%), breast (17%) and melanoma (11%), half are single and half are multiple. Progression of brain disease is the cause of death in 50% and progression of the systemic disease in 50%.

- Treatment depends on the site of the metastasis, the number of metastases, the age of the patient, the Karnofsky performance score and the extent and activity of extracranial disease.
- Better outcome if:
  - age < 65 years
  - Karnofsky performance score ≥ 70
  - controlled primary without other systemic metastases
  - single metastasis in operable site.

Pre-treatment evaluation

- MRI brain scan with gadolinium to identify whether single or multiple lesions.
- Thorough history and examination, including breasts, testes, rectum and skin.
- Chest and abdominal CT to look for widespread disease, or primary tumour site (or chest X-ray and abdominal ultrasound).
- Full blood count, urea and electrolytes, liver function, calcium and alkaline phosphatase.
- Alpha-fetoprotein and beta-HCG (germ cell tumour), CA-125 (ovary), prostatic acid phosphatase (prostate) and serum CEA (colon/lung).

Management

- Around 10% of patients with a known primary tumour and a single lesion on brain CT thought to be a metastasis are found to have a *different* condition on biopsy/resection of the cerebral lesion.
- Surgery should be considered if there is diagnostic doubt.
- Solitary brain metastasis (< 3 cm) in operable site and stable disease elsewhere:
  - resection of metastasis confirms diagnosis, or
  - stereotactic radiotherapy.
- Single brain metastasis > 3 cm in operable site and stable disease elsewhere:
  - resection of metastasis confirms diagnosis.
- Multiple brain metastases with good Karnofsky performance score:
  - whole-brain radiotherapy
  - or stereotactic radiosurgery if only 2–3 lesions.
- Multiple brain metastases in elderly with poor performance score, comorbid disorders or with widespread systemic metastases:
  - palliative care without local treatment.
- The value of whole-brain radiotherapy following resection/stereotactic radiotherapy is uncertain.
- Chemosensitive tumours (e.g. small-cell lung cancer, breast and germ cell tumours) may benefit from chemotherapy relevant to the primary tumour type.

RARE INTRACRANIAL TUMOURS

Primary CNS lymphoma

- Accounts for 2% of brain tumours and is often associated with immunosuppression (especially human immunodeficiency virus (HIV)).

- Slit lamp examination of the eyes for cells in vitreous. CSF analysis for lymphoma cells. CT chest/abdomen for any systemic disease.
- Median survival is about 6 months in HIV patients (highly immuno-suppressed) and 2 years in non-immunosuppressed treated patients.
- Tumours appear slightly high signal on non-contrast-enhanced CT scan and enhance highly following contrast.
- Corticosteroids often cause the CT changes to disappear (rarely for more than a year).
- Biopsy to diagnose (resection not required and associated with complications).
- Many patients respond to chemotherapy (high-dose methotrexate-based regimens or CHOP).
- Radiotherapy can result in tumour disappearance and resolution of symptoms and signs for years; avoid radiation to eyes (unless vitreous disease).
- Radiation induced leukoencephalopathy occurs in late survivors (especially if concomitant chemotherapy has been given).

Medulloblastoma

- Rare tumour in the brainstem/cerebellum, usually in children, and which commonly seeds through the craniospinal axis.
- MRI of the brain and spine are necessary in the diagnostic work-up, along with examining the cerebrospinal fluid (CSF) for malignant cells.
- Standard management:
  - maximum safe tumour resection
  - radiotherapy to the whole neuroaxis
  - chemotherapy in children, although optimum regimen is unclear at present; uncertain role in adults.

Pineal tumours

- Present with visual symptoms or obstructive hydrocephalus and the tumours often seed to CSF.
- Serum or CSF tumour marker studies may help diagnose germ cell tumours.
- Standard management:
  - shunting of any hydrocephalus, or endoscopic fenestration with biopsy
  - biopsy of lesion and intraoperative diagnosis; if germinoma then no further surgery, otherwise resect tumour if possible
  - craniospinal radiotherapy for pineoblastoma/metastatic germ cell tumours

- stereotactic radiation for incompletely resected pineocytoma, astrocytomas, as per other astrocytoma (see above)
- chemotherapy for germ cell tumours.

Pituitary and pituitary region tumours

■ Pituitary tumours are usually benign adenomas (95%), and may be functioning (hypersecretion of prolactin, growth hormone, TSH, ACTH) or non-functioning mass lesions.

■ Craniopharyngiomas are the most common peripituitary tumours in children. They may be associated with pituitary failure, obstructive hydrocephalus and visual impairment.

■ Meningiomas and epidermoid/dermoid/Rathke's pouch cysts can also occur at this site.

Once imaging and any endocrine diagnosis has been made (e.g. hyperprolactinaemia), patients should be referred to a specialist centre. Endocrinologists usually take responsibility for treatment and follow-up, with a multidisciplinary team including an ophthalmologist, neurosurgeon and radiation oncologist.

■ Assessment should include:
  - formal tests of visual acuity and visual fields
  - pituitary imaging (contrast-enhanced MRI, coronal images)
  - pituitary function testing.

Management

■ Reverse any pituitary failure.
■ If hyperprolactinaemia, dopamine agonists (e.g. cabergoline, bromocriptine).
■ Surgery not required for prolactin-secreting microadenomas that respond to drug treatment.
■ Surgery for patients with visual or cranial nerve problems if no improvement with dopamine agonists within 7 days.
■ Large tumours and tumours outwith the pituitary fossa require surgery.
■ Craniopharyngiomas may need insertion of reservoirs to drain cyst fluid and shunting of obstructive hydrocephalus, or other CSF-diversion procedures.
■ Postoperative diabetes insipidus is common, but frequently transient, and is best managed with endocrinology support.
■ Radiotherapy reduces the likelihood of long-term recurrence.
■ Stereotactic radiotherapy or radiosurgery may assist in the management of tumours that continue to secrete hormones.

Acoustic neuroma

- Base-of-skull multidisciplinary team meeting to decide management plan.
- Surgical removal by specialist skull base multidisciplinary team in fit younger patients, but complete excision is not always possible.
- Fractionated stereotactic radiotherapy or radiosurgery as first line is now not uncommon and can halt growth. However, symptomatic benefit may take months, or may not occur at all.
- Radiotherapy for an incompletely resected tumour is useful if it is symptomatic or imaging shows tumour regrowth. Subacute and late effects of radiation may occur if the brainstem is included in the treatment field.
- Conservative management is justified in elderly patients with extensive comorbidity and no brainstem compression.

Meningioma

- Surgical resection in fit younger patients is the norm with easily accessible tumours, but complete excision is not always possible.
- Some tumours can be embolised to reduce their vascularity prior to surgery.
- Radiotherapy is given for incompletely resected tumours if histology shows atypical or anaplastic changes, but symptomatic benefit may take many months.
- Conservative management is justified in elderly patients with extensive comorbidity.
- Chemotherapy is ineffective.

Spinal cord tumours

Tumours involving the spinal cord can be divided into:
- Extradural (common): e.g. metastatic carcinoma, lymphoma, plasma cell tumours.
- Intradural/extramedullary (rare): e.g. meningioma, neurofibroma.
- Intramedullary (very rare): e.g. glioma, metastasis.

The incidence of metastatic extradural spinal cord compression is 8–10 per 100,000 population per year, most commonly from breast, lung, prostate, lymphoma, sarcoma and kidney.

Management

General points

- Management depends on:
  - primary site and type of tumour, if already known
  - extent of systemic involvement
  - extent of spinal disease.
- Corticosteroids may improve neurological impairments, reduce pain and temporarily prevent progression (for dose and gastrointestinal protection see intracranial tumours, above).
- Laxatives reduce the need for straining, which increases intraspinal pressure.
- Deep venous thrombosis prophylaxis (see intracranial tumours, above).
- Urinary catheter if incontinent or urinary retention.

Indications for surgery

- Diagnosis in doubt.
- Bony compression or spinal instability, and limited disease elsewhere.
- Radiotherapy fails to improve symptoms.
- Single-level lesion.

Indications for radiotherapy

- Primary site of tumour known and multilevel disease.
- Widespread systemic disease.
- Significant comorbid disease that is a contraindication to surgery.

Indications for chemotherapy or hormonal therapy

- Mildly affected patients with a chemoresponsive/hormonal responsive tumour (e.g. myeloma, prostate and breast).

Malignant meningitis

- Malignant meningitis is due to tumour cells in the leptomeningeal coverings which cause focal or multifocal cranial or spinal root involvement, or cognitive problems usually due to non-obstructive hydrocephalus.
- The cells can come from a primary tumour within the CNS (e.g. medulloblastoma) or more often spread from a haematological (acute leukaemia, non-Hodgkin's lymphoma) or systemic malignancy (breast, lung, melanoma, gastrointestinal).

- It affects approximately 5% of patients with cancer, and usually there is a known history of cancer at neurological presentation.
- The prognosis is poor, with the exception of leukaemia and lymphoma.
- Treatment is seldom effective and should only be considered in certain situations with limited neurological involvement, limited systemic disease and chemoresponsive systemic disease:
  - Radiotherapy to symptomatic areas with MRI evidence of tumour deposits.
  - Systemic high-dose iv methotrexate (e.g. in lymphoma/leukaemia) and via an intraventricular reservoir in cases with cranial nerve involvement, or via lumbar intrathecal route in cases with spinal leptomeningeal involvement: 12 mg intrathecally 2–3 times weekly in preservative-free saline, or cytarabine 40–50 mg 2–3 times weekly, or thiotepa 10 mg 2–3 times weekly.

Adverse effects of radiotherapy

Brain and spinal cord
Acute radiation reactions

- Symptoms appear within days of starting treatment to large tumours of the brain or spinal cord; radiation causes significant oedema and swelling, particularly if large fraction size, high total dose and large treatment volume.
- Causes temporary worsening of pre-existing neurological symptoms (e.g. headache, raised intracranial pressure, worsening myelopathy).
- Treat with high-dose iv corticosteroids.

Early delayed radiation reactions

- Starts within 1–2 weeks of completion of radiotherapy and can last for 2–4 months.
- Causes fatigue, sleepiness, and possibly worsening focal symptoms due to demyelination in the region of the tumour.
- On imaging it is indistinguishable from tumour progression.
- Treatment by increasing corticosteroids temporarily for a few weeks, and then slowly taper the dose.

Late radiation reactions

- Radiation necrosis can start 4 months to several years after completion of radiation. MRI appearances are similar to tumour progression, with microvascular damage and necrosis. Single photon emission tomography (SPECT) or positron emission tomography (PET) may help distinguish between the two conditions.

■ Treatment is with corticosteroids, occasionally surgical resection for diagnosis and treatment if the patient is steroid dependent.

■ Leukoencephalopathy characteristically comes on years after effective treatment of a primary tumour or after prophylactic cranial irradiation in small-cell lung cancer:
  – slow cognition, short-term memory impairment, unsteadiness due to apraxia, incontinence, slowly progressive subcortical dementia
  – brain MRI shows diffuse white-matter change with ventricular dilatation
  – a slowly progressive myelopathy occurs, with high signal on T2-weighted images and cord atrophy
  – there is no effective treatment.

Local radiation effects on non-target structures within the field

■ Early:
  – alopecia
  – erythema
  – deafness due to wax.

■ Late:
  – pituitary insufficiency (adults, gonadotrophins first then thyroid, later corticotrophins)
  – cataract
  – optic neuropathy
  – nerve deafness
  – stroke due to radiation-induced occlusive vasculopathy of large vessels occurs years to decades after treatment.

Peripheral nerves and plexuses

■ Peripheral nerves are remarkably tolerant to radiation, but plexopathies do occur many years after therapy, most likely due to fibrosis of surrounding tissues within the plexus.

■ Plexopathies can be painful, and distinguishing them from tumour involvement or other causes of plexopathy can be difficult.

■ Radiation-induced vascular occlusion of vessels supplying the plexus or nerves can cause nerve infarction.

■ Most cases are treated symptomatically for neuropathic pain (see Chapter 18).

Radiation-induced tumours

- These are a rare complication of radiation.
- The tumour occurs within the previous radiation field (usually 10–20 years later) and is of a different histology from the original (e.g. meningioma, sarcoma, glioma).

Adverse effects of chemotherapy

Direct effects on neural tissue

Brain and cranial nerves

- Intravenous or intra-arterial methotrexate: encephalopathy.
- Intra-carotid BCNU or cisplatin: optic neuropathy, focal encephalopathy.
- High-dose cytosine arabinoside: reversible cerebellar syndrome.
- 5-Fluorouracil: cerebellar syndrome.
- Intrathecal Ara-C, methotrexate: encephalopathy.
- Cisplatinum: deafness.

Spinal cord

- Cisplatinum: Lhermitte's symptom.
- Intrathecal Ara-C, methotrexate: myelopathy.

Muscle and nerve

- Cisplatinum: sensory neuropathy.
- Vincristine: neuropathy/myopathy.
- Taxol, paclitaxol, docetaxel: neuropathy/myopathy.
- Cyclosporin, interferon-α, interleukin-2: sensorimotor neuropathy.

Myelosuppression

- Leukopenia and resulting opportunistic infections (bacterial, fungal, etc.).
- Low platelets, resulting in haemorrhage.
- Anaemia, resulting in tiredness, heart failure, dyspnoea and syncope.

Organ-specific complications

- Nitrosoureas: pulmonary fibrosis, heart failure.
- Cisplatinum: renal failure.
- Procarbazine: hepatic failure.

Paraneoplastic syndromes

The incidence of neurological paraneoplastic syndromes is < 0.5 per 100,000 population per year. These syndromes present subacutely, with fairly characteristic neurological symptoms and signs reflecting damage in both the central and peripheral nervous systems.

- The most common association is with small-cell lung cancer.
- Not all patients have or are destined to have cancer – about 40% have a non-cancer-related autoimmune disorder.
- Of all cases associated with cancer, approximately 50% are known to have cancer at neurological presentation, and in 50% it is the first manifestation of cancer.
- Investigations may identify the responsible tumour at a very early stage of its growth.

Potentially important tests when investigating possible paraneoplastic syndromes

- MRI brain/spinal cord with gadolinium to exclude direct cancer effects.
- CSF to exclude malignant meningitis, infection and Creutzfeld–Jakob disease.
- Electroencephalogram (EEG) to exclude herpes simplex encephalitis and non-convulsive status epilepticus.
- Dementia screen: serum thyroid autoantibodies, ACE, ANCA, vasculitis screen, vitamin B_{12}, folate.
- Cerebellar ataxia screening: genetics.
- Leber's optic neuropathy: genetics and electroretinogram.
- Nerve conduction studies.
- Electromyogram.

Looking for the primary tumour

- CT of chest and abdomen.
- CT, pelvic ultrasound, pelvic examination.
- Mammogram.
- Bronchoscopy (smoker with anti-Hu antibodies).
- Exploratory laparotomy.
- Whole-body PET scan.

Management

If paraneoplastic antibody positive, known cancer but brain metastases and malignant meningitis excluded, or characteristic presentation and paraneoplastic antibody negative but no other likely differential diagnosis:

- Methylprednisolone, 1 g/day iv for 3 days followed by oral prednisolone taper.
- Intravenous immunoglobulin (IVIg) 0.4 g/kg body weight per day for 5 days, usually starting at ultraslow flow rates (see Chapter 11) and building up quickly, assuming no adverse reactions. Give two treatments separated by 4 weeks.
- Plasmapheresis if allergic response to IVIg.
- Treatment of the underlying tumour will occasionally lead to improvement in the neurological syndrome.

Further reading

Bataller L, Dalmau J. Paraneoplastic neurologic syndromes. Neurol Clin 2003; 21: 221–247.

Grant R (ed). Treating central nervous system tumours. In: Evidence based oncology. BMJ Publishing, 2003, pp 559–578.

Stewart LA. Chemotherapy in adult high-grade glioma: a systematic review and metaanalysis of individual patient data from 12 randomised trials. Lancet 2002; 359: 1011–1018.

Stupp R, Mason WP, van den Bent MJ et al. Radiotherapy plus concomitant and adjuvant Temozolomide for glioblastoma. N Engl J Med 2005; 352: 987–996.

Van den Bent MJ. Management of metastatic (parenchymal, leptomeningeal and epidural) lesions. Curr Opin Oncol 2004; 16: 309–313.

van den Bent MJ, Afra D, de Witte O, Ben Hassel M, Schraub S, Hoang-Xuan K, Malmstrom PO, Collette L, Pierart M, Mirimanoff R, Karim AB. Long-term efficacy of early versus delayed radiotherapy for low-grade astrocytoma and oligodendroglioma in adults: the EORTC 22845 randomised trial. Lancet 2005; 366(9490): 985–990.

Verstappen CC, Heimans JJ, Hoekman K, Postma TJ. Neurotoxic complications of chemotherapy in patients with cancer: clinical signs and optimal management. Drugs 2003; 63: 1549–1563.

16 METABOLIC, ENDOCRINE AND TOXIC DISORDERS

Lionel Ginsberg

This chapter begins with a description of the management of acquired metabolic, nutritional and endocrine conditions, many of them common, which have neurological manifestations. This is followed by an account of some much rarer inherited metabolic diseases that have prominent neurological features. Discussion is restricted to those genetic metabolic disorders that may present in adult life and for which treatment, beyond supportive measures, is available. Finally, the effects of various toxins on the nervous system are outlined, along with the management of the resulting disorders.

Acquired metabolic disease

LIVER FAILURE

Hepatic encephalopathy is the cerebral dysfunction which results from liver failure. It may be:

- Acute, as in fulminant liver failure caused by hepatitis or paracetamol poisoning, which has a high mortality unless treated by liver transplantation.
- The consequence of 'decompensation' in a patient with cirrhosis (acute-on-chronic liver failure), which is potentially reversible.

The treatment of hepatic encephalopathy depends on understanding the underlying pathophysiological mechanisms. The success or otherwise of treatment is monitored both clinically and from the results of investigations.

The most widely accepted pathophysiology for hepatic encephalopathy is that it arises from a disorder of nitrogen metabolism:

- Ammonia is formed in the bowel by the action of urease-producing microbes on dietary protein.
- The ammonia reaches the liver via the portal circulation.
- The liver then fails to metabolise ammonia to urea because of hepatocellular failure and/or portal–systemic shunting of blood.
- Excess ammonia therefore reaches the systemic circulation where it interferes with brain metabolism by mechanisms that may include neurotransmitter dysfunction.

Neurological findings in hepatic encephalopathy usually coexist with jaundice and other signs of chronic liver disease. The severity of hepatic encephalopathy is graded as:

I   Change of mood, personality, behaviour.
II   Disorientation, delirium, drowsiness, dysarthria.
III Incoherent speech, agitation, restlessness or stupor.
IV   Coma.

With deepening coma, limb rigidity, upgoing plantar responses, primitive reflexes and seizures may appear. Asterixis, the characteristic movement disorder of hepatic encephalopathy, is also seen in other metabolic and toxic encephalopathies.

Investigations

- Psychometric testing in low-grade encephalopathy may show prominent visuospatial dysfunction.
- The EEG slows and characteristic triphasic waves appear.
- Hyperammonaemia (ideally an arterial sample) correlates approximately with the degree of encephalopathy.

Management

In a cirrhotic patient encephalopathy can be triggered or exacerbated by numerous factors, which should be identified and corrected (Box 16.1). Despite recent critiques of the limited evidence base, standard therapy consists of attempting to lower the blood ammonia concentration by:

- Low protein diet.
- Enemas to clear the bowel.
- Lactulose 30–50 ml oral tds, subsequently adjusted to produce 2–3 soft stools daily. This was originally thought to act by acidifying the colon, thereby trapping ammonia in the lumen in its non-absorbable ionised form. However, it is more likely that it interferes directly with bacterial ammonia production. Lactitol (1 sachet bd) is an alternative to lactulose.
- In resistant cases, a poorly absorbed antibiotic, such as neomycin (up to 4 g/day oral in 4 divided doses), may be given in combination with lactulose, to reduce the gut population of urease-producing micro-organisms. This should be used cautiously, however, as small amounts may be absorbed from the gut in patients with liver failure and if there is coexistent renal failure, neomycin may then accumulate, with the risk of ototoxicity.

Although hepatic encephalopathy is potentially completely reversible, repeated or prolonged bouts may lead to fixed or progressive neurological disability (non-Wilsonian hepatocerebral degeneration) with a varying combination of dementia, ataxia, dysarthria, extrapyramidal signs and myelopathy.

Box 16.1   Factors that may precipitate or aggravate encephalopathy in cirrhosis of the liver

- High dietary protein intake.
- Gastrointestinal haemorrhage.
- Constipation.
- Infection.
- Sedative drugs.
- Surgery.
- Hypoxia.
- Hypokalaemia.
- Electrolyte depletion.
- Excessive diuresis.
- Hyper- or hypoglycaemia.
- Hepatocellular carcinoma.

RENAL FAILURE

Uraemic encephalopathy

This occurs late in the evolution of chronic renal failure and is characterised by progressive drowsiness, confusion, twitching, myoclonus, asterixis and, ultimately, seizures and coma – the 'uraemic twitch–convulsive syndrome'. Dialysis and transplantation may reverse the encephalopathy, but bring their own neurological complications.

For dialysis, these complications have become rarer with modern techniques, but still include:

- Dialysis disequilibrium syndrome:
  - Occurs acutely, during or immediately after dialysis, due to osmotic shifts of water causing cerebral oedema. These shifts are a result of the delay between the removal of free water and solutes from the vascular compartment andre-establishment of osmotic equilibrium in the brain.
  - Mildly affected patients experience headache, nausea, fatigue, blurred vision, muscle cramps and tremulousness.
  - In severe cases, coma with epileptic seizures develops.
  - Improved techniques, with slower haemodialysis and haemofiltration (where there is no osmotic gradient) have made the severe form of the syndrome rare.
- Dialysis dementia syndrome:
  - This chronic condition is characterised by cognitive impairment, personality change, dysarthria, gait disorder, myoclonus and seizures.
  - It is caused by aluminium toxicity to the brain, but again, with current technology, in this case reducing aluminium levels in the dialysate, the full-blown syndrome has become rare.

Neurological complications of renal transplantation include:

- Adverse effects of ciclosporin and related drugs (tremor, ataxia, neuropathy, epileptic seizures and posterior leukoencephalopathy). The seizures may respond to parenteral magnesium.
- Rejection encephalopathy (headache, confusion, convulsions) occurs typically in the first 3 months after transplantation and may respond to corticosteroids.
- Opportunistic infections secondary to immunosuppression.

Management of epileptic seizures in a patient with renal failure

This partially depends on recognising and treating potential causes, such as:

- uraemic encephalopathy
- dialysis disequilibrium syndrome
- infection
- stroke, which is common in uraemic patients, many of whom are diabetic and/or hypertensive.

The choice of antiepileptic drug may be difficult. Although parenteral phenytoin is central to acute seizure control in general, its use in patients with renal failure is complicated by its altered pharmacokinetics in uraemia. Furthermore, phenytoin toxicity is awkward to manage in these patients, because the drug is not removed by dialysis. Alternative parenteral agents for uraemic seizures include phenobarbital and sodium valproate (see Chapter 2).

Uraemic neuropathy

This is a predominantly sensory length-dependent process, sometimes painful, which accompanies advanced renal failure and may be exacerbated by drugs that are often used in this clinical setting, such as nitrofurantoin. The neuropathy is potentially reversible, at least in part, with dialysis and transplantation.

Neurological complications of the underlying cause of renal failure

Other neurological problems in patients with renal failure may be complications of the underlying cause of the kidney disease, such as diabetes, hypertension or systemic lupus erythematosus, which require their own specific treatments.

ELECTROLYTE ABNORMALITIES

Hyponatraemia

Severe hyponatraemia (< 120 mM) may remain asymptomatic, if gradual in onset. If more sudden, symptomatic patients progress through headache, nausea, muscle cramps and fatigue, to drowsiness, confusion, coma and epileptic seizures. Hyponatraemia may also accentuate the effects of any underlying neurological disease.

In the context of the syndrome of inappropriate antidiuretic hormone secretion (SIADH), hyponatraemia is associated with many neurological conditions, including:

- meningitis and encephalitis

- head injury
- stroke
- subarachnoid haemorrhage
- Guillain–Barré syndrome
- acute intermittent porphyria
- carbamazepine and oxcarbazepine therapy.

Some of these same conditions, notably head injury and subarachnoid haemorrhage, may *also* lower the serum sodium by a different mechanism, known as 'cerebral salt wasting', where blood volume is decreased, unlike the case in SIADH. It is important to establish whether a patient with one of these neurological diagnoses and hyponatraemia has true SIADH by determining whether the urine is inappropriately concentrated in the absence of factors that normally stimulate ADH release. This is because the standard treatment of SIADH (by fluid restriction, see below) is potentially hazardous in a patient with salt wasting, where further volume reduction may lead to cerebral ischaemia.

There are many other, non-neurological, causes of hyponatraemia that may occur in the context of normal, increased or decreased extracellular fluid volume. Of these, hyponatraemia associated with alcoholism is particularly important in view of the possible neurological complications of treatment in this patient group (see below).

Correction of dilutional hyponatraemia should be gradual; restriction of water intake is all that is required in mild and moderate cases. Indeed, over-rapid correction of the serum sodium may cause the serious complication of *central pontine myelinolysis*, particularly in alcoholic patients, but also following liver and renal transplantation among other severe systemic disorders. This is characterised by non-inflammatory demyelination in the centre of the basis pontis, and sometimes more extensively in the brainstem and elsewhere. The classical clinical picture is of pseudobulbar palsy and tetraplegia, evolving within days after overzealous correction of hyponatraemia. The prognosis is variable but the damage is often permanent.

Management of a hyponatraemic patient can therefore be difficult. If the patient is already encephalopathic from the hyponatraemia, there are conflicting needs to correct the sodium, yet avoid central pontine myelinolysis. Although there is uncertainty, certain general comments may be made:
- Where possible, treatment should consist solely of water restriction and discontinuation of any diuretics.

- If intravenous saline is used (e.g. in patients who are very agitated or convulsing), the rate of serum sodium correction should not exceed 12 mM in the first 24 hours and 20 mM in the first 48 hours. Hypertonic saline is probably best avoided, but central pontine myelinolysis may occur even with isotonic saline.
- Loop diuretics may be required in combination with saline administration to correct the serum sodium concentration and normalise intravascular volume.
- Electrolytes should be monitored frequently (every 2 hours) to guard against overrapid correction and indeed overshooting into hypernatraemia.
- Demeclocycline 600–900 mg/day oral in 2–3 divided doses may be used to treat chronic SIADH. It is thought to block the action of ADH on the renal tubules. Patients should be warned about the risk of photosensitivity.

Hypernatraemia

Hypernatraemic encephalopathy may progress through agitation and restlessness to confusion, coma and seizures. There may also be intracranial bleeding from veins bridging the space between the brain and dural sinuses as a consequence of cerebral shrinkage. Causes of hypernatraemia include:

- diabetes insipidus
- non-ketotic diabetic coma
- severe diarrhoea, or excessive fluid loss from burns or sweating
- fluid-deprived confused or comatose patients.

In fluid-deprived patients, the water deficit may be estimated using the following approximation:

$$\text{Deficit in litres} = 0.6 \times \text{body weight (kg)} \times (1 - 140/\text{serum sodium})$$

As for hyponatraemia, correction should be gradual, not exceeding 12 mM change in serum sodium in 24 hours. Water replacement should be given orally whenever possible. If intravenous fluids are necessary, 5% dextrose, dextrose saline or normal saline can be used.

Other electrolytes

The neurological effects of other electrolyte abnormalities, their major causes and the principles of treatment are summarised in Table 16.1.

Table 16.1   Neurological effects of electrolyte abnormalities and their treatment*

Electrolyte abnormality	Examples of causes	Neurological effects	Principles of treatment
Hypokalaemia	Gut loss Alkalosis Diuretics Hyperaldosteronism	Weakness, rhabdomyolysis	Potassium chloride
Hyperkalaemia	Acute renal failure Acidosis Addison's disease	Weakness, paraesthesia	Calcium gluconate, iv glucose/insulin, iv calcium resonium
Hypocalcaemia	Hypoparathyroidism Vitamin D deficiency Renal failure	Paraesthesia, tetany, seizures, chorea, parkinsonism	Calcium gluconate, iv then oral calcium and vitamin D
Hypercalcaemia	Hyperparathyroidism Bone metastases Myeloma Sarcoidosis	Lethargy, depression, weakness, drowsiness	Rehydration, bisphosphonates, corticosteroids (for sarcoid or malignancy)
Hypomagnesaemia	Dietary deficiency Malabsorption Alcoholism	Weakness, tremor, tetany, epileptic seizures	Magnesium sulphate
Hypermagnesaemia	Magnesium infusion in eclampsia or renal failure	Weakness, drowsiness, confusion	Discontinue magnesium

*See text for hypo- and hypernatraemia.

Nutritional and gastrointestinal disorders

VITAMIN DEFICIENCY

Vitamin B$_1$

Thiamine deficiency polyneuropathy (beriberi) is still seen in developing countries. In developed countries, thiamine deficiency occurs in four important clinical contexts:

- alcoholic, malnourished patients
- hyperemesis gravidarum
- cachexia
- gastrointestinal disease.

In all cases, the neurological features of the vitamin deficiency may be precipitated or exacerbated by carbohydrate intake (including intravenous dextrose administration) if there is no concomitant thiamine replacement, because thiamine is an essential coenzyme in carbohydrate metabolism. This still happens all too frequently when thiamine-deficient patients are admitted to hospital and the early features, or indeed the risk, of the condition are not recognised.

The clinical features of thiamine deficiency, as usually encountered in industrialised nations, constitute the Wernicke–Korsakoff syndrome. Many patients also have a polyneuropathy, and are deficient in other B vitamins (see below). Wernicke's encephalopathy is characterised by the classical triad of:

- confusion
- ataxia
- ophthalmoplegia.

It is potentially reversible with early thiamine replacement. If replacement is delayed, Korsakoff's psychosis, characterised by a chronic amnesic syndrome with prominent confabulation, is likely to be permanent, as are nystagmus and gait ataxia.

- Treatment with parenteral thiamine (at least 100 mg/day iv, usually given in a multivitamin preparation) should start immediately on any clinical suspicion of the Wernicke–Korsakoff syndrome, and continue until the patient is taking a normal diet.
- Anaphylaxis has been reported with parenteral B vitamins: the injection should therefore be given slowly (over 10 minutes), with resuscitation facilities available.

- The relevant biochemical investigations in thiamine deficiency, blood pyruvate level and erythrocyte transketolase enzyme activity, are rarely offered routinely by hospital laboratories. Even when they are, treatment should begin on clinical suspicion, and not be delayed for these, or any other, investigations.
- Prevention is the best policy, so thiamine should be given to alcoholic malnourished patients, and to women with hyperemesis gravidarum, from the time of admission.

Vitamin B$_{12}$

The classical neurological manifestation of vitamin B$_{12}$ deficiency, subacute combined degeneration of the cord, along with other neurological deficits such as polyneuropathy, optic atrophy and cognitive impairment, may occur in the absence of haematological disease.

- As with vitamin B$_1$, the longer vitamin B$_{12}$ deficiency is left untreated, the less likely the neurological deficits will recover.
- There should, therefore, be a high index of suspicion of vitamin B$_{12}$ deficiency and, if suspected, treatment should not be delayed. In urgent cases, replacement may have to begin before the results of the vitamin assay are available.
- The common cause of vitamin B$_{12}$ deficiency, pernicious anaemia, requires parenteral therapy, because patients lack the intrinsic factor required for the vitamin's absorption.
- Other patients who have dietary vitamin B$_{12}$ deficiency (e.g. vegans) may be treated with oral replacement (cyanocobalamin 100 µg/day).
- Hydroxocobalamin is the form of vitamin B$_{12}$ of choice for parenteral therapy. It is retained in the body longer than cyanocobalamin. The recommended dosing schedule is 1 mg im on alternate days until no further clinical improvement, then 1 mg im every 2 months.
- With rapid replacement of vitamin B$_{12}$ in a severely deficient patient, there is a risk of initial hypokalaemia; serum potassium should be monitored closely.

Other vitamins

- Vitamin B$_6$ (pyridoxine) deficiency in adults is associated with polyneuropathy. This is a well-known development during isoniazid administration, and occasionally other drugs such as hydralazine and penicillamine. To avoid this complication, pyridoxine (10–20 mg/day oral) should always be given to patients with tuberculosis receiving long-term isoniazid. Paradoxically, excessive pyridoxine is also associated with neurological complications, in the form of a sensory ganglionopathy. Mega-dose therapy (> 100 mg/day) should therefore be avoided.

- Folic acid deficiency is a rare and rather uncertain cause of a cord syndrome resembling that in vitamin B_{12} deficiency. Folic acid replacement for megaloblastic anaemia should not be given without first knowing whether vitamin B_{12} levels are normal or, failing that, without concomitant vitamin B_{12} therapy. This is because large doses of folic acid can correct the haematological features of pernicious anaemia without influencing the neurological dysfunction. Folic acid replacement may even precipitate neuropathy in these circumstances.

- Niacin (nicotinic acid) deficiency with the classical triad of pellagra – dementia, diarrhoea and dermatitis – is rare nowadays in developed countries because of widespread consumption of bread and cereals fortified with the vitamin, but it may be seen in the context of multiple vitamin deficiency (see below).

- Vitamin D deficiency may lead to a proximal myopathy in association with osteomalacia. Replacement therapy rapidly relieves muscle pain but weakness improves more slowly and sometimes only partially. Vitamin D has physiological roles other than in bone metabolism, including a contribution to normal macrophage differentiation and function. This becomes relevant in the treatment of certain infections. In particular, patients of Asian origin, who are immigrants to the UK and other countries with temperate climates, may have subclinical vitamin D deficiency and are also at risk of tuberculosis, with all its neurological manifestations. Care should be taken to ensure that these patients receive adequate vitamin D replacement in combination with antituberculous chemotherapy.

- Vitamin E deficiency presents neurologically as a spinocerebellar degeneration and polyneuropathy. It may be acquired in malabsorption states or arise on a genetic basis. Replacement therapy is with oral tocopherol 200–600 mg/day. If there is no improvement, higher oral doses or parenteral therapy may be required. With treatment, the syndrome is likely to be at least partially reversible.

- Alcoholic, malnourished patients are at risk of multiple vitamin deficiencies, especially of the B group, which may lead to a combination of optic atrophy and painful sensory neuropathy. Alcoholic cerebellar degeneration is also likely to be caused by vitamin deficiency. These patients may be treated with oral vitamin B compound, or simply an adequate diet with avoidance of alcohol.

■ Vitamin A toxicity is more likely to present to the neurologist than deficiency. It occurs when mega-doses of multivitamin preparations are consumed, or with unusual foods such as polar bear liver or halibut liver. The clinical picture resembles idiopathic intracranial hypertension.

GASTROINTESTINAL DISEASES

Diseases of the gastrointestinal tract may have neurological complications through various potentially treatable mechanisms, including:
■ Malabsorption of vitamins and other essential nutrients (e.g. in Crohn's and coeliac disease).
■ Prothrombotic tendency, leading to stroke, notably intracranial venous thrombosis, in association with inflammatory bowel disease.
■ Autoimmune and vasculitic processes in extraintestinal tissues, including the nervous system, in association with inflammatory bowel disease.

Coeliac disease

Coeliac disease is a special case, in that a relatively distinctive encephalopathy has been described in association with the gut disorder, apparently unrelated to any dietary deficiency.
■ The clinical features comprise a progressive, and potentially lethal, cerebellar ataxia, with eye movement disorder, and sometimes myoclonus and epilepsy.
■ Treatment with a gluten-free diet does not always help.
■ Other treatment options include vitamin supplementation.
■ There are anecdotal reports of a cerebral vasculitis and response to corticosteroids and immunosuppression.

Endocrine disorders

DIABETES MELLITUS

Diabetes affects the nervous system in three principal ways:
■ coma, for many reasons (Box 16.2)
■ risk factor for ischaemic stroke
■ peripheral neuropathy.

Diabetic coma

Apart from stroke, the only cause of diabetic coma for which neurologists may regularly take primary acute management responsibility is hypoglycaemia,

> ## Box 16.2   Causes of coma in diabetic patients
>
> - Diabetic ketoacidosis.
> - Non-ketotic diabetic coma.
> - Hypoglycaemia from insulin or oral medication.
> - Uraemic encephalopathy.
> - Stroke.
> - Lactic acidosis may also contribute to coma.

secondary to insulin or oral hypoglycaemic drugs. Hypoglycaemic coma also occurs outside the context of diabetes and its treatment, in patients with:

- pancreatic islet cell tumour
- severe liver disease
- alcohol toxicity
- hypopituitarism, hypoadrenalism
- malaria
- factitious disorder or poisoning with hypoglycaemic drugs
- childhood causes (glycogen storage diseases, Reye's syndrome, idiopathic).

The emergency treatment of hypoglycaemic coma consists of:

- Intravenous 50% dextrose 50 ml, repeated as necessary. Less concentrated solutions may be used, but larger volumes are then needed.
- Intravenous thiamine 100 mg, preceding dextrose in malnourished patients where there is a risk of the Wernicke–Korsakoff syndrome (see above).
- Glucagon 1 mg by sc, im or iv injection may be given for insulin-induced hypoglycaemic coma, for example by close family members of insulin-treated diabetic patients in an emergency in the community. If there is no response within 10 minutes, intravenous dextrose should be given.

Any patient with coma of unknown cause should receive a bolus of intravenous dextrose to cover the possibility of hypoglycaemia (see Chapter 8).

Diabetic neuropathy

- Optimal glycaemic control reduces the risk of developing neuropathy, and reduces the severity of the neuropathy in those who are mildly affected.

- Once established, diabetic sensory polyneuropathy and autonomic neuropathy are largely irreversible.
- Treatment of these conditions is therefore predominantly symptomatic (Table 16.2).
- Initiation of hypoglycaemic treatment in a diabetic patient may trigger an acute painful neuropathy ('insulin neuritis'), attributed to axonal sprouting consequent on the improvement in glycaemic control.
- Proximal diabetic neuropathy may be caused by inflammatory changes in nerves, including vasculitis. Various immunomodulatory regimes have therefore been tried, but corticosteroids in diabetic patients are problematic. Assessment of any benefit is difficult because these forms of diabetic neuropathy tend to improve spontaneously, albeit slowly.

THYROID DISEASE

Hyperthyroidism

- Hyperthyroidism may present to neurologists in many ways (Box 16.3).
- Treatment with a thionamide and a beta-blocker (and Lugol's iodine solution in the emergency situation of thyrotoxic crisis, in combination

Table 16.2 Symptomatic treatment for the complications of diabetic neuropathy	
Complication	**Treatment**
Neuropathic pain	See Chapter 18
Foot ulceration	Remove callus, treat infection
Arthropathy	Bed rest, bisphosphonates
Gustatory sweating	Propantheline
Postural hypotension	Elevate head of bed Fludrocortisone (see Chapter 6)
Gastroparesis	Metoclopramide, domperidone Erythromycin
Diarrhoea	Codeine phosphate, loperamide Tetracycline
Bladder dysfunction	See Chapter 17
Erectile dysfunction	See Chapter 17

Box 16.3   Neurological features of hyperthyroidism

- Confusion, coma (in thyrotoxic crisis – 'thyroid storm').
- Anxiety, psychosis.
- Lethargy, depression (apathetic hyperthyroidism in the elderly).
- Headache.
- Stroke, secondary to atrial fibrillation.
- Chorea.
- Tremor.
- Hyperreflexia.
- Dysthyroid eye disease.
- Myopathy.
- Association with myasthenia gravis.
- Thyrotoxic periodic paralysis.

---

with hydration, cooling and corticosteroids) may need to be initiated urgently before an endocrinologist can be involved.
- Treatment options for dysthyroid eye disease (Graves' ophthalmopathy) include corticosteroids, radiotherapy and surgical decompression.
- Thyrotoxic periodic paralysis is triggered by physical activity and high carbohydrate intake. It responds acutely to potassium, given whenever possible as oral supplements of effervescent potassium chloride, the dose depending on plasma potassium concentration, and in the longer term to antithyroid drugs. The hyperthyroidism may be clinically silent apart from the periodic paralysis and this condition is seen particularly in patients of south-east Asian origin.

Hypothyroidism

The neurological complications of hypothyroidism usually recover with thyroxine replacement. They include encephalopathy, ataxia, hearing loss and other cranial nerve involvement, carpal tunnel syndrome, sensory polyneuropathy and myopathy.

Hashimoto's encephalopathy

A relapsing encephalopathy with seizures, myoclonus, tremor and stroke-like episodes has been described in association with high titres of antithyroid antibodies, usually antimicrosomal. Corticosteroids are the mainstay of treatment and the prognosis is generally good.

OTHER ENDOCRINE DISORDERS

The neurological features and principles of treatment of other endocrine disorders are summarised in Table 16.3.

Inherited metabolic disease

In addition to the specific treatments outlined for the diseases in this section, genetic counselling is important in all cases.

WILSON'S DISEASE

Wilson's disease is a rare autosomal-recessive disorder of copper metabolism which presents in adolescence or early adult life with tremor, rigidity, dystonia, chorea and/or psychosis. Presentation in childhood is usually with cirrhosis. Kayser–Fleischer rings (copper deposits in the cornea) are found on slit-lamp examination in all Wilson's disease patients presenting neurologically.

The diagnosis is made by detecting low or absent serum copper and ceruloplasmin. Supplementary investigations include 24 hour urinary copper excretion (increased) and liver biopsy.

Untreated, the condition is fatal. Early diagnosis and treatment are vital to prevent and indeed reverse clinical manifestations which would otherwise be permanent and lethal:

- A low copper diet should be followed (< 1 mg/day), although some debate this.
- Penicillamine (1–2 g/day oral, in 2–4 divided doses), a copper-chelating drug, has been the principal treatment for many years, but has a poor adverse-effect profile:
  - skin reactions
  - thrombocytopenia
  - leukopenia and indeed pancytopenia
  - haemolytic anaemia
  - nephrotic syndrome
  - Goodpasture's syndrome
  - syndromes resembling systemic lupus erythematosus and myasthenia.
- Alternatives for patients intolerant of penicillamine include:
  - trientine 1.2–2.4 g/day oral in 2–4 divided doses
  - ammonium tetrathiomolybdate is another chelating agent but is not yet widely available.

Table 16.3 Neurological consequences and treatment of endocrine disorders*

Endocrine disorder	Neurological features	Treatment
Acromegaly	Chronic encephalopathy, bitemporal hemianopia, carpal tunnel syndrome, obstructive sleep apnoea, headache, myopathy	Hypophysectomy, radiotherapy, somatostatin analogues, dopamine agonists
Hypopituitarism	Encephalopathy (acute and chronic), fatigue, apathy Pituitary apoplexy: headache, visual loss, diplopia	Hormone replacement
Prolactinoma	Bitemporal hemianopia	Surgery, dopamine agonists
Cushing's syndrome	Anxiety, depression, myopathy, intracranial hypertension	Surgery, metyrapone, ketoconazole
Addison's disease	Depression, lethargy, weakness, acute encephalopathy	Rehydration, glucose, hydrocortisone, fludrocortisone
Phaeochromocytoma	Paroxysmal headache, anxiety, tremor, hypertensive encephalopathy, intracranial haemorrhage	Alpha- and beta-blockade, surgery

*See text for thyroid disorders, diabetes and hypoglycaemia; se Table 16.1 for parathyroid disorders.

■ Zinc prevents the absorption of copper in Wilson's disease and may be given as zinc acetate 50 mg oral tds (expressed as elemental zinc). The onset of action is slow: initial treatment with a chelating agent is therefore required. Some use zinc as maintenance therapy.

Patients with established Wilson's disease may improve significantly on therapy (50%) or stabilise (15%). The remainder deteriorate initially and some of these patients do not recover to pretreatment levels. Indeed, severely disabled patients may progress despite treatment. Improvement, if it is to occur, begins approximately 6 months after starting treatment and is usually complete by 2 years.

- The effects of treatment must be monitored clinically and by measuring urinary copper excretion.
- Treatment should be lifelong; sudden deterioration is likely if therapy is discontinued.
- Liver transplantation is curative in Wilson's disease and is indicated in patients with severe liver damage.

PORPHYRIA

Porphobilinogen and δ-aminolevulinic acid are virtually always present in the urine during a neurovisceral attack of acute porphyria; their absence effectively excludes porphyria as the cause of the patient's symptoms.

Management of an acute attack of porphyria consists of:

- Supportive care and elimination of potential triggers (e.g. discontinuing offending drugs (Table 16.4) and treating any intercurrent infection).
- High carbohydrate diet (> 400 g/day, or equivalent glucose infusion) to inhibit hepatic δ-aminolevulinic acid synthase activity and reduce porphyrin precursor production.
- If there are persistent symptoms or neurological deficits that progress for 24 hours after carbohydrate loading, haem treatment is indicated in the form of haem arginate 3 mg/kg iv once daily for 4 days. This preparation is less likely to cause thrombotic complications than standard haematin.

Prevention of recurrent attacks requires an adequate carbohydrate intake and avoidance of potential triggers (see Table 16.4). Prophylactic haem arginate has been used in resistant patients.

The large number of unsafe drugs in porphyria limits the choice of treatments for the neurological problems in an acute attack. Neuropathic pain may be treated with morphine, gabapentin and chlorpromazine, but not tricyclic antidepressants. Seizures may be controlled with intravenous diazepam.

HOMOCYSTEINAEMIA

Severe hyperhomocysteinaemia and homocystinuria develop in children who are homozygous for mutations of the gene for cystathionine synthase. Among other features, these children are at risk of arterial and venous thromboses.

Table 16.4   Examples of safe and unsafe drugs in porphyria

Drug class	Probably safe	Unsafe
Antiepileptics	Diazepam, lorazepam, magnesium sulphate, gabapentin	Barbiturates, phenytoin, carbamazepine, sodium valproate, ethosuximide, clonazepam
Psychiatric	Chlorpromazine, lithium, fluoxetine	Tricyclic antidepressants, sulpiride, monoamine oxidase inhibitors, thioridazine
Endocrine	Insulin	Oestrogens, progestogens, danazol, tamoxifen, anabolic steroids, sulphonylureas
Analgesics	Aspirin, codeine, morphine, ibuprofen	Oxycodone, pentazocine
Antimicrobials	Penicillin, aminoglycosides	Sulphonamides, trimethoprim, erythromycin, nitrofurantoin, isoniazid, pyrazinamide, dapsone, griseofulvin
Other	Allopurinol, furosemide (frusemide), warfarin	Ergot derivatives, statins, amiodarone, baclofen, chlorambucil, hydralazine, ranitidine, nifedipine, verapamil

More moderate elevation of serum homocysteine is seen in adult patients who are heterozygous for mutations of this gene, or who have mutations of genes for other enzymes involved in the metabolism of sulphur-containing amino acids.

Another group of patients has moderate hyperhomocysteinaemia because of mild nutritional deficiency of cofactors (vitamins B_6 and B_{12}) or substrate (folic acid) for these enzymes.

Hyperhomocysteinaemia is a risk factor for vascular disease and patients with moderately or severely elevated serum homocysteine levels should therefore be treated:

■ Pyridoxine-responsive patients may normalise serum homocysteine levels with low doses of vitamin B_6 (25 mg/day oral) but larger doses may be needed. Folic acid (5 mg/day oral) is also given.

- Pyridoxine-resistant patients may be tried on a low methionine diet, but this is relatively unpalatable.
- Betaine 6–9 g/day may be used to recycle homocysteine to methionine.
- Antiplatelet therapy should be prescribed (see Chapter 4).
- Vitamin B_{12} replacement is only indicated if there is actual deficiency, or if the serum level is at the lower end of the normal range.

REFSUM'S DISEASE

The neurological and other features are a consequence of accumulation of phytanic acid, a branched-chain fatty acid derived solely from dietary sources. Restriction of dietary phytanic acid, and its precursor phytol, prevents disease progression, and may even lead to significant improvement. Plasma exchange may also be used at the time of diagnosis to lower serum phytanic acid concentration acutely.

ADRENOLEUKODYSTROPHY

- Adrenal insufficiency in this condition is controlled with corticosteroid replacement, but this has no effect on the neurological complications.
- The success of *Lorenzo's oil* (a mixture of glyceryl trioleate and glyceryl trierucate) in normalising plasma very long-chain fatty acids (which accumulate in adrenoleukodystrophy) has not been matched by any effect on the neurological features of the disease.
- Bone marrow transplantation may stabilise the neurological manifestations, but only when the disease is still mild. The risks of transplantation probably outweigh the benefits in patients with the usual adult presentation (adrenomyeloneuropathy).

FABRY'S DISEASE

Fabry's disease is an X-linked lysosomal storage disorder caused by deficiency of α-galactosidase A. The neurological manifestations are a painful small fibre neuropathy and an increased risk of ischaemic stroke, with an early age of onset. Non-neurological features include cardiac dysfunction and renal failure, along with skin and eye lesions.

Until recently, treatment was purely symptomatic, with standard measures for neuropathic pain and control of vascular risk factors. The development of enzyme replacement therapy has provided a more specific approach:

- Two formulations are available – agalsidase alfa and agalsidase beta. Both are given as intravenous infusions, and both are well tolerated. The two preparations are roughly equivalent.

- Agalsidase alfa has been shown to improve features of the neuropathy, including pain, thermal sensation, sweating and quality of life.
- In view of the extreme expense of this treatment, its long-term availability will depend on whether any impact on the life-threatening complications of the disease can be demonstrated.

METACHROMATIC LEUKODYSTROPHY

Metachromatic leukodystrophy may present in adult life with dementia, psychosis and polyneuropathy. Bone marrow transplantation has been reported to stabilise the condition.

AMYLOIDOSIS

- Familial amyloid polyneuropathy is an autosomal-dominant condition which presents in adult life. The most severe form is caused by mutations in the gene for the plasma protein transthyretin. Amyloid deposition in peripheral nerves leads to a painful sensory neuropathy with prominent autonomic involvement. There is associated cardiomyopathy and nephropathy. The disease progresses remorselessly, death occurring 10–15 years after onset.
- Transthyretin is largely synthesised in the liver, providing a rationale for liver transplantation as treatment. Unfortunately, although transplantation may reverse some of the neuropathic symptoms, it does not arrest progression of the systemic features.
- Among the acquired causes of amyloid, only primary systemic (AL) amyloidosis, with deposition of immunoglobulin light chain fragments, is regularly associated with polyneuropathy. As with the genetic form, there is a painful sensory neuropathy, with autonomic features, and systemic involvement of the heart and kidney. The prognosis is poor, with a median survival of only 20 months from diagnosis, and 40 months for patients with neuropathy but no cardiac or renal disease at presentation. Oral melphalan and prednisolone may prolong survival but do not reverse the neuropathy.

MITOCHONDRIAL DISORDERS

Molecular defects of the mitochondrial respiratory chain and associated enzymes show clinical, biochemical and genetic heterogeneity. Three of the most characteristic syndromes are:

- Kearns–Sayre syndrome: progressive external ophthalmoplegia, cardiac conduction block, pigmentary retinopathy and dementia. Other features include hearing loss, ataxia and endocrine dysfunction.

■ MELAS: **M**itochondrial **E**ncephalomyopathy with **L**actic **A**cidosis and **S**troke-like episodes.
■ MERRF: **M**yoclonic **E**pilepsy with **R**agged **R**ed **F**ibres. These patients have myoclonus, generalised seizures, ataxia and dementia. Although the muscle biopsy shows the characteristic finding of mitochondrial myopathy, weakness may not be marked.

To these syndromes, many other clinical patterns may be added, with varying combinations of encephalopathic features, myopathy and other protean neurological and non-neurological problems.

Despite advances in understanding the biochemistry and genetics of these conditions, treatment is unsatisfactory:
■ General supportive measures for endocrine complications, epilepsy and cardiac arrhythmias are important.
■ There are anecdotal reports of benefit from vitamins, cofactors and substrates of the electron transport chain.
■ The largest literature is for coenzyme Q_{10} (ubiquinone), given at doses of 2–4 mg/kg/day oral.
■ Some patients with respiratory chain disease have secondary carnitine deficiency: carnitine supplements (1–3 g/day oral) have therefore been used in combination with coenzyme Q_{10}.
■ Prednisolone has been reported to help some patients with MELAS.
■ The experimental drug dichloroacetate (25 mg/kg/day oral or iv) may help cases with prominent lactic acidosis, but has significant adverse effects including peripheral neuropathy.

Leigh's syndrome – subacute necrotising encephalomyelopathy – has a mitochondrial basis: coenzyme Q_{10}, carnitine, thiamine and dichloroacetate have therefore been used, but with little effect on the course of the disease.

Toxic disorders

ALCOHOL

The management of many of the neurological complications of alcoholism has already been outlined in the preceding sections on hepatic encephalopathy, hyponatraemia and vitamin deficiency.

Alcoholic coma is treated primarily by general supportive measures for respiratory depression, aspiration pneumonia and other complications of the unconscious state. Care should be taken to diagnose and treat any coexistent drug intoxication, head injury or liver disease.

Alcohol withdrawal syndrome is characterised by tremulousness, hallucinations, epileptic seizures ('rum fits') and a confusional state (*delirium tremens*), occurring within hours or days after a habitual drinker abstains from alcohol. The management comprises:

- Fluid and electrolyte correction (cautious correction of sodium).
- Sedative drugs, used carefully. Benzodiazepines may calm tremor, irritability and insomnia, and protect against seizures. Clomethiazole has a similar effect and is given as a course of capsules or syrup, tapering over 6–9 days.
- Thiamine prophylaxis against Wernicke–Korsakoff syndrome (see above).

OTHER TOXINS

The nervous system is the primary target of numerous chemical poisons and biological toxins. Table 16.5 summarises some examples for which there are specific treatments beyond general supportive measures.

Table 16.5   Actions of poisons and toxins on the nervous system and their treatment*

Toxin	Neurological effects	Treatment
Carbon-containing poisons		
Carbon monoxide	Coma, seizures, pyramidal and extrapyramidal signs	Oxygen (100% or hyperbaric)
Cyanide	Coma	Dicobalt edetate, sodium nitrite with sodium thiosulphate, oxygen, hydroxocobalamin
Organophosphates (acute poisoning)	Headache, tremor, weakness, convulsions, coma	Atropine, pralidoxime
Metals		
Arsenic	Collapse, confusion, subacute neuropathy	Chelating agents: dimercaprol, penicillamine
Lead	Encephalopathy (children), neuropathy (adults)	Chelating agents: dimercaprol with sodium calcium edetate, penicillamine

Continued

Table 16.5 *Continued*

Toxin	Neurological effects	Treatment
Metals – continued		
Mercury	Personality change, tremor, weakness, confusion	Chelating agents: dimercaprol
Drugs		
Opioids	Coma, respiratory depression, pinpoint pupils	Naloxone
Benzodiazepines	Drowsiness, ataxia, dysarthria	Flumazenil (only under expert guidance)
Bacterial toxins		
Diphtheria	Descending motor and autonomic neuropathy	Antitoxin, penicillin
Botulism	Descending paralysis, autonomic failure	Antitoxin
Tetanus	Trismus, risus sardonicus, opisthotonos, respiratory paralysis	Wound toilet, antibiotics, human tetanus immune globulin, active immunisation
Animal toxins		
Snake toxins	Paraesthesia, weakness, fasciculations, rhabdomyolysis	Antivenom
α-Latrotoxin (black widow spider venom)	Pain, spasms, weakness, autonomic symptoms	Antivenom (in life-threatening poisonings)
Scorpion toxin	Pain, paraesthesia, autonomic symptoms, spasms, seizures, coma, paralysis	Antivenom
Ixodid ticks	Paralysis, paraesthesia	Tick removal
Marine toxins		
Ciguatera	Headache, paraesthesia, ataxia, weakness	Mannitol acutely

Continued

Table 16.5 *Continued*		
Toxin	**Neurological effects**	**Treatment**
Plant and fungal toxins		
Jimson weed (anticholinergic alkaloids)	Blurred vision, delirium, hallucinations, seizures, coma, autonomic failure	Physostigmine in severe cases
Mushrooms	Cholinergic activity, euphoria, ataxia, seizures, coma	Pyridoxine, atropine or physostigmine, depending on species

*Toxins are only included in the table if there is an antidote or other specific treatment, beyond simply discontinuing exposure to the toxin and symptomatic therapy. Patients poisoned with toxins listed in the table also need general supportive measures, usually on an intensive care unit. Even when an antidote is available, it is only likely to be effective if given early.

Further reading

Bolton CF, Young GB. Nephrology. In: Hospitalist neurology (Samuels MA, ed) (Blue books of practical neurology). Butterworth Heinemann, Boston, 1999, pp 231–253.

Ginsberg L. Inherited metabolic storage diseases. In: Contemporary treatments in neurology (Scolding N, ed). Butterworth Heinemann, Oxford, 2001, pp 249–263.

Laureno R. Electrolyte disorders. In: Hospitalist neurology (Samuels MA, ed) (Blue books of practical neurology). Butterworth Heinemann, Boston, 1999, pp 159–173.

Shawcross D, Jalan R. Dispelling myths in the treatment of hepatic encephalopathy. Lancet 2005; 365: 431–433.

Taylor RW, Turnbull DM. Mitochondrial diseases. In: Contemporary treatments in neurology (Scolding N, ed). Butterworth Heinemann, Oxford, 2001, pp 283–301.

Thomas PK. Diabetic peripheral nerve disease. In: Contemporary treatments in neurology (Scolding N, ed). Butterworth Heinemann, Oxford, 2001, pp 236–248.

17 NEUROGENIC PELVIC ORGAN DYSFUNCTION

Clare J. Fowler

During human evolution, the control of bladder, bowel and sexual function has become integrated into our complex social behaviour. Higher order cortical processing influences more primitive neuronal systems which are organised largely in the midbrain and brainstem, and which in turn require intact connections to the sacral segments of the spinal cord from where afferent and efferent nerves travel through roots and nerves to innervate pelvic organs (Fig. 17.1). Because large parts of the nervous system are required to effect proper physiological control, it is not surprising that dysfunction of the pelvic organs is common in neurological disease.

BLADDER

Physiology

- The bladder has only two functions – storage and voiding of urine. Depending on fluid intake, the frequency of micturition of an individual with a bladder capacity of approximately 500 ml is once every 3–4 hours. As voiding only takes a few minutes, the bladder is in the storage mode for more than 98% of life.
- Control of the two mutually exclusive activities, storage and voiding, requires intact central and peripheral neural pathways. To accomplish voiding, the pontine micturition centre, situated in the dorsal tegmentum of the pons, is activated. The conscious decision to switch from storage to voiding is determined by the perceived state of bladder fullness, and an assessment of the social appropriateness to do so.
- There are many different levels within the nervous system where disease can result in bladder dysfunction (see Fig. 17.1), but despite this the range of symptoms is limited. Patients with neurological disease most often complain of frequency and urge incontinence.

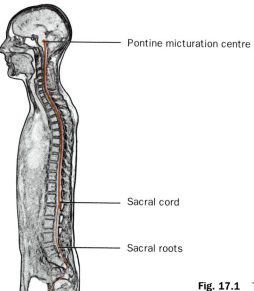

Fig. 17.1   The pathways involved in the control of the bladder.

Pontine micturation centre

Sacral cord

Sacral roots

Neurological causes of bladder dysfunction

Spinal cord lesions

- Damage to spinal tracts between the pontine micturition centre and the sacral spinal cord allows a sacral segmental reflex to emerge, the afferent limb of which is mediated by unmyelinated C fibres, formerly quiescent but now mechanosensitive to bladder filling. It is this reflex which gives rise to detrusor overactivity, the pathophysiological basis for involuntary bladder contractions at low volumes – and so frequency of micturition.
- The consequences for bladder function of a spinal lesion are shown in Table 17.1. In the UK, the commonest non-traumatic cause of spinal cord disease causing bladder dysfunction is multiple sclerosis.

Suprapontine lesions

- Damage to the complex higher controlling neurological processes affecting bladder control most commonly results in detrusor overactivity but without the process of bladder emptying being affected (Table 17.2). The neural process underlying the detrusor overactivity is thought to be lack of appropriate inhibition of the pontine micturition centre rather

Table 17.1   Consequences for bladder function of spinal cord lesions

	Dysfunction	Symptoms
Detrusor overactivity	Detrusor muscle develops involuntary contractions at low filling volumes	Urgency Frequency Urge incontinence
Detrusor-sphincter dyssynergia	Contraction of the sphincter as the detrusor contracts	Interrupted stream Incomplete bladder emptying
Upper motor neuron lesion of sphincter and pelvic floor	Loss of central connections	Difficulty with voluntary initiation Inability to suppress urge and so urge incontinence

Table 17.2   Consequences for bladder function of suprapontine lesions

	Dysfunction	Symptoms
Detrusor overactivity	Detrusor muscle develops involuntary contractions at low filling volumes	Urgency Frequency Urge incontinence

than the emergence of a new driving reflex, but the bladder's limited repertoire of expression means that detrusor overactivity and incontinence are likely to result.

- Table 17.3 lists those suprapontine disorders which are commonly associated with detrusor overactivity and urge incontinence. In the majority of these conditions the degree of impaired bladder control can be predicted from the severity of the overall neurological disease.
- But multiple system atrophy is unusual in that urinary incontinence may be the first symptom. Unlike Parkinson's disease, when urinary symptoms should only be attributed to the neurological disease if it has been present for more than 10 years, bladder symptoms are amongst the earliest of multiple system atrophy; Table 17.4 shows the sites affected and which are involved with bladder control. The combination of an overactive bladder together with incomplete emptying and sphincter weakness may explain why bladder symptoms can be so severe in this disease.

Table 17.3 Suprapontine diseases associated with bladder symptoms

Disease type	Diseases
Basal ganglia disease	Parkinson's disease Multiple system atrophy (but see Table 17.4)
Frontal lobe damage	Vascular Trauma Tumour Hydrocephalus
Dementia	Alzheimer's disease Vascular
Diffuse cerebral damage	Trauma Vascular Anoxic

Table 17.4 Bladder dysfunction in multiple system atrophy

Site of cell loss	Pathophysiology	Symptoms
Brainstem	Detrusor overactivity	Urgency, frequency, urge incontinence
Descending parasympathetic	Impaired detrusor contractions	Incomplete emptying
Intermediolateral spinal columns	Open bladder neck	Incontinence
Onuf's nucleus	Sphincter denervation	Stress incontinence in both women and men

Subsacral and peripheral lesions

- Damage to the sacral roots (S2–S4) within the spinal canal, as occurs with a cauda equina lesion (Table 17.5), and damage to the peripheral innervation, may occur with lesions within the pelvis or a generalised small fibre neuropathy. Pathologies at this level are likely to produce pelvic organ dysfunction affecting more than just the bladder (Table 17.6).

Table 17.5 Sacral root or peripheral lesions affecting pelvic organ function

Lesion	Causes
Cauda equina lesion	Prolapsed intervertebral disc Trauma Tumour Spinal dysraphism
Injury to peripheral innervation, pelvic plexus	Sacral trauma Extensive pelvic surgery
Corporeal nerves	Radical prostatectomy
Generalised small fibre neuropathy	Diabetes Amyloidosis Immune-mediated neuropathies Inherited neuropathies

Table 17.6 Consequences of cauda equina (S2–S4) damage

Pathophysiology	Symptoms
Bladder 'decentralised' (usually causing failure of emptying but may sometimes cause detrusor overactivity)	Impaired voluntary bladder emptying, incontinence
Lower motor neuron damage to sphincter innervation	Stress incontinence and anal incontinence
Loss of rectal parasympathetic innervation	Constipation
Loss of genital innervation	Erectile, ejaculatory and orgasmic dysfunction
S2–S4 sensory impairment	Saddle anaesthesia and erotic sensory loss

- Damage to the cauda equina leaves the detrusor 'decentralised' rather than denervated since the postganglionic parasympathetic innervation is unaffected. This may explain why bladder dysfunction following a cauda equina lesion is unpredictable and detrusor overactivity can occur.

Investigations

- If bladder dysfunction is an expected consequence of an established disease, only investigations which determine management are necessary. However, it may sometimes be necessary to carry out investigations to demonstrate the existence of a suspected but previously unrecognised neurological disease, although in general terms tests of bladder symptoms in that context are rarely helpful. It is in fact unusual for bladder symptoms to be part of a presenting symptom complex without any other neurological features, the exception being multiple system atrophy (see Table 17.4).

- Urodynamic tests involve measuring pressure–volume relationships during bladder filling and micturition to assess detrusor behaviour. As shown in Tables 17.1 to 17.6, urinary incontinence due to detrusor overactivity is the commonest symptom of neurological disease and, although this may be demonstrated by cystometry, it is usually reasonable first to give symptomatic treatment (i.e. anticholinergics) to a patient with a neurological disease on the basis of their complaints of urgency, frequency and urge incontinence.

- One exception to this advice is troublesome urinary symptoms in a man with idiopathic Parkinson's disease – cystometry in these patients may detect obstructed voiding due to the common condition of benign prostatic hypertrophy.

- There is, however, one investigation that is mandatory in most cases of incontinence in a neurological patient and that is the measurement of post-void residual volume. This is particularly the case in patients with spinal cord dysfunction where the neural process for voiding may be as affected as the pathways that normally inhibit the detrusor (see Table 17.1). Such patients may be unaware that they have incomplete bladder emptying except from their own observation that they may pass urine again within a few minutes of supposedly emptying their bladder.

- An anticholinergic is likely to exacerbate incomplete emptying (Fig. 17.2) which in turn can precipitate contractions of the overactive detrusor. For this reason the recommended algorithm for management is shown in Fig. 17.3.

- Microscopy and urine culture are indicated if there is any suggestion of a urinary tract infection. Recurrent urinary tract infections are an indication for referral to a urologist, as are the other problems shown in Box 17.1.

- Following spinal cord trauma, and in patients with spina bifida, there may be damage to the upper urinary tract due to constant high bladder

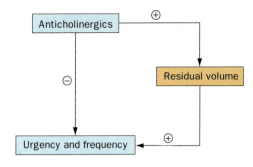

Fig. 17.2 An anticholinergic is likely to exacerbate incomplete emptying, which in turn can precipitate contractions of the overactive detrusor.

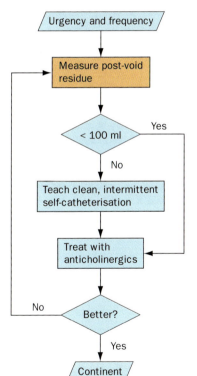

Fig. 17.3 Recommended algorithm for the management of neurogenic incontinence.

pressures. Patients with such conditions should be under the care of a urologist, who will arrange annual surveillance of the kidneys and ureters. In chronic spinal disorders such as multiple sclerosis, although the extent of neurological disability may be as severe as after traumatic spinal cord lesion, upper tract involvement is extremely uncommon. It is only likely to occur if the patient has had recurrent urinary tract infections and an indwelling catheter.

■ In general, therefore, investigations in patients with progressive neuro-logical disease should be aimed at improving bladder management.

Management

Incontinence

■ The first-line treatment of detrusor overactivity is with an oral anticholinergic. There are a number available, mostly of comparable efficacy, but all limited by the adverse effects expected from their mode of action (Table 17.7), most commonly a dry mouth but also dry eyes and constipation. With the range of medication available it is reasonable to change the drug if adverse effects are troublesome since the exact profile of muscarinic blockade produced by each is different and this may be the determining factor of the reported adverse effects. Drugs that do not cross the blood–brain barrier, such as trospium, darifenacin and tolterodine, may be preferred on theoretical grounds in patients with cognitive impairment.

■ Desmopressin has an antidiuretic effect. It increases reabsorption of water by the kidney and temporarily decreases urine production. It therefore circumvents the problem of volume-determined detrusor overactivity and can be given either as a nasal spray (10–40 µg) or orally (200–400 µg). It must however be stressed to the patient that it should only be used once in 24 hours and it should not be prescribed to those over 60 years of age because it may precipitate heart failure. Although most often used to treat night-time frequency, a dose can be taken during the day to provide a period of some hours relatively free from urinary symptoms without a subsequent compensatory period of troublesome frequency. Patients should be warned about the symptoms of hyponatraemia, which include general malaise, headache and oedema.

Table 17.7   Oral anticholinergics for treating symptoms of an overactive bladder

Generic name	Trade name	Dose (mg)	Doses per day	Elimination half-life of drug (hours)
Propantheline	Pro-Banthine	15	3	< 2
Tolterodine tartrate	Detrusitol	2	2	2.4
Tolterodine tartrate	Detrusitol XL	4	1	8.4
Trospium chloride	Regurin	20	2	20
Oxybutynin chloride	Ditropan	2.5–5	2–4	2.3
Oxybutynin chloride XL	Lyrinel XL	5–30	1	13.2
Propiverine hydrochloride	Detrunorm	15	1–4	4.1
Darifenacin	Emselex	7.5–15	1	3.1
Solifenacin	Vesicare	5–10	1	40–68

- Second-line therapies aimed at lessening detrusor overactivity have been largely based on the principle of deafferenting the bladder. But, despite work over the last 10 years to devise intravesical agents that primarily effect the afferent innervation of the bladder, none are now clinically available.
- Injection of botulinum toxin into the detrusor muscle, although as yet unlicensed for this indication, is emerging as a highly effective treatment for severe detrusor overactivity. The injections are given through a cystoscope at 20–30 different sites in the detrusor muscle wall, avoiding the trigone. The introduction of injections through a flexible cystoscope has meant the entire process can be achieved as a 20-minute outpatient procedure. Bladder capacity is increased for 6–9 months. Fortunately the efficacy of second and subsequent injections does not seem to diminish. As with botulinum toxin injections at other sites very few adverse events, other than occasional flu-like symptoms, have been reported. The range of patients for whom this treatment will be suitable remains to be defined, but neurological patients must be prepared to self-catheterise following the treatment, since bladder emptying may be further compromised.

Incomplete emptying

- There is no effective oral medication for improving neurogenic incomplete bladder emptying. A physical method of achieving elimination is necessary if the patient has a raised postmicturition residual volume of more than 100 ml or one-third of their total bladder capacity. Residual volumes vary during the day so that a single measurement may not be representative and a series of estimates is ideal, although not always possible.
- A permanent indwelling catheter can be used, or the patient can be taught to perform clean intermittent self-catheterisation. The latter is the treatment of choice in most patients.
- This technique is highly beneficial in controlling or alleviating urinary incontinence, and is suitable for those who have a significant residue as a result of impaired voiding. Patients should be instructed by a nurse continence adviser, who provides follow-up support. There are various types of catheter available and expert advice will help the patient identify the type that suits them best. Usually a size of 10–14 F is sufficient for bladder drainage. In general, intermittent self-catheterisation should be performed three to five times per 24 hours.

Complete retention

- Complete urinary retention may occur in a number of different disorders (Table 17.8). If of neurogenic origin, the underlying neurological disorder is usually obvious. If no neurological condition is apparent a urologist must exclude a bladder-outlet problem.
- An indwelling catheter is usually required in the acute phase, but this should be replaced by a suprapubic catheter in the long term if the problem persists and the patient or their carer cannot perform intermittent catheterisation.
- The commonest cause of acute urinary retention in a young woman is Fowler's syndrome, a primary abnormality of the striated urethral sphincter in the absence of any urological or general neurological disorder. Of the conditions listed in Table 17.8, sacral neuromodulation using an implanted stimulator to restore voiding is probably only effective in Fowler's syndrome.
- Proven recurrent urinary tract infections are an indication for referral to a urologist (see Box 17.1), who will be able to exclude a nidus for infection such as a stone. Patients performing self-catheterisation may have persistent bacteriuria, but this is not grounds for treatment with

Table 17.8   Causes of complete urinary retention

Condition type	Causes
Acute neurological condition	Spinal injury
	Cauda equina lesion
	Inflammatory neuropathy
Chronic neurological condition	Advanced multiple sclerosis and other causes of chronic spinal dysfunction
	Multiple system atrophy
Urological conditions	Prostatic hypertrophy
	Urethral stricture
	Isolated urinary retention in young women (Fowler's syndrome)

antibiotics unless there is additional clinical evidence of frank infection such as dysuria, fever, and change in colour and odour of the urine. If a urinary tract infection is suspected, after taking a specimen for culture and sensitivity, a short course of antibiotics should be started. The choice should be determined by the sensitivity of a previous specimen if available. Although long-term antibiotics are in general inadvisable because of the risk of antibiotic-resistant organisms emerging, some patients with recurrent infections may be helped by a long-term daily dose of a urinary antiseptic such as nitrofurantoin 50–100 mg oral at night.

BOWEL

Physiology

- Control of faecal continence depends on the smooth muscle tone of the internal anal sphincter, tonic contraction of the puborectalis muscle maintaining the acute anorectal angle, and the activity of the striated external sphincter, which can delay defaecation until the situation is socially acceptable.
- Like the bladder, the rectum is mainly in storage mode, and the process of elimination is started in response to a conscious sensation of a full rectum, filled by faeces that have been propelled distally by colonic contractions.
- The efficient passage of stool requires a combination of propulsive factors and the removal of continence-maintaining barriers.

■ Since the process is under voluntary control, intact spinal connections are necessary from higher centres (still largely undefined) to the sacral spinal cord, as well as an intact intrinsic recto-anal inhibitory reflex, which causes appropriate relaxation of the internal anal sphincter in response to rectal distension.

Neurological causes of bowel disorders

■ Patients with neurological disease commonly complain of constipation (Box 17.2) and some have faecal incontinence (Table 17.9).
■ Slow transit time causing constipation can be a troublesome problem in patients with Parkinson's disease or multiple system atrophy.
■ Constipation in patients with mild multiple sclerosis seems to be a symptom similar to the fatigue that many of these patients experience, in that neither complaint can be clearly attributed to a neurological lesion at a known particular site in the nervous system.
■ With severe spinal dysfunction the ability to voluntarily initiate and coordinate defaecation may be lost as well as the ability to postpone bowel emptying, both because of impaired sensation of impending defaecation and the inability to voluntarily contract the anal sphincter. Faecal incontinence is a great worry to many patients following spinal cord injury and may become increasingly a problem for patients with multiple sclerosis if they become disabled and then chair- or bed-bound.

Investigations

■ Establishing the cause of the bowel complaint is the first step in management.
■ Table 17.10 lists the investigations that may be carried out and what may be learnt from them.

Box 17.2　Neurological causes of constipation

- Slow transit:
  - multiple sclerosis
  - Parkinson's disease
  - multiple system atrophy.

- Difficulty with defaecation:
  - spinal cord dysfunction, including advanced multiple sclerosis
  - cauda equina lesion.

Table 17.9   Neurological causes of faecal incontinence

Symptom	Cause
Intrinsic sphincter weakness	Childbirth injury
External anal sphincter weakness	Childbirth injury Cauda equina lesion
Loss of voluntary sphincter activation	Advanced spinal cord dysfunction including multiple sclerosis
Loss of sensation of rectal filling	Small fibre neuropathy
Overflow incontinence following faecal impaction	Severe constipation

Table 17.10   Anorectal investigations

Investigation	What is tested
Constipation	
Transit studies	Slow transit
Defaecating proctogram	Ability of rectum to retain a volume of faeces Incoordination of process Intussusception
Faecal incontinence	
Anorectal manometry	Rectal sensitivity and anal sphincter competency
Endoanal ultrasound	Damage to internal and external anal sphincter
Sphincter EMG	Denervation of anal sphincter

Management

Constipation

■ This is a complaint of patients with neurological disease on which there has been almost no medical research. Laxatives, suppositories and enemas are of course all possible treatments and Table 17.11 lists the various preparations. Most are available over the counter, and patients are likely to have discovered what helps them. It should be noted that patients with slow-transit constipation are not likely to be helped by a high-fibre diet, nor laxative bulking agents, since these will merely result in worsening bowel distension.

■ Intussusception, involution of one segment of bowel into a distal one, is a surgically correctable cause of severely obstructed defaecation and should be excluded in patients with advanced multiple sclerosis who have difficulty with defaecation.

Faecal incontinence

■ Faecal incontinence in multiple sclerosis may occur if the patient becomes unable to inhibit bowel emptying as a result of severe spinal cord disease. This only occurs in those who are chair bound or unable to stand; faecal incontinence in less severely affected patients should be investigated separately by a colorectal surgeon.

■ Faecal incontinence in the severely disabled can be exacerbated by constipation so the aim of management is to achieve regular bowel emptying at a set time. Suppositories and enemas (see Table 17.11), administered by a carer if necessary, are most effective in this situation.

■ Striated anal sphincter weakness following a cauda equina lesion can result in impaired bowel control and incontinence of flatus. The principle of management is the same as above – to empty the rectum at a predictable time – but manual evacuation may be necessary long term. Additionally, denervation of the anal sphincter can result in incontinence of flatus or liquid motions. Loose motions are avoided by use of loperimide 4 mg/day oral in 2 divided doses, increasing if necessary to 16 mg/day.

■ Weakness of the intrinsic anal sphincter (smooth) muscle causes faecal seepage rather than loss of formed motions. This type of damage is commonest following difficult childbirth and can be demonstrated by ultrasound. Referral for this investigation should be arranged in ambulant women with multiple sclerosis complaining of faecal incontinence.

SEXUAL DYSFUNCTION

Physiology

■ There are similarities in the neurological control of sexual function in men and women (Tables 17.12 and 17.13), although that of women is less well understood. As is evident from these tables, extensive and intact neural pathways are necessary for normal physiological responses.

■ In health, psychogenic and reflexogenic erectile types of response reinforce one another to produce an erection adequate for intercourse.

Table 17.11 Agents used to treat constipation		
Type of drug	**Generic name**	**Trade names**
Bulking agents to increase faecal mass	Bran	–
	Ispaghula husk	Fybogel, Isogel, Knosyl, Regulan
	Sterculia	Normacol
Stool softeners for difficulty with defaecation	Castor oil	Non-proprietary
	Docusate	Dioctyl, Docusol
Osmotics for slow transit	Magnesium salts	Milpar
	Lactulose	Non-proprietary
	Macrogols	Movicol
Colonic stimulants for more severe slow transit	Senna	Manevac, Senokot
	Bisacodyl	Dulco-lax
Rectal stimulants to promote evacuation	Glycerine or bisacodyl suppositories	Glycerol Suppositories, BP or Dulco-lax suppositories
	Enemas 'mini-dose' or phosphate	Micralax Micro-enema or Fleet Ready-to-use Enema

Provided one form of erection response is preserved it seems that phosphodiesterase inhibitors (see below) can be effective.

■ The neurology of nocturnal penile erections has not yet been elucidated, but these may be preserved in men with spinal cord transection as well as in men with multiple sclerosis.

■ In women, the analogous response to penile erection is vaginal lubrication, a process also mediated by the transmitter nitric oxide. It is due to transudation through the vaginal walls as well as fluid from Bartholin's glands.

Neurological causes of sexual dysfunction

■ Table 17.14 lists the range of sexual dysfunction that can affect men and women with neurological disease. The commonest and most evident problem in men is erectile dysfunction, but problems with libido, desire

Table 17.12	Neurological control of the male sexual response	
Penile erection	**Neural pathway**	**Physiological result**
Reflexogenic, resulting from direct genital stimulation	S2–S4 genital innervation	Increased penile blood flow
Psychogenic	Spinal cord and thoraco-lumbar sympathetic outflow Sacral parasympathetic genital innervation through pelvic and cavernosal nerves Neurotransmitter: nitric oxide (NO)	Increased penile blood flow
Ejaculation	Sympathetic control	Closure of bladder neck, emission of semen
Orgasm	Pudendal nerve	Contraction of pelvic floor accompanied by acute pleasurable penile sensation
Detumescence	Sympathetic control	Resolution of genital engorgement

and orgasmic response can also occur. In women these problems have been loosely grouped as 'female sexual dysfunction'.

■ Theoretically a lesion below spinal level L2 leaves psychogenic erections intact, but in practice it is uncommon for men with such a lesion to have erections adequate for intercourse. Psychogenic erections are more likely to be preserved in incomplete lesions.

■ Preserved ejaculation function following a spinal cord lesion is unusual.

■ About 60% of men with multiple sclerosis have erectile dysfunction, often in conjunction with urinary symptoms, reflecting the common spinal cord dysfunction responsible for both problems. In the early stages of the disease the chief complaint is of difficulty sustaining an erection for intercourse despite preservation of normal nocturnal penile tumescence. With advancing neurological disability there may be total failure of erectile function and difficulty with ejaculation.

Table 17.13 Neurological control of the female sexual response		
Vaginal lubrication and clitoreal erection	**Neural pathway**	**Physiological result**
Reflexogenic, resulting from direct genital stimulation	S2–S4 genital innervation	Increased genital blood flow
Psychogenic	Spinal cord and thoraco-lumbar sympathetic outflow Sacral parasympathetic genital innervation through pelvic nerves Neurotransmitter: nitric oxide (NO)	Increased genital blood flow
Orgasm	Pudendal nerve	Contraction of pelvic floor accompanied by acute pleasurable pelvic sensation
Detumescence	Sympathetic control	Resolution of genital engorgement

- Sexual dysfunction in women with multiple sclerosis is likewise a common problem. Presumed neurogenic problems with intercourse include decreased lubrication and reduced orgasmic capacity. In women with advanced disease there may be the additional problems of lower limb spasticity, loss of pelvic sensation, genital dysaesthesia and fear of incontinence.

Investigation

Andrologists have not reached a consensus as to what investigations are required routinely to investigate erectile dysfunction in the general population. Therefore, it would seem appropriate only to initiate investigations in neurological patients if sexual dysfunction is an unexpected aspect of their disease.

Table 17.14   Neurological causes of sexual dysfunction in men and women

Neurological disorder	Nature of sexual dysfunction
Temporal lobe damage	Erotic apathy and lack of sexual interests
Prolactinoma	Loss of libido and impaired sexual sensations
Multiple system atrophy	Erectile dysfunction in some, probably also female sexual dysfunction
Parkinson's disease	Early erectile dysfunction, sometimes hypersexuality
Spinal cord lesions (e.g. trauma, multiple sclerosis)	Erectile dysfunction and female sexual dysfunction Inability to sustain an erection Failure of orgasm in both genders
Cauda equina lesion	Loss of genital sensation Inability to sustain an erection Failure of orgasm in both genders
Injury to peripheral innervation including pelvic plexus and corporeal nerves	Complete erectile dysfunction Less known about female sexual dysfunction
Generalised small fibre neuropathy	Erectile dysfunction and female sexual dysfunction Often orgasmic function preserved

Management

- The management of erectile dysfunction has been transformed by sildenafil citrate, the first oral phophodiesterase-5 (PDE-5) inhibitor. The action is to enhance nitric oxide that has been released in response to sexual stimulation. There are now several PDE-5 inhibitors available (Table 17.15). Important information to give the patient when prescribing this medication is about the timing of onset and duration of action, and also that the medication will be ineffective unless sexual stimulation

Table 17.15   Phophodiesterase-5 (PDE-5) inhibitors for treatment of erectile dysfunction

Generic name	Trade name	Daily dose (mg)	Frequency in 24 hours	Time dose administered prior to sexual activity (hours)	Elimination half-life of parent drug (hours)
Sildenafil	Viagra	25–100	1 dose	1	4
Tadalafil	Cialis	10–20	1 dose	0.5–12	17.5
Vardenafil	Levitra	5–10	1 dose	0.25–1	4

occurs. Common adverse effects include headache and nasal stuffiness, and occasionally symptoms of gastric reflux.

- The only complete contraindication to PDE-5 inhibitors is the concurrent use of nitrates to treat angina, since the combination can induce severe postural hypotension. An additional precaution is in multiple system atrophy, where pre-existing, possibly unrecognised, postural hypotension can be exacerbated. Checking the lying and standing blood pressure is recommended in such patients.
- In women with multiple sclerosis, sildenafil citrate has only a marginal effect on vaginal lubrication and does not restore lost orgasmic sensation.
- Other measures to assist erection include injection of the corpora with prostaglandin (Caverject), and the use of a vacuum pump. These methods should be introduced if full dosages of PDE-5s are ineffective and a man wishes to remain sexually active. Referral to an andrology clinic is recommended.
- Failure of ejaculation and orgasmic response, for which there is as yet little effective treatment, are distressing complaints for patients with neurological disease. Yohimbine 5–20 mg taken 1–2 hours before intercourse may help a small proportion of men, but otherwise advice about access to sex (vibratory) aids may be helpful for both men and women.

Further reading

Corcos J, Schick E (eds). Textbook of the neurogenic bladder. Martin Dunitz, London, 2004.

Fowler CJ (ed). Neurology of bladder, bowel and sexual dysfunction (Blue book series for neurologists, vol 23). Butterworth-Heinemann, Oxford, 1999.

Fowler CJ (ed). Neurologic bladder, bowel and sexual dysfunction (World Federation of Neurology seminars in neurology, vol 1). Free downloadable PDFs available from: http://www.wfneurology.org/wfnseminars.htm#vol%201

Fowler's syndrome website: http://www.ion.ucl.ac.uk/fowlersyndrome

Pemberton JH, Swash M, Henry M (eds). The pelvic floor. Its function and disorders. WB Saunders, London, 2002.

18 NEUROPATHIC PAIN

John Scadding

Neuropathic pain is caused by damage to the somatosensory pathways of the peripheral (Box 18.1) and central nervous systems (CNS) (Box 18.2): for peripheral nerves, particularly damage to small nociceptive neurons, and in the CNS damage to the spinothalamic tract and thalamus. Unlike nociceptive pain, neuropathic pain serves no useful bioprotective function. It is often debilitating and is relatively refractory to treatment in many patients.

A recent change in the terms used to refer to these pains is potentially confusing:

- Neurogenic pain, an old term, refers to pain caused by *either* peripheral *or* CNS lesions. It is now used infrequently, although it remains acceptable.
- Neuropathic pain, the preferred term, is 'pain initiated or caused by a primary lesion or dysfunction of the nervous system'. It refers to all central and peripheral nervous system causes of pain. The complex regional pain syndrome type 1, formerly known as reflex sympathetic dystrophy, is included as a neuropathic pain. Some authorities question the validity of this because the initiating event is not a neurological lesion. What this terminological difficulty emphasises is the limited understanding of the pathophysiology of pain in these conditions.
- Neuralgia is 'pain arising in the distribution of a nerve or nerves'. This perfectly good term has been inexplicably relegated to refer to a few particular pains, for example trigeminal neuralgia.
- Central pain, an older term that has been retained, can be used to refer to pain due to CNS lesions.

Box 18.1   Causes of peripheral neuropathic pain

Mononeuropathies

- Traumatic mononeuropathies:
  - transection, partial or complete, including limb amputation
  - nerve entrapment syndromes
  - post-thoracotomy

- Non-traumatic mononeuropathies and multiple mononeuropathies:
  - diabetic mononeuropathy
  - borreliosis
  - vasculitic
  - neuralgic amyotrophy
  - diabetic amyotrophy
  - malignant plexus invasion
  - radiation plexopathy

Polyneuropathies

- Metabolic/nutritional:
  - alcoholic
  - amyloid
  - beriberi
  - burning feet syndrome
  - Cuban neuropathy
  - pellagra
  - Tanzanian neuropathy

- Drugs:
  - antiretroviral drugs
  - cisplatin
  - disulfiram
  - ethambutol
  - isoniazid
  - nitrofurantoin
  - thalidomide
  - vincristine

- Hereditary:
  - amyloid
  - Fabry's disease (angiokeratoma corporis diffusum)
  - hereditary motor and sensory neuropathy type V
  - hereditary sensory and autonomic neuropathy type 1

- Malignant:
  - paraneoplastic
  - myeloma

- Infective/postinfective:
  - human immunodeficiency virus (HIV)
  - acute inflammatory polyradiculoneuropathy
  - borreliosis

- Toxic:
  - acrylamide
  - arsenic
  - clioquinol
  - thallium

- Other polyneuropathies:
  - idiopathic small fibre neuropathy
  - cold injury (trench foot)

- Causalgia means burning pain and is defined as 'a syndrome of sustained burning pain, allodynia and hyperpathia after a traumatic

Box 18.2 Causes of central neuropathic pain

Spinal root/dorsal root ganglion
- Prolapsed disc
- Arachnoiditis
- Postherpetic neuralgia
- Surgical rhizotomy
- Root avulsion
- Tumour
- Trigeminal neuralgia

Spinal cord
- Trauma including compression
- Syringomyelia
- Dysraphism
- Infarction, haemorrhage, vascular malformation
- Anterolateral cordotomy
- HIV
- Multiple sclerosis
- Vitamin B_{12} deficiency
- Syphilis

Brainstem
- Lateral medullary syndrome
- Syrinx
- Multiple sclerosis
- Tumour
- Tuberculoma

Thalamus
- Infarction
- Haemorrhage
- Tumour
- Surgical thalamotomy

Subcortical and cortical
- Infarction
- Vascular malformation
- Tumour
- Trauma

nerve lesion, often combined with vasomotor and sudomotor dysfunction and later trophic changes' (now referred to as complex regional pain syndrome, type 2).

The use of these terms, with overlapping meanings, can lead to difficulties. For example, when a drug is effective in neuropathic pain of peripheral origin and is then licensed for the treatment of 'neuropathic pain', this suggests it is also effective in central pain, which is not necessarily the case. The qualification of neuropathic pain as 'peripheral' or 'central' would help resolve this ambiguity.

CLINICAL FEATURES OF NEUROPATHIC PAIN

The major clinical features can be summarised as:
- Pain quality: burning pain, cold pain.
- Associated sensory symptoms: paraesthesia, numbness, itching.
- Paroxysmal pains: stabbing, electric-shock-like pains.
- Immediate or delayed onset after injury.
- Sensory impairment in an anatomical distribution.

- Frequently associated:
  - allodynia, pain due to a stimulus that does not normally produce pain
  - hyperalgesia, heightened sensation of pain to a stimulus that is normally painful
  - hyperpathia, symptom complex in which there is a raised sensory threshold, delay in perception of a stimulus, an abnormally painful reaction to a stimulus, often with summation (increasing pain) to a repetitive stimulus and a painful after-sensation.
- Sometimes associated vasomotor and sudomotor changes.
- Comorbidities are common:
  - depression
  - sleep disturbance
  - job loss
  - financial, marital, domestic and social problems
  - motor and other neurological deficits due to the underlying neurological disease.

Complex regional pain syndrome

This replaces the older term 'reflex sympathetic dystrophy', discarded because it implies a pathogenic role for the sympathetic nervous system that is neither supported by clinical evidence nor by any long-term response to sympatholytic treatments.

- Type 1 describes a variety of painful conditions that usually (Box 18.3):

Box 18.3   Causes of the complex regional pain syndrome

Type 1
- Peripheral tissues:
  - fractures and dislocations
  - soft tissue injury, including tendonitis, fasciitis, ligamentous injury
  - arthritis
  - deep venous thrombosis
  - prolonged limb immobilisation
- Viscera:
  - myocardial infarction
  - abdominal disease
- Idiopathic

Type 2
- Peripheral nerve:
  - trauma, including postganglionic plexus lesions
- Dorsal root:
  - postherpetic neuralgia
  - root trauma, including avulsion
- Central nervous system:
  - myelopathies, particularly spinal cord injury
  - head injury
  - cerebral infarction, haemorrhage, tumour

- follow injury
- occur regionally
- have a distal predominance of abnormal findings
- exceed in both magnitude and duration the expected course of the inciting event
- result in marked impairment of motor function
- are associated with oedema, abnormal skin blood flow or sudomotor activity in the region of the pain at some time during the course of the illness
- result in the development of soft tissue and bone dystrophic changes, of variable severity.

Previously described syndromes now considered part of type 1 include reflex sympathetic dystrophy, algodystrophy, Sudeck's atrophy and the shoulder–hand syndrome.

■ Type 2 is usually caused by partial damage to a major limb peripheral nerve, also confusingly called 'causalgia' (Box 18.3). Type 2 may occasionally be caused by CNS lesions.

THE GENERAL MANAGEMENT OF NEUROPATHIC PAIN

Diagnostic problems in neuropathic pain that may affect treatment

■ When pain is partly neuropathic and partly nociceptive (somatic), for example in cervical and lumbar spine disease, the relative contributions of the two components can be difficult to disentangle. Differentiation on the basis of pain description, including radiation, may be misleading. Imaging and electrophysiological testing may resolve whether the pain is likely to be neuropathic or a widely radiating pain of musculoskeletal origin.

■ There are other situations in which there may be multiple sources of pain. For example, in patients with diabetes a neuropathy may coexist with lower limb ischaemia causing intermittent claudication. And in patients with central post-stroke pain (thalamic pain), or with multiple sclerosis, there are often additional pains with a musculoskeletal basis, including pain due to spasticity.

■ The guiding principle is that meticulous clinical assessment, supported by investigation, is needed in all patients. Inappropriate treatment may result if the diagnosis of pain type and its cause is incorrect, notwithstanding the difficulty in defining this in many patients.

General considerations

■ Pain due to compression of peripheral nerves, spinal roots (radicular pain) and occasionally the spinal cord (myelopathic pain) may be relieved by appropriate surgery.

■ Ablative neurosurgery, either to the peripheral nervous system or CNS, to relieve neuropathic pain should no longer be performed, except in a very few patients (see treatment of central neuropathic pain, below). A surgical lesion in the somatosensory pathway may itself lead to neuropathic pain.

■ For patients with neuropathic pain associated with allodynia and hyperalgesia in relatively restricted areas, local measures (Box 18.4) may be helpful and obviate the need for drug therapy (an advantage particularly in older patients, in whom adverse effects of systemic therapy are often dose limiting and outweigh any therapeutic effect).

■ Nerve blocks and epidural injection with local anaesthetic, with or without corticosteroid or opioid, may be helpful diagnostically, and for short-term pain relief, but this rarely lasts.

■ Many patients with chronic neuropathic pain are best treated in a multidisciplinary setting, where they benefit from cognitive–behavioural psychotherapeutic methods, physiotherapy and occupational therapy.

■ For selected patients, in whom all 'medical' treatments have failed, pain management programmes offer a way forward, through adjustment, coping and pacing strategies.

DRUG TREATMENT OF PERIPHERAL NEUROPATHIC PAIN

The quality of the clinical trials of systemic drug treatment has improved substantially over the past 20 years or so. Prior to this, many trials were inadequately controlled, involved small numbers of patients and were

---

Box 18.4   Local interventions to relieve neuropathic pain

- Topical local anaesthetic (impregnated patches or ointment)
- Topical capsaicin (may be limited by initial burning pain)
- TENS (transcutaneous electrical nerve stimulation)
- Acupuncture
- Hot or cold packs
- Vibration
- Massage

conducted over very short periods, thus not reflecting the chronic nature of neuropathic pain. There are now several excellent systematic reviews.

- Increasingly, the measure of clinical efficacy is the 'number-needed-to-treat': the number of patients who need to be treated to achieve a defined level of pain relief in one patient and which would not have been achieved if the patients had taken placebo. The level of pain relief is usually defined as 50% or 30% reduction, the latter equating to the value patients describe as at least moderate pain relief.
- Although the aim of drug treatment should always be to find a single effective agent for an individual patient, often several drugs need to be used in combination. Even so, partial pain relief is the usual outcome, and multiple drug therapy inevitably brings with it a high risk of adverse effects.

Evidence from randomised trials of systemic drugs for the treatment of peripheral neuropathic pain is summarised in Table 18.1 and Box 18.5. Where there is insufficient evidence from trials, it is justifiable to use drugs on the basis of extrapolation of evidence gained in other conditions causing neuropathic pain at the same anatomical level. However, it is important to note that:

- In most countries, very few drugs are licensed specifically for the treatment of neuropathic pain.
- The use of a drug not licensed for the treatment of neuropathic pain should only be undertaken after careful discussion with the patient

---

Box 18.5   Recommendations for the drug treatment of peripheral neuropathic pain

The following sequence of drugs in individual patients is suggested (excluding trigeminal neuralgia, see Chapter 7). Whenever possible, each drug should be given singly to assess effectiveness, but many patients end up taking combinations of two or more drugs.

- Nortriptyline
- Gabapentin (first choice in older patients)
- Amitriptyline or other tricyclic
- Pregabalin
- Duloxetine
- Venlafaxine
- Paroxetine
- Tramadol
- Carbamazepine
- Oxycodone
- Morphine or fentanyl

Table 18.1   Oral drug treatments for peripheral neuropathic pain

Drug	Daily dose range (mg)	Condition	Number-needed-to-treat
Tricyclic antidepressants			
Imipramine	100–200	Diabetic neuropathy	1–3
Nortriptyline	30	Diabetic neuropathy	1
Nortriptyline/desipramine	89/63*	Postherpetic neuralgia	4
Amitriptyline	75–105	Diabetic neuropathy	2–6
Amitriptyline	75	Polyneuropathy	2
Amitriptyline	100	HIV neuropathy	14
Desipramine	200	Diabetic neuropathy	2–3
Desipramine	111	Diabetic neuropathy	5
Clomipramine	75	Diabetic neuropathy	2
Selective serotonin reuptake inhibitors			
Paroxetine	40	Diabetic neuropathy	3
Fluoxetine	40	Diabetic neuropathy	15
Citalopram	40	Diabetic neuropathy	8
Serotonin and noradrenaline reuptake inhibitors			
Venlafaxine	75	Diabetic neuropathy	16
Venlafaxine	150–225	Diabetic neuropathy	4
Duloxetine	20–120	Diabetic neuropathy	4–6
Antiepileptic drugs			
Gabapentin	900–3600	Diabetic neuropathy	4–5
Gabapentin	2400–3600	Postherpetic neuralgia	5–6
Pregabalin	75–600	Diabetic neuropathy	3–104
Pregabalin	75–600	Postherpetic neuralgia	3–31
Carbamazepine	200–600	Diabetic neuropathy	3
Lamotrigine	300–400	HIV neuropathy	No effect
Lamotrigine	400	Diabetic neuropathy	4
Opioids			
Morphine/methadone	91/15*	Postherpetic neuralgia	3
Tramadol	100–400	Diabetic neuropathy	3
Tramadol	100–400	Polyneuropathy	4
Oxycodone	40	Diabetic neuropathy	3
Oxycodone	60	Postherpetic neuralgia	2

Continued

Table 18.1   Continued

Drug	Daily dose range (mg)	Condition	Number-needed-to-treat
NMDA antagonists			
Dextromethorphan	381–960*	Diabetic neuropathy	2–4
Dextromethorphan	960	Postherpetic neuralgia	7
Memantine	58	Diabetic neuropathy	12
Antiarrhythmics			
Mexiletine	675	Diabetic neuropathy	10
Mexiletine	600	HIV neuropathy	46

*Ranges based on averages from several studies.

about the possible benefits and risks, particularly the potential for serious adverse effects with some drugs.

Antidepressants (see Chapter 13)

- Tricyclic antidepressants are thought to exert an analgesic effect by their serotonergic action, leading to enhanced activity in descending analgesia pathways from the brainstem to the dorsal horn of the spinal cord. However, this is unlikely to be the sole or even the main mechanism of action, as the selective serotonin reuptake inhibitors (SSRIs) have a greater serotonergic action, yet are less potent as analgesics.
- There is little to choose between the different tricyclics, but nortriptyline may be preferred as it tends to cause fewer anticholinergic adverse effects.
- Tricyclics are effective both at low and high dosage.
- Their analgesic and antidepressant actions can be separated, the former usually coming on more quickly than the latter.
- Some patients report pain relief with doses as low as 10 mg/day amitryptiline; it is sensible to start with a low dose and increase gradually, to minimise the adverse effects that so often limit the use of tricyclics (dry mouth, blurred vision, drowsiness, urinary retention, etc.).
- SSRIs are less effective than the tricyclics; paroxetine has greater analgesic effects than either citalopram or fluoxetine.
- Of the serotonin and noradrenaline reuptake inhibitors (SNRIs), venlafaxine, at adequate dose, has an analgesic effect in painful diabetic neuropathy, though not at low dose. Recently, duloxetine has shown promise in patients with painful diabetic neuropathy.

Antiepileptic drugs (see Chapter 2)

- Phenytoin, carbamazepine and lamotrigine have little or no effect, in marked contrast to the benefit of carbamazepine in trigeminal neuralgia.
- Sodium valproate has rather uncertain effects.
- Gabapentin and pregabalin are effective in diabetic neuropathy and postherpetic neuralgia and there is probably little to choose between them, but experience with pregabalin is limited. The adverse effects (most commonly drowsiness and dizziness) are usually mild, and thus many clinicians opt to try one of these drugs in preference to a tricyclic, particularly in the elderly.

Opioids

- Opioids were for many years regarded as ineffective. There was understandable concern about adverse effects, particularly habituation and addiction. But several trials have now demonstrated efficacy.
- Although adverse effects (particularly sedation, dysphoria and constipation) limit therapy in many patients, there are undoubtedly some who benefit from long-term opioid treatment.
- However, opioids should not be considered as first-line treatment.
- Clinical experience suggests that fentanyl, via the transdermal route, is often at least as effective as morphine, and may be associated with fewer adverse effects, particularly sedation and dysphoria.

NMDA antagonists

- Parenteral ketamine temporarily relieves both nociceptive and neuropathic pains, but is limited by adverse effects (typically marked sedation, nausea and psychological disturbances, including hallucinations).
- Current evidence with oral agents is inconclusive: dextromethorphan may be more effective in painful diabetic neuropathy than in postherpetic neuralgia, and memantine has a very weak action in peripheral neuropathic pain.

Antiarrhythmics

- Intravenous infusions of lignocaine often temporarily relieve peripheral neuropathic pain. However, the oral analogue mexiletine is ineffective.

Complex regional pain syndrome type 1

The pathophysiology is poorly understood. By definition, it is not provoked by a primary neurological lesion, but many of the clinical features are exactly similar to those of neuropathic pain (severe pain, allodynia, hyperalgesia, hyperpathia, loss of motor function, and variable vasomotor and sudomotor disturbances). There is some evidence for an inflammatory pathology in the earlier stages. Once established, it is extremely difficult to treat. In addition to the pain, dystrophic changes may develop and sometimes become severe.

- In the absence of good evidence, it is reasonable to recommend systemic drug therapy along the same lines as for peripheral neuropathic pain (see Table 18.1).
- The effect of spinal cord stimulation is unpredictable, but occasionally the pain may be markedly reduced.
- A major challenge in treatment is restoration of function; physiotherapy should take advantage of periods of even partial analgesia.
- There is evidence that disuse compounds the problem and indeed it is an aetiological factor in some patients.

Complex regional pain syndrome type 2 (causalgia)

- Despite the sometimes prominent vasomotor and sudomotor disturbances, the response to sympatholytic treatment is unpredictable and unsustained. Although partial analgesia occasionally results from temporary blocks, surgical sympathectomy rarely produces long-term analgesia.
- Treatment is usually with local measures (see above) and systemic drugs for peripheral neuropathic pain (see Table 18.1).

CENTRAL NEUROPATHIC PAIN

- The three commonest causes of central neuropathic pain are spinal cord injury and other myelopathies, multiple sclerosis and central post-stroke pain.
- The mechanisms of central neuropathic pain are even less well understood than those of peripheral neuropathic pain. Lesions in the spinothalamic tract and the ventroposterior thalamus are the usual responsible sites, although subcortical and cortical lesions may rarely lead to pain.
- The evidence base for the drug and other types of treatment of central neuropathic pain is much smaller than for peripheral neuropathic pain. Table 18.2 lists the treatments used.
- Attempts to relieve the pain with drugs are all too often unsuccessful; partial analgesia is achieved in relatively few patients using combinations of treatments.
- Realistic goals of treatment need to be set in discussion with patients.

Table 18.2 Treatments for central neuropathic pain	
Treatment type	**Treatments**
Systemic drugs	See text
Multidisciplinary clinic	Physiotherapy
	Occupational therapy
	Psychological measures
Sensory stimulation	Transcutaneous electrical stimulation (TENS)
	Spinal cord stimulation
	Deep brain stimulation
	Motor cortex stimulation
Neuroablative	Dorsal root entry zone lesions

Drug treatments for central neuropathic pain

- Controlled trials in spinal cord injury pain have shown that intravenous lignocaine, alfentanil and propofol produce temporary analgesia. Intrathecal morphine and clonidine (but not morphine alone), and intrathecal baclofen are also effective. Oral drug treatments are not helpful.
- In multiple sclerosis, painful paroxysms may respond to carbamazepine and, less often, to phenytoin or sodium valproate. Tricyclic antidepressants have a weak effect on non-paroxysmal pains.
- In central post-stroke pain, trials indicate weak analgesic actions of amitriptyline and lamotrigine.

Non-drug treatments for central neuropathic pain

- Transcutaneous electrical nerve stimulation (TENS):
  - Usually has a very weak analgesic effect, largely because of the wide area over which the pain is often felt and the small area over which TENS exerts its action.
  - Can be effective if the dorsal column–lemniscal pathway is at least partly intact (i.e. only in patients with preservation of some spinal cord sensory function).
- Spinal cord stimulation:
  - Is effective in only a small minority of patients, for similar reasons as TENS; the wider area in which stimulation may be felt with spinal cord stimulation is sometimes associated with partial analgesia.

- Displacement of electrodes away from the dorsal columns over time is a problem, even when electrodes are fixed in place at open operation.
- Gradual loss of effectiveness over several months is frequently reported, probably due to central adaptive physiological changes.
- It may help a few selected patients with the failed back surgery syndrome, where there is a combination of neuropathic and nociceptive musculoskeletal pain.

■ The place of deep brain stimulation is not yet established, although it is used for intractable central post-stroke pain:
- Targets in the ventroposterior thalamus are reported as being effective in some patients, but the results are unpredictable.
- Even when initial deep brain stimulation provides effective analgesia, long-term results are frequently disappointing.

■ Surface stimulation of the motor cortex has recently been reported to be effective and requires further evaluation.

Neuroablative treatments

■ Many sites in the CNS have been lesioned for the treatment of central neuropathic pain, including anterolateral cordotomy, commissural myelotomy, mesencephalic tractotomy, thalamotomy targeting various nuclei in the thalamus itself, cingulotomy, and cortical ablation. None has been associated with reliable long-term analgesia.

■ Anterolateral cordotomy has a very limited place in the treatment of cancer pain, as part of terminal care, when analgesia may last weeks to months.

■ Surgical lesions at many sites may themselves give rise to central neuropathic pain after months or even years.

■ Dorsal root entry zone lesioning partly relieves deafferentation pain in up to half of patients with brachial plexus avulsion. It has also been reported to produce good analgesia, below the level of the lesion, in up to 80% of patients with spinal cord injury.

Further reading

Kingery WS. A critical review of controlled clinical trials for peripheral neuropathic pain and complex regional pain syndromes. Pain 1997; 73: 123–139.

McMahon SB, Koltzenburg M (eds). Wall and Melzack's textbook of pain, 5th edn. Elsevier Science, London, 2005.

McQuay HJ, Carroll D, Jadad AR, Wiffen PJ, Moore RA. Anticonvulsant drugs for management of pain: a systematic review. BMJ 1995; 311: 1047–1052.

McQuay HJ, Tramer M, Nye BA, Carroll D, Wiffen PJ, Moore RA. A systematic review of antidepressants in neuropathic pain. Pain 1996; 68: 217–227.

Perez RS, Kwakkel G, Zuurmond WW, de Lange JJ. Treatment of reflex sympathetic
    dystrophy (CRPS type 1): a research synthesis of 21 randomized clinical trials. J Pain
    Symptom Manage 2001; 21: 512–526.
Sindrup SH, Jensen TS. Efficacy of pharmacological treatments of neuropathic pain: an
    update and effect related to mechanism of drug action. Pain 1999; 73: 389–400.

19 ANAESTHESIA FOR PATIENTS WITH NEUROLOGICAL DISEASE

Nicholas Hirsch

Patients with neurological disease often pose a challenge for anaesthetists but, common to all anaesthetic techniques, success depends on careful preoperative assessment and meticulous perioperative and postoperative care.

PREOPERATIVE ASSESSMENT

This aims to assess the risk to the patient of surgery, to determine the best technique of anaesthesia, and to optimise the patient's general condition prior to surgery. The need for an intensive care bed for postoperative care is also considered. Increasingly, a preliminary assessment is being performed in pre-admission clinics. The following areas should be covered:

- Full general medical history to define coexisting conditions, and a surgical history including details of the proposed procedure:
  - any cardiac dysfunction, including cardiac failure, cardiomyopathy and conduction defects commonly seen in muscular dystrophies and dystrophia myotonica
  - any respiratory symptoms suggestive of defects in central control of breathing (e.g. multiple system atrophy), the neural pathway to the respiratory muscles (e.g. motor neuron disease), the neuromuscular junction (e.g. myasthenia gravis) or of the muscles themselves (e.g. primary muscle disease), and any symptoms of obstructive sleep apnoea (e.g. in acromegaly, multiple system atrophy)
  - any gastrointestinal symptoms such as indigestion, gastro-oesophageal reflux and constipation suggesting delayed gastric emptying (e.g. in autonomic dysfunction due to spinal cord injury)
  - any endocrine dysfunction suggesting hypothalamic or pituitary disease (e.g. Cushing's disease, acromegaly).

- Full neurological history:
  - the nature and severity of the underlying condition and degree of disability or deficit
  - the presence of symptoms associated with cerebrovascular disease (e.g. stroke, transient ischaemic attacks)
  - the presence of associated autonomic dysfunction (e.g. parkinsonian syndromes, Guillain–Barré syndrome, spinal cord injury)
  - the presence of associated bulbar dysfunction (e.g. myasthenia gravis, motor neuron disease), including vocal cord dysfunction (e.g. multiple system atrophy), which predisposes to aspiration of gastric contents on induction of anaesthesia and in the postoperative period.
- Previous anaesthetic history:
  - previous adverse reactions
  - postoperative nausea and vomiting
  - details of any family history of anaesthetic problems (e.g. malignant hyperpyrexia, which may be associated with central core disease).
- Drug history (including complementary remedies) and drug allergies.
- Tobacco and alcohol intake.
- Condition of teeth (especially in patients taking phenytoin).
- Examination should include:
  - routine examination of the cardiovascular system (including listening for carotid bruits)
  - examination of the respiratory system, including assessment of diaphragmatic function (paralysis is suggested by paradoxical in-drawing of the abdomen on early inspiration with the patient supine)
  - examination of the airway, teeth, temporomandibular function and any other factors that may be associated with difficulty in tracheal intubation.
- Neurological examination should concentrate on:
  - Glasgow Coma Score
  - cranial nerve examination, particularly of the lower cranial nerves (preoperative tracheostomy must be considered if bulbar dysfunction is severe)
  - full examination of motor and sensory systems
  - examination of autonomic nervous system looking for postural drop in systemic blood pressure, effect of Valsalva manoeuvre on R–R interval of electrocardiogram (ECG), etc.
- Suitability for regional anaesthesia (e.g. look for contractures, kyphoscoliosis).
- Suitable veins for cannulation.

Preoperative investigations

These must be tailored to the individual's need and include:

- Routine preoperative haematology and biochemistry testing, plasma levels of antiepileptic drugs if indicated.
- Blood cross-matching if necessary.
- Chest X-ray if patient has cardiovascular or respiratory disease and there is no recent film, or if there is a possibility of metastases or tuberculosis.
- ECG in patients > 45 years old; earlier in smokers or if neurological disease is associated with cardiovascular abnormalities.
- Other investigations if suggested by history and examination:
  - formal autonomic nervous system testing
  - echocardiography, carotid ultrasound
  - respiratory function tests may include serial measurement of forced vital capacity (normal 75 ml/kg), formal spirometry and arterial blood gas analysis
  - videofluoroscopy to assess bulbar function
  - formal assessment by physiotherapists and treatment preoperatively if indicated (e.g. with bronchodilators, incentive spirometry).

Explanation of the forthcoming anaesthesia

- Confirm patient consent.
- Premedication if appropriate, but generally avoid unless the patient is particularly anxious, when an oral benzodiazepine is appropriate (e.g. temazepam 10 mg 2 hours preoperatively).
- H_2 receptor antagonist (e.g. ranitidine 150 mg oral 2 hours preoperatively) or a proton pump inhibitor (e.g. omeprazole 40 mg oral the night before and 40 mg on the day of surgery) for patients with upper gastrointestinal symptoms.
- Anticholinergic drugs should be avoided if autonomic dysfunction is present.
- Patients being treated with long-term corticosteroids should receive hydrocortisone 50–100 mg with their premedication, or at induction of anaesthesia.
- Medication taken regularly by the patient must generally be continued preoperatively (e.g. antihypertensive, antiparkinsonian, antiepileptic drugs).

REGIONAL VERSUS GENERAL ANAESTHESIA

Many operations, especially those involving the extremities, can be performed under regional anaesthesia.

■ Advantages:
  - conscious, cooperative patient able to warn of adverse effects (e.g. during carotid artery surgery)
  - extradural/spinal anaesthesia prevents autonomic hyperreflexia in spinal cord injury patient
  - affords good postoperative analgesia
  - reduction of certain postoperative complications (e.g. pulmonary atelectasis, deep venous thrombosis).
■ Absolute contraindications:
  - patient refusal
  - anaesthetist's inexperience
  - localised infection.
■ Relative contraindications:
  - abnormal anatomy (e.g. kyphoscoliosis)
  - coagulation disorder
  - neurological conditions that may vary considerably over time (e.g. multiple sclerosis), because neurological deterioration occurring even some time after regional anaesthesia may be erroneously attributed to it and lead to medico-legal distractions.

GENERAL ANAESTHESIA

Anaesthetists use balanced anaesthesia, which provides adequate analgesia, anaesthesia and muscular relaxation using a combination of drugs whilst maintaining adequate oxygenation and cerebral perfusion. Maintenance of the latter is especially important in those patients with critically impaired cerebral blood flow (e.g. severe carotid artery stenosis or occlusion).

The choice of drugs used in patients with neurological disease requires great care and many must be avoided.

Following establishment of routine monitoring and intravenous access, induction of anaesthesia is most commonly achieved using either thiopental or propofol (Table 19.1).

Following induction, tracheal (and nasogastric if indicated) intubation is achieved using either a depolarising (suxamethonium) or a non-depolarising neuromuscular blocking drug (e.g. vecuronium, atracurium). Suxamethonium must be avoided in certain neurological conditions (Table 19.2).

Table 19.1 Induction of general anaesthesia

Agent	Dose	Comments
Thiopental	3–6 mg/kg	Contraindicated in porphyria
		May result in severe hypotension if autonomic dysfunction present
		Reduces cerebral perfusion pressure and intracranial pressure
Propofol	1.5–2.5 mg/kg	Hypotension and respiratory depression more profound than with thiopental
		May produce myoclonic type jerks but not thought to be epileptogenic

Table 19.2 Contraindications to the use of suxamethonium

Condition	Possible effect of suxamethonium
Chronic spinal cord injury, denervation and demyelinating diseases	Massive hyperkalaemia due to denervation hypersensitivity
Raised intracranial pressure	Increases pressure by 7–10 mmHg transiently, so avoid unless rapid tracheal intubation necessary
Neuromuscular disorders:	
Myasthenia gravis	Relative resistance to action of suxamethonium, extreme sensitivity to non-depolarising relaxants
Lambert–Eaton myasthenic syndrome	Prolonged paralysis with suxamethonium and non-depolarising relaxants
Muscular dystrophies	Hyperkalaemia may occur due to loss of muscle membrane integrity
Myotonic syndromes	Sustained muscular contraction resulting in difficulty performing tracheal intubation and ventilating lungs
Malignant hyperpyrexia	Suxamethonium is a major trigger – contraindicated

Following tracheal intubation, anaesthesia is maintained with a combination of volatile anaesthetic agents in air or nitrous oxide, and intravenous opioids (Table 19.3).

POSTOPERATIVE CARE

At the end of the operation neuromuscular blockade is reversed and the patient's trachea extubated when ventilation is adequate. Oxygen (5 l/min) is administered by mask until the patient is fully awake. Depending on the procedure, the patient will be recovered in a dedicated recovery area or in a high-dependency area. The two main functions of these areas are to:

- Perform routine postoperative observations (Box 19.1).
- Provide effective postoperative analgesic and antiemetic medication. Often this is inadequately managed, and suggested drug regimens for adults are given in Tables 19.4 and 19.5.

Table 19.3 Maintenance of general anaesthesia	
Agent	**Comments**
All volatile anaesthetic agents	Use at lowest effective concentrations to maintain cerebral autoregulation
	Potent triggers of malignant hyperpyrexia, contraindicated in this condition
Enflurane	Avoid in epilepsy, causes EEG abnormalities at high concentrations in the presence of hypocarbia
Sevoflurane	Most suitable pharmacodynamic profile for patients with neurological disease

Box 19.1   Routine postoperative observations

- Observations to be performed every 15 minutes for the first 2 hours, and then:
  - every 30 minutes for 2 hours, then
  - every hour until stable
- Observations (depending on surgery performed) include:
  - temperature, heart rate, blood pressure, respiratory rate, oxygen flow rate, oxygen saturation, blood glucose
  - Glasgow Coma Score, pupil size and reaction, limb power
  - pain, sedation and nausea scores

Table 19.4	Postoperative analgesia	
Magnitude of pain	**Regular oral analgesia to be considered**	**Additional analgesia if required**
Minor	• Paracetamol 1 g qds • NSAIDs (e.g. diclofenac 75 mg bd)	• Dihydrocodeine 30 mg qds
Intermediate	• Paracetamol 1 g qds • Dihydrocodeine 30 mg qds • NSAIDs (e.g. diclofenac 75 mg bd)	• Morphine 7.5–10 mg im, 2-hourly, prn
Major	• Paracetamol 1 g qds • Dihydrocodeine 30 mg qds • NSAIDs (e.g. diclofenac 75 mg bd)	• Morphine 7.5–10 mg im, 2-hourly, prn or • Regular oral morphine or • After discussion with the anaesthetist, patient-controlled analgesia with morphine

Table 19.5	Control of postoperative nausea and vomiting	
	Drug	**Dose**
First-choice drug	Cyclizine 50 mg im or iv 6-hourly	Maximum 150 mg in 24 hours. Rapid iv injection causes tachycardia and pain at the site of injection
Second-choice drug (to be given if first choice ineffective after 30 minutes)	5-HT$_3$ receptor antagonist (e.g. granisetron 1 mg iv 12-hourly)	Maximum 2 mg in 24 hours

All analgesia regimens should be reviewed after 2 days and, if the patient is receiving opioid drugs, regular laxatives (e.g. lactulose 20 ml bd) must be given.

Postoperative nausea and vomiting is common, especially in female patients, those with a past history and the obese. If it occurs postoperatively, the drugs in Table 19.5 can be given.

Postoperative intravenous fluid therapy

- Maintenance fluids for adults should be given at approximately 1.5 ml/kg body weight per hour: 0.9% sodium chloride or compound sodium lactate solution should be used.
- Glucose-containing solutions must be avoided in patients with cerebral ischaemia as high intracellular glucose levels worsen ischaemic damage.
- In general, blood transfusion is unnecessary if the haemoglobin level is above 8 g/dl; the threshold for transfusion may be lower in patients with ischaemic heart disease.

Further reading

Hirsch NP. Advances in neuroanaesthesia. Anaesthesia 2003; 58: 1162–1165.
Yentis SM, Hirsch NP, Smith GB. Anaesthesia and intensive care A–Z: an encyclopaedia of principles and practice. Butterworth-Heinemann, London, 2004.